DATE DUE

MAY 0 3 1994		
~~MAY 2 7 1996~~		
JUN 0 4 1996		
7981277	NOV 2 5 1997	
GAYLORD		PRINTED IN U.S.A.

Methodological Issues in AIDS Behavioral Research

AIDS Prevention and Mental Health

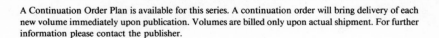

A Continuation Order Plan is available for this series. A continuation order will bring delivery of each new volume immediately upon publication. Volumes are billed only upon actual shipment. For further information please contact the publisher.

Methodological Issues in AIDS Behavioral Research

Edited by

David G. Ostrow, M.D., Ph.D.

and

Ronald C. Kessler, Ph.D.
University of Michigan
Ann Arbor, Michigan

Plenum Press • New York and London

Library of Congress Cataloging-in-Publication Data

Methodological issues in AIDS behavioral research / edited by David G.
 Ostrow and Ronald C. Kessler.
      p.   cm. -- (AIDS prevention and mental health)
    Includes bibliographical references and index.
    ISBN 0-306-44439-9
    1. AIDS (Disease)--Social aspects--Research--Methodology. 2. AIDS
 (Disease)--Psychological aspects--Research--Methodology. 3. AIDS
 (Disease)--Epidemiology--Research--Methodology.   I. Ostrow, David
 G., 1947-   . II. Title: Kessler, Ronald C. III. Series.
    [DNLM: 1. Acquired Immunodeficiency Syndrome. 2. Sex Behavior.
 3. Research--methods. 4. Research Design.   WB 25 M592 1993]
 RA644.A25M48   1993
 616.97'92'0072--dc20
 DNLM/DLC
 for Library of Congress   93-30675
                                                                   CIP

RA
644
.A25
M48
1993

ISBN 0-306-44439-9

Published 1993 by Plenum Press
A Division of Plenum Publishing Corporation
233 Spring Street, New York, N.Y. 10013

Printed in the United States of America

Contributors

Diane Binson • Center for AIDS Prevention Studies, Department of Medicine, University of California, San Francisco, California 94143

Robert F. Boruch • Graduate School of Education, University of Pennsylvania, Philadelphia, Pennsylvania 19104-6216

Joseph A. Catania • Center for AIDS Prevention Studies, Department of Medicine, University of California, San Francisco, California 94143

Robert T. Croyle • Department of Psychology, University of Utah, Salt Lake City, Utah 84112

Robyn M. Dawes • Department of Social and Decision Sciences, Carnegie Mellon University, Pittsburgh, Pennsylvania 15213

Victor De Gruttola • Department of Biostatistics, Harvard School of Public Health, Boston, Massachusetts 02115

Dorothy De Moya • Correctional Health Solutions, Chalfont, Pennsylvania 18914

Mindy Thompson Fullilove • HIV Center for Clinical and Behavioral Studies, New York State Psychiatric Institute and Columbia University, New York, New York 10027

Robert E. Fullilove, III • HIV Center for Clinical and Behavioral Studies, New York State Psychiatric Institute and Columbia University, New York, New York 10027

Eve Golden • Center for AIDS Prevention Studies, Department of Medicine, University of California, San Francisco, California 94143

Nicholas P. Jewell • Program in Biostatistics and Department of Statistics, University of California, Berkeley, California 94720

Graham Kalton • Westat, Inc., Rockville, Maryland 20850-3129.

John M. Karon • Division of HIV/AIDS, National Center for Infectious Diseases, Centers for Disease Control, Atlanta, Georgia 30333

Ronald C. Kessler • Institute for Social Research, University of Michigan, Ann Arbor, Michigan 48106-1248

Elizabeth F. Loftus • Department of Psychology, University of Washington, Seattle, Washington 98195

Karen Mast • Center for AIDS Prevention Studies, Department of Medicine, University of California, San Francisco, California 94143

David G. Ostrow • Department of Psychiatry, University of Michigan School of Medicine, Ann Arbor, Michigan 48109-0704

Marcello Pagano • Department of Biostatistics, Harvard School of Public Health, Boston, Massachusetts 02115

Willo Pequegnat • AIDS Research Program, National Institute of Mental Health, National Institutes of Health, Rockville, Maryland 20857

Robert C. Pierce • Center for AIDS Prevention Studies, Department of Medicine, University of California, San Francisco, California 94143

James M. Robins • Departments of Epidemiology and Biostatistics, Harvard School of Public Health, Boston, Massachusetts 02115

Stephen C. Shiboski • Department of Epidemiology and Biostatistics, University of California, San Francisco, California 94143-0560

Howard C. Stevenson • Graduate School of Education, University of Pennsylvania, Philadelphia, Pennsylvania 19104-6216

Carol Stocking • Center for Clinical Medical Ethics, University of Chicago, Chicago, Illinois 60637

Ellen Stover • AIDS Research Program, National Institute of Mental Health, National Institutes of Health, Rockville, Maryland 20857

Heather Turner • Department of Sociology and Anthropology, College of Liberal Arts, Horton Social Sciences Center, University of New Hampshire, Endura, New Hampshire 03824-3586

Richard A. Zeller • Department of Sociology, Bowling Green State University, Bowling Green, Ohio 43403

Series Preface

We are pleased to introduce a new series, *AIDS Prevention and Mental Health,* with the publication of this volume on methodology issues in AIDS mental health research. The objective of the series is to publish high-quality and up-to-date volumes that HIV prevention and mental health researchers, clinicians, policymakers, and educators will find useful and that will thus contribute significantly to their work in these important areas. While there has been an enormous increase in research on the prevention and mental health aspects of AIDS and HIV infection, there is no book series on AIDS with a prevention or mental health focus. The creation of this series represents a high level of commitment from the publisher, Plenum, and the series editors to this important area of scientific research. It is especially fitting that the series' inaugural volume focuses on methodological issues that are crucial to the future of HIV-related mental health research.

The *AIDS Prevention and Mental Health* series comes at a pivotal time in the history of the AIDS epidemic and the responses of mental and public health systems. For the past two years, we have met regularly with Mariclaire Cloutier at Plenum to discuss the burgeoning interest among mental health and prevention professionals in AIDS and HIV, as evidenced by the response to prior Plenum publications on the topic. At the same time, we have been increasingly aware of the need to support and stimulate the authorship of books by leading authorities in this rapidly growing field that go beyond collections of articles based on conference proceedings and allow authors to lay out a comprehensive view of their area of work and expertise. With the recent explosion of research and applied work in the area of HIV/AIDS mental health and prevention, we feel that it is time to create a book series that will provide timely communication of emerging ideas, practical experiences, and science.

The series will focus primarily on books that address current issues in HIV prevention and the psychological, psychiatric, and social aspects of HIV/AIDS. Volumes will reflect the highest scholarly standards while exploring clinical applications of interest to a broad range of mental health, public health, and community professionals. Series topics include HIV prevention approaches with various populations, including adolescents, gay men, women, and the chronically mentally ill; assessment of psychiatric disorders in persons with HIV/AIDS; psychotherapy and psychopharmacological interventions; stress and coping issues; HIV research methodologies; support and prevention of burn-out among caregivers; and bereavement issues. We hope that this monograph on research methodological issues serves as a fitting inaugural volume in the series and that future volumes will continue to meet the needs of our target audiences.

David G. Ostrow
Jeffrey A. Kelly

Ann Arbor and Milwaukee

Preface

Any methodological review needs to successfully resolve the issues of timeliness and detail in order to maximize its relevancy and usefulness to the target audience. When the subject is AIDS behavioral research, these problems are accentuated by the rapid explosion of interest among scientists from many different disciplines. We began to discuss the need for a systematic review of the methodological problems confronting survey research efforts in AIDS prevention and mental health in 1987; six years later we have this collection of reviews as the concrete result of the process begun with the simple question: How can quantitative behavioral research best contribute to the battle against AIDS and its recently discovered etiologic agent, HIV? Our goals were to produce a monograph that would be timely and useful to a broad audience working in both research and prevention efforts; to present a selection of methodological issues that would be of interest to both experienced and beginning researchers; and to present examples that illustrate innovative methodological approaches that would be relevant to persons working with the diverse populations affected by the multiple epidemics of AIDS.

If we have been successful in meeting the objectives of the AIDS Research Methodology Project, it is due to the involvement of many colleagues and associates who found the initial question of interest and contributed generously to the Project. That list is extensive and at the risk of omitting someone due to the passage of time, we wish to acknowledge those persons who helped make this book a reality. First, our colleagues at the Institute for Social Research and School of Public Health who participated in the Survey Research Methodology Group (SRMG) of the Midwest AIDS Biobehavioral Research Center: Charles Cannell, Robert Groves, Jill Joseph, James Koopman, Howard Schuman, and Michael Trauggott. Meeting bimonthly between 1987 and 1990, the SRMG identified the initial set of critical survey research issues facing the behavioral and mental health AIDS research communities. Those meetings were enhanced by visits to the University of Michigan from colleagues at other institutions, including John Gagnon from SUNY Stony Brook, Edward Lauman and Stuart Michaels from the National Opinion Research

Center of the University of Chicago, Eleanor Levy from Columbia University, June Reinisch and colleagues from the Kinsey Institute, and Gail Wyatt from UCLA. By early 1989, those meetings and discussions led directly to the proposal for a conference on the methodological issues identified by the MABRC SRMG as crucial to AIDS behavioral research.

Also starting in 1988, the National Institutes for Mental Health (NIMH) AIDS Program began sponsoring meetings of methodological working groups, including the Workgroup for Psychosexual Assessment (chaired by Heino Meyer-Bahlburg of the Columbia HIV Center) and the Workgroup for Psychosocial Assessment (chaired by Susan Folkman from the UCSF Center for AIDS Prevention Studies). Each of these working groups was charged by the NIMH AIDS Program Director (Ellen Stover) and staff (primarily then Deputy Director Anita Eichler and Willow Pequenot) with identifying state-of-the-art descriptive research methodologies and critical gaps which might be the focus of collaborative research efforts involving the growing number of NIMH-sponsored AIDS Research Centers. Through membership on the NIMH working groups the MABRC SRMG members were able to incorporate those identified areas into the proposal for a Midwest AIDS Behavioral Research Symposium. That proposal called for the commissioning of up to fifteen background issue papers in five general areas: Sampling, Study Design, Measurement, Analysis, and Ethical Issues.

On August 10, 1990, the NIMH AIDS Program convened an *ad hoc* Methodology Steering Committee to consider priorities and recommend potential solutions to the methodological issues deemed most crucial to the AIDS prevention and mental health effort. Members of the Steering Committee were Robert Boruch of the University of Pennsylvania and the NRC Committee on AIDS Research, Joseph Catania of the University of California at San Francisco Center for AIDS Prevention Studies, Judith Rabkin and Robert Fullilove of the Columbia HIV Center, Ellen Stover, Anita Eichler, and William Narrow, NIMH, Lydia Temoshok of the Henry M. Jackson Foundation, and ourselves, as proposers of the AIDS Mental Health Research Methodology Conference. The Steering Committee ended up recommending that three AIDS Mental Health Methodology Conferences and monographs be developed: a mental health treatment research volume, a prevention volume, and the present volume on observational/survey research. We hope that ongoing efforts will soon lead to the publication of additional volumes in the broad area of AIDS/HIV Behavioral and Mental Health Research.

Of course, this volume exists because of the authors who contributed so much of their time and effort in writing the fifteen chapters. To all of the contributors, our deepest thanks and gratitude for creating clear and straightforward reviews that, we hope, will be accessible and useful to both experienced and beginning AIDS/HIV researchers.

A special thanks goes to our steadfast editor at Plenum Publishing, Mariclaire Cloutier, who early on pursuaded Plenum to publish a collection of papers that were in the public domain. She became involved in the project during its planning stages and provided an enormous incentive in the recruitment of potential contributors. We hope that this monograph and the process that led to its development can serve as a model for methodological improvement in AIDS and other chronic diseases mental health research.

David G. Ostrow
Ronald C. Kessler

Ann Arbor

Contents

Part I: Design and Sampling Issues

Chapter 2. Sampling Considerations in Research on HIV Risk and Illness

Graham Kalton

Chapter 3. Quasiexperimental Designs in AIDS Psychosocial Research

Ronald C. Kessler

Part II: Measurement Issues

Chapter 4. Combining Qualitative and Quantitative Techniques to Develop Culturally Sensitive Measures

Richard A. Zeller

Chapter 5. Understanding Sexual Behaviors and Drug Use among African-Americans: A Case Study of Issues for Survey Research

Mindy Thompson Fullilove and Robert E. Fullilove, III

Chapter 6. Response Bias in Surveys of AIDS-Related Sexual Behavior

Joseph A. Catania, Heather Turner, Robert C. Pierce,
Eve Golden, Carol Stocking, Diane Binson, and Karen Mast

Chapter 7. Recollection in the Kingdom of AIDS

Robert T. Croyle and Elizabeth F. Loftus

Comments on Croyle and Loftus's Recollections in the Kingdom
Robyn M. Dawes

Part III: Analysis and Modeling Issues

Chapter 8. Using Surveillance Data for Assessing and Projecting the AIDS Epidemic

Victor De Gruttola and Marcello Pagano

Comment on De Gruttola and Pagano's Using Surveillance Data for
Assessing and Projecting the AIDS Epidemic
John M. Karon

Chapter 9. Analytic Methods for Estimating HIV-Treatment and Cofactor Effects

James M. Robins

Chapter 10. The Design and Analysis of Partner Studies of HIV Transmission

Nicholas P. Jewell and Stephen C. Shiboski

Design, Measurement, and Analysis Issues in AIDS Mental Health Research

DAVID G. OSTROW, RONALD C. KESSLER, ELLEN STOVER, and WILLO PEQUEGNAT

1. INTRODUCTION

Since the beginning of the AIDS epidemic, researchers have faced a number of methodological problems that have hampered efforts to understand, control, and ultimately eliminate AIDS and infection by the human immunodeficiency virus (HIV*). While some of these problems are particular to research on the behavioral and mental health aspects of AIDS, others are generic issues that apply more broadly to sexually transmitted diseases and health behavior research. The papers collected in this monograph are the result of a 5-year process of defining the most important methodological issues, identifying persons actively attempting to resolve those issues, and working with these individuals to create a document that would be of practical use to researchers

---

* Throughout this monograph, the abbreviation "HIV" will be used to indicate the human immunodeficiency virus type 1 or HIV-1, the strain of retrovirus that is responsible for all but a few cases of AIDS in the United States and most of the world with the exception of parts of western Africa, where HIV-2 appears to be more prevalent.

DAVID G. OSTROW • Department of Psychiatry, University of Michigan School of Medicine, Ann Arbor, Michigan 48109-0704.   *RONALD C. KESSLER* • Institute for Social Research, University of Michigan, Ann Arbor, Michigan 48106-1248.   *ELLEN STOVER and WILLO PEQUEGNAT* • AIDS Research Program, National Institute of Mental Health, National Institutes of Health, Rockville, Maryland 20857.

Methodological Issues in AIDS Behavioral Health Research, edited by David G. Ostrow and Ronald C. Kessler. Plenum Press, New York, 1993.

and would-be researchers in the behavioral/mental health aspects of HIV and AIDS. As that process included various groups and constituencies involved with AIDS behavioral research, and the final document reflects their activities over several years, it is useful to begin with a brief summary of the history of the "AIDS Survey Research Methodology Monograph Project," or SRMC as we have affectionately called it. Preceding the historical narrative, we discuss several of the overall organizing principles and objectives that guided the later stages of the project and we conclude with brief overviews of the three book sections. We hope that this introduction will help the intended audience better to understand and utilize the diverse methodological approaches represented in this final product of the SRMC.

2. BALANCING SCIENTIFIC RIGOR WITH URGENCY IN AIDS RESEARCH

The epidemics of AIDS and HIV first recognized in 1981 have produced crises not only in the public health and policy arenas but also in the behavioral, mental health, and social science research communities. A number of review processes have examined the history and problems associated with the scientific research communities' response to the AIDS epidemic; each concluded that efforts to "fast track" scientific studies have inevitably resulted in difficulties in validating and interpreting the results of those studies (Reinisch *et al.,* 1988; Gagnon, 1989; Turner *et al.,* 1989). Certainly the ever-unfolding magnitude of the multiple epidemics of AIDS, HIV infection, stigmatization, fear, and panic justifies the need for mobilizing resources and streamlining the process of research planning, funding, and implementation of studies designed to curtail those epidemics. What is less certain is just how to modify and expedite the conduct of scientific research so it responds to the urgent needs of the AIDS crisis without sacrificing the scientific rigor necessary to ensure the validity and applicability of the resulting research outcomes.

3. CENTRALITY OF SOCIAL AND ETHICAL ISSUES TO PROCESS

Key to understanding and overcoming barriers to the timely conduct of AIDS/HIV prevention-oriented research is the recognition that social stigma and taboos concerning the behaviors and populations that are the focus of that research effort continue unabated in our society. The same stigma and taboos that led to the almost complete halting of sexual behavior research in the United States during the 1950s and 1960s today result in the halting of efforts to conduct national surveys of sexual behavior among adults and adolescents. It is not surprising, given the widespread climate of distrust of sexual and drug use behavior researchers that exists in our society, that research in these areas is undervalued and underfunded and that methodological research is rarely, if ever, seen as a priority for the use of scarce resources (Catania *et al.*, 1990; Gagnon, 1989). Similarly, survey researchers have long been wary of conducting methodological studies among unfamiliar populations or concerning "sensitive" questions of sexual or drug use practices. As a result, most of the survey research instruments available to early entrants into AIDS/HIV research were developed using readily available white, middle-class populations of students or gay men. Few, if any, included the broad range of social and sexual behaviors subsequently recognized as important to the transmission of HIV and other cofactors of infection or disease progression. And none was available in a form that was adequately field-tested for valid use in populations other than well-educated men and women living outside of the environments of poverty and social deprivation that are the increasing focus of AIDS/HIV prevention efforts.

The traditional approach of scientific research in dealing with socially "sensitive" research topics and populations, at least during the latter half of the 20th century, has been to analyze the research benefits and risks from an ethical perspective. Driven by the primary ethical concerns of *primum non nocere* (or "above else, do no harm") and respect for individual autonomy and privacy, AIDS behavioral and mental health researchers have, for the most part, made enormous strides through ethical approaches for solving the complex social issues surrounding the epidemic. But ethical concerns can sometimes be as inhibiting of creative solutions to problematic but urgent research issues as historical examples of unethical research practices. For example, out of concern for the unethical exploitation of pregnant women and incarcerated persons, prison inmates were systematically excluded from AIDS/HIV therapeutic trials until advocates for women and prison inmates engaged the scientific and policy-making communities on their behalf. And certain political leaders are not above appropriating ethical issues, such as privacy concerns, in their efforts to block urgently needed research to ascertain the prevalence and determinants of the behaviors that inhibit or facilitate HIV transmission. As a result of recognition of these social and ethical concerns, AIDS researchers and policymakers are increasingly involving both ethicists and representatives of the target communities in the design, planning, and implementation of their research activities. Similarly, early on in the planning processes that resulted in this monograph, we decided that ethical and social concerns had to be integral to the review of research methodological issues and the development of innovative solutions.

4. HISTORY OF PROJECT

The SRMC was the result of the intersection of two independent research planning and review processes that began in late 1987. One was the planning and implementation of the Midwest AIDS Biobehavioral Research Center (MABRC) including a core Survey Research Methods Group, or SRMG. That group, organized by Michael Traugott of the Center for Political Studies of the Institute for Social Research (ISR) at the University of Michigan, was composed of various survey research experts from ISR and other MABRC collaborating organizations, such as the National Opinion Research Center. The MARBC SRMG had as one of its central objectives the identification of critical AIDS survey research issues that could be addressed through targeted reviews and meta-analyses of both published and unpublished methods experiments, small pilot studies, and incorporation of methodological experiments into planned MABRC research studies. Meeting bimonthly over a period of 2 years, the SRMG identified a set of critical survey research issues facing the behavioral and mental health AIDS research communities. These issues ranged from the problems involved in minimizing biases in answering "sensitive" questions in general population surveys to designing ways to sample relatively rare populations defined in terms of sexual or drug use behaviors, to ascertaining the effects of gender, race, and sexual preference matching of interviewers and respondents in surveys of AIDS risk behaviors. By early 1989, the MABRC SRMG proposed the organization of a conference focusing on the methodological issues they had identified as crucial to the planned research activities of MABRC.

Also starting in 1988, the NIMH AIDS Research Centers [then composed of MABRC, the Miami AIDS Research Center, the UCSF Center for AIDS Prevention Studies (CAPS), and the Columbia HIV Center] formed a number of methodology working groups, including the Workgroup for Psychosexual Assessment (chaired by Heino Meyer-Bahlburg of the Columbia HIV Center) and the Workgroup for Psychosocial Assessment (chaired by Susan Folkman from the UCSF CAPS). Each of these working groups was charged by the NIMH AIDS Program staff with identifying state-of-the-art descriptive research methodologies and critical gaps that might be the focus of collaborative methodological research activities involving the NIMH Centers. The NIMH AIDS Research Center ad hoc working groups systematically catalogued available methods in each specific area of psychosexual and psychosocial assessment deemed critical to AIDS behavioral and mental health research efforts and, in so doing, identified a number of critical gaps or unresolved controversies that impeded ongoing and future research.

By early 1990, the NIMH AIDS Program staff began the process of reviewing the MABRC proposal, reports from the AIDS Center ad hoc working groups, and summary statements from recent research proposal reviews in order to identify Program priorities for methodological development related to AIDS behavioral/mental health research needs. On August 10, 1990, the NIMH AIDS Program convened an ad hoc steering committee composed of researchers from both within and outside of the NIMH AIDS Research Centers* to consider those priorities and recommend practical approaches to resolving those methodological issues deemed most crucial. The steering committee both endorsed the list of critical methodological issues that had been assembled by NIMH AIDS Program staff and the concept of developing several series of background issue papers that could serve both as technical assistance tools and as the basis of methodological conferences as proposed by the MABRC SRMG. It was agreed that Kessler and Ostrow, who had previously made a proposal for a survey research methodology conference through the MABRC SRMG, should take the lead in this area and that this should be the first NIMH-sponsored AIDS research methodology conference.

Soon after the ad hoc steering committee's recommendations were combined with the earlier efforts and a report issued by NIMH AIDS Program staff, we began the process of selecting expert authors for each of the ten high-priority topic areas in survey/observational research methodology directly relevant to AIDS behavioral and mental health research. This was perhaps the most difficult part of the entire 5-year process. As each paper was to be authored by a senior expert in the relevant field of survey research who could combine basic methodological insights with concrete examples related to AIDS research, the field of potential authors was relatively limited. The tight schedule that we and NIMH staff set for the implementation phase of this project further limited the available potential authors who had both the experience and time to participate. It is no secret that the best researchers and methodologists are extremely busy conducting, analyzing, and writing up their own research efforts and that methodological reviews are not among the highest priorities for such individuals. We were helped considerably in this difficult task by the offer of Plenum Medical Publishing to publish the final monograph as part of their publishing commitment to the areas of AIDS and human behavior. Still, we were happily surprised to find that some of the very best people in the field were willing to commit to this project even though there

---

* The ad hoc NIMH methodology issues steering committee members were Ronald Kessler and David Ostrow (University of Michigan, MABRC), Judith Rabkin and Robert Fullilove (Columbia HIV Center), Robert Boruch (University of Pennsylvania and the NRC Committee on AIDS Research), Lydia Temoshok (Henry M. Jackson Foundation for the Advancement of Military Medicine), and Joseph Catania (UCSF CAPS). NIMH program staff included Ellen Stover and Anita Eichler, AIDS Program, William Narrow, Epidemiology/Biometry Branch, and Peter Muehrer, Prevention Research Branch.

was so little money and time and so much work. Each author was asked to address a concrete set of methodological problems within their specific area of AIDS mental health and/or survey observational research expertise and to include in their reviews the following information:

- Critique of the key methodological problems in their topic area
- Case examples of ongoing AIDS mental health research projects that exemplify specific methodological obstacles, including cultural and ethnic-specific issues
- An analysis of methodological problems, successes, and strategies for improving study designs
- Consideration of the ethical issues related to both the methodological problems and their proposed innovative solutions
- The latest developments in relevant research methodologies as well as their own proposals for innovative solutions to the key methodological problems they identified

At the AIDS Survey Research Methods Conference, which took place July 11–12, 1991, in Rockville, Maryland, all of the chapter authors as well as a dozen invited discussants, plus NIMH AIDS Program Staff and other interested staff members from ADAMHA, NIH, and CDC AIDS research programs, met to continue the process of conversion of the Conference paper drafts into this monograph. Each discussant was chosen in order to provide an optimal level of feedback between survey research methodologists and AIDS researchers actually working in the field settings where the recommended innovative methodological approaches would be ultimately tested. The resulting discussions were both extremely animated and productive of new insights into the key AIDS behavioral/mental health research questions and creative approaches to answering those questions.

It can be said that everyone left the conference with a renewed sense of what could be accomplished in bringing together methodological experts and front-line researchers in this most challenging and urgent field. What remained for us was the challenge of getting the excitement and creativity of the Conference discussion into a form that would make our insights available to the target audiences of researchers in both substantive and methodological fields related to AIDS and HIV and their behavioral and mental health implications. Working from transcripts of the Conference, we recommended specific revisions and additions to each author. Several of the invited discussants agreed to incorporate their own and other discussants' remarks into brief Discussion papers that follow several of the chapters. By early 1992, we had received the revised chapters and discussions and began the process of final editing and preparation of this Introduction.

We hope that out of this long process a cohesive and up-to-date monograph has emerged that will provide the state-of-the-art technical assistance to the target audience that was intended when we first began discussing the issues of AIDS survey research methodology in 1987. In that time, AIDS research priorities have changed dramatically as clinical, epidemiological, and prevention efforts have achieved notable successes as well as experienced major setbacks. But we believe that the major methodological obstacles that confronted us in 1987 are still relevant as researchers turn their attention to newly emerging at-risk populations and behavioral/mental health questions. We know that as researchers and administrators dedicated to bringing innovative methodology to the urgent public health issues of the AIDS and HIV epidemics, we are still confronted daily with the challenge of balancing methodological rigor with the urgency of fighting those epidemics with accurate and useful information. And we hope that the successful completion of this project will encourage our colleagues to pursue similar endeavors in the fields of behavioral and mental health intervention research.

The rest of this chapter outlines some of the major methodological problems that still confront the field in meeting this challenge. These issues are based on participation in AIDS review committee meetings and site visits and reviewing summary statements of AIDS research applications. While these topics are not exhaustive, they can be broadly categorized into the following areas:

- Theoretical considerations
- Research design
- Recruitment and sampling
- Control or comparison group
- Instrumentation and related measurement issues
- Criteria for establishing change
- Intervention issues
- Data analysis
- Ethical issues

The contributions from relevant chapters are highlighted in the appropriate topical sections.

5. THEORETICAL CONSIDERATIONS

Summary statements, which represent the product of a peer review, frequently identify the lack of a theory or model to frame the study as a fatal flaw in research applications (Herek, 1992). AIDS has been hindered by a paucity of theoretical frameworks that specify relationships among the multiple biomedical and psychosocial variables that are usually measured in studies of HIV. Even when a theory has been adopted, it has been poorly used to provide a conceptual framework to guide the development of testable hypotheses (Dawes, 1992) and the data analysis (Taylor, 1992). Clearly, development of explanatory models and constructs that yield testable models is a high priority in improving AIDS research.

6. RESEARCH DESIGN

AIDS is a rapidly changing area of clinical study that has created unprecedented design problems. In developing a study it has often been unclear which treatments to test and what should be controlled, because of the rapidity of the introduction of different pharmacological treatments. Both the external and internal validity of studies have been threatened by the fact that new drugs and treatments have come on-line in the middle of studies. Because of the urgency of the disease, many cross-sectional studies have been conducted without a longitudinal component. While this has resulted in important work, it has not allowed certain questions that have long-term implications to be asked (and answered).

A major problem has been the difficulty of using random samples and of random assignment to treatment groups. One potentially useful strategy for dealing with the great difficulty in obtaining the random assignment we would ideally like to have in AIDS behavioral research is to use quasiexperimental designs that take advantage of naturalistic opportunities to approximate randomization. Ron Kessler's chapter focuses on quasiexperimental designs and achieving control through the design of data collection. He reviews the use of time-series designs in evaluating treatments in nonrandomized clinical trials or comparable institutions. He discusses the use of a regression discontinuity design for samples from communities or institutions. The regression point displacement design provides a potent tool for AIDS researchers who are introducing a communitywide AIDS educational program. Kessler discusses other designs and recommends the use of LISREL and EQS methods rather than a regression approach.

Although Nicholas P. Jewell and Stephen C. Shiboski appear in the section directed to issues of data analysis, they also address some special design concerns. There are sparse data about the probability of transmission of HIV and the associated cofactors. They discuss the myriad of issues in modeling transmission in both retrospective and prospective designs and the procedures to analyze these results.

Richard A. Zeller outlines a strategy to combine quantitative and qualitative methods in a design that can enhance the data that are collected. This is a particularly important discussion in the context of AIDS behavioral research because many of the behaviors that are of concern are very private. In designing cross-cultural studies, an ethnographic design may be the only strategy that is effective in collecting reliable and valid data. In a related chapter, Mindy and Robert Fullilove suggest that focus group methodology may be the only way to tap the rich nuances of language with Afro-American populations.

7. RECRUITMENT AND SAMPLING ISSUES

Another area that peer review groups often highlight as a criticism of research applications is the sampling plan. Selecting appropriate sampling strategies for the specific populations at risk for HIV presents some unique problems. For example, subgroups (e.g., Afro-American and Hispanic teenage males) may not participate in the institutions from which researchers generally recruit their subjects (e.g., schools, hospitals, community groups). For the subgroups that do participate in these institutions, there may be problems of parental and community consent when the study involves examining private behaviors associated with a socially stigmatized disease. Even when a good sampling plan has been developed, there has been concern that the sampling of moderator variables may not have been adequately addressed.

Selection criteria for research subjects can be difficult to specify because of the vast number of variables associated with the staging of HIV disease. Currently, the traditional way to stage the disease is using CDC classifications. However, these criteria were established to provide disease prevalence data and there is a question whether this is an appropriate system to use in defining asymptomatic and symptomatic patients. And, since the CDC classification system was originally established on the basis of experience, whether this system underdiagnoses women's problems associated with HIV.

In designing a study, the investigator selects a target sample size based on considerations of statistical power. The latter, in turn, is based on estimates of the seroprevalence rate in the sample prior to the time of enrollment. Many studies have subsequently suffered from problems of low statistical power because the actual rate of HIV disease was less than expected in a recruitment area during the period of the study or researchers were not successful in recruiting from the study population. Even when adequate samples have been enrolled in studies, retention and attrition have been a major threat. Some of these problems are unavoidable because of the chronic and life-threatening nature of the disease, but better recruitment and sampling strategies may ameliorate some of them.

Generalizability and external validity have been difficult to establish for studies conducted on one small sample in a single locale because of faulty sampling. There have been concerns about biases because of the reliance on convenience samples (e.g., methadone maintenance facilities, STD clinics). Self-selection biases may contribute to unreliable results in studies that rely on convenience samples or do not permit random assignment to treatment groups.

Graham Kalton's chapter reviews sampling strategies that might be used to address these problems. He indicates that either standard area probability sampling or random digit dialing may be used with general population surveys or client surveys of particular AIDS-related services. However, in a survey of high-risk groups, he suggests that obtaining a hidden, socially stigmatized group requires a range of techniques such as screening in conjunction with other techniques (e.g., multistage sampling, location sampling, snowballing). Kalton discusses each technique as well as its limitations and provides a number of useful suggestions for future sampling efforts.

8. CONTROL OR COMPARISON GROUP

While there have been problems in defining the population to be studied, determining what constitutes a satisfactory control or comparison group is even more difficult in designing studies of the effects of HIV-1 infection on the central nervous system (CNS). For example, finding a group of HIV-1 seropositive and symptomatic gay men who are not receiving some type of pharmacological treatment is not realistic. While this might be ideal, given the treatment environment of HIV disease, there might be a myriad of treatment biases to which such a study would be vulnerable. Therefore, with what is a group of seropositive, symptomatic persons who are receiving a treatment compared? In a clinical trial, different strategies may be adopted: (1) a seropositive symptomatic group receiving another treatment; (2) a group of chronically ill persons receiving treatment for a disease that does not affect the CNS; or (3) a population-based group matched on age, SES, and other sociodemographic variables. There is, as yet, no clear consensus on the best strategy to use in these situations. The problem of appropriate comparison groups is likely to remain with us for some time and it is critical that AIDS behavioral researchers are sensitive to it and that they evaluate the sensitivity of their results to differences in decisions about appropriate comparisons.

9. INSTRUMENTATION AND RELATED MEASUREMENT ISSUES

Currently, gay and bisexual men and injection drug users (IDUs) are the majority of subjects in most studies; however, the number of HIV-infected heterosexual women and adolescents, especially those in urban areas among ethnically diverse groups, is increasing rapidly. Each of these populations differs in social culture and behavioral norms. Since health behavior research has historically focused on middle-class populations, and because Afro-Americans and Hispanics have traditionally been underserved in prevention and health research initiatives, little is known about the social context of the populations most imminently threatened by the HIV epidemic in the second decade and the variables that are most critical to evaluate. Mindy and Robert Fullilove suggest that qualitative methods can be used to learn about these issues.

Therefore, assessing multicultural populations across the age span may require different measurement strategies. Remien (1992) has suggested a strategy of adapting instruments that has worked relatively well with gay populations. The instruments most frequently used in AIDS research may be culturally biased in unknown ways and there are no norms that can be used to correct this problem. There are many variables associated with instruments that may need to be noted: terminology or wording of question, order of the questions, level of language, connotation of words.

In addition to suggesting that combining quantitative and qualitative methods may contribute to a more culturally sound approach, Richard Zeller suggests a measurement effort to develop valid, reliable, and culturally sensitive measures of risk perceptions, social support, and coping strategies. This strategy can be used to remedy the problems associated with existing instruments.

The validity of the data can be affected by aspects of the behaviors or experience that are being assessed by the instrument. For example, there may be less reliable data if there is great complexity about what must be recalled, the meaningfulness of the experience to the person, the person's memory for events and people which may be paired with the context of the event and the associated emotional state, and whether the event is of low or high frequency.

Robert T. Croyle and Elizabeth F. Loftus explore the utility of theories and methods of cognitive psychology associated with these recall problems in HIV (e.g., number of partners or number of times a condom was used). They explore the relationship between episodic (events or life experiences) and semantic (general factual knowledge) types of memory. They review memory errors associated with reporting health-related behaviors and discuss some research needs in theories and methods of cognitive psychology associated with high-risk behavior.

While many traditional psychological instruments are appropriate for AIDS research, there has been a lack of valid instruments that index specific areas of AIDS behavioral research. For example, there have been few instruments to collect sexual data that have established validity and reliability. While there are instruments that are valid and reliable to assess neuropsychological and neuropsychiatric problems associated with HIV, they are time-consuming and may present undue patient burden with persons who are sick and have limited energy.

Joseph A. Catania and his colleagues discuss measurement issues related to bias in surveys of sexual behavior. Specifically, they discuss participation bias, systematic measurement error, and the effect of attrition in longitudinal surveys. This chapter provides data from several telephone surveys that clarify the effect that these issues can have on results in a study of sensitive issues.

10. INTERVIEWING TECHNIQUES

There has been concern about whether the interviewing techniques used in face-to-face or telephone interviews have been effective. There may be feasibility and reliability issues related to the use of these techniques in studying sexual behavior in the general population. Questions have been raised about the difference in data collected from same-gender or same-ethnic pairs of interviewer and subject. Catania and his colleagues report that many Hispanic women may not be willing to discuss sex with a man who is a stranger.

In addition to the traditional interviewer variables (gender, age, ethnicity, sexual orientation), the interviewer can provide other confounds to the data collection if the person is not comfortable with the questions being asked or if the person changes the meaning of the question by intonation or changes the order of questions or words.

There has been controversy about whether structured and standardized interview procedures or unstructured methods yield better data. While one might provide more comparable data using the same metric, it may miss issues that are most salient to the study questions. There are problems and benefits encountered when using a member of the community to interview the subjects, especially if it is a hard-to-reach population. While it might facilitate access, it may blunt honesty if the subject feels that confidentiality may be violated.

11. INTERVENTION AND TREATMENT ISSUES

While extensive knowledge, attitude, and behavior (KAB) studies have been conducted, there are still only limited data about populations at high risk for whom interventions are needed. Some data on interventions were gathered early when little KAB data were available and so it may not be clear how to apply this work to other populations. In some instances, random assignment to treatment was not possible, which biased the findings on efficacy of different treatments. Many treatments were confounded or contaminated by other treatments that the subjects were receiving but that were not the focus of the study. In some instances, persons were self-medicating or seeking additional social support beyond that provided by the intervention.

The variation in the time of the assessment periods may have contributed to the efficacy of the treatment in unknown ways. There is also difficulty in maintaining the research and service boundary when studying populations who are dependent on the study site for clinical care.

12. CRITERIA FOR ESTABLISHING CHANGE

Identifying the variables associated with behavior change in multifaceted interventions has been hampered by the problems discussed in the previous section. In addition, there are concerns associated with psychometrics and defining outcomes.

In studies of HIV infection there may be persons at different stages of the disease who will score at both the high and low end of the instrument. In assessing change, the range of the metric of the instrument can have a profound and unintended effect on the results. When subjects score near the ceiling of an instrument, missing an item may dramatically influence a test score and similarly if subjects near the floor of the instrument complete a single extra item the score may be strongly affected.

Variables appropriate for HIV studies generally involve constructs that are unidimensional and that can be measured in a continuous, quantitative fashion. Raw score metrics or vertically equated scale scores are necessary in order to establish the process of change. That is, when a person's score goes up or down a point, that translates into gaining or losing a specified amount of ability. When data are standardized according to an age criterion, information concerning the process of true change may be masked by restandardization of the data at each age point. This may be more pronounced with children where standard score indicators may suggest decline in intelligence while using raw scores may provide evidence that the child is capable of learning and is actually improving on each assessment. This is because the child is actually acquiring new skills at a slower rate than his or her age cohort, which means that the standardized IQ score declines even though the child is actually continuing to develop.

In addition to problems of instrumentation in predicting aspects of HIV disease, there is a problem in specifying and evaluating outcomes. Most outcomes in AIDS research are self-report measures that are subject to many problems.

There are major methodological problems associated with relying solely on self-report measures but there may not be any biological marker or objective measure to cross-validate the information. Sexually transmitted diseases may provide only a rough index of penetrative sexual activity while correlation of the number of partners may be subject to selective recall. Because these are private behaviors, it may not be possible to confirm by direct observation. Under some circumstances, it may be possible to have them corroborated by the partner or other participants in the event that may also be vulnerable to participant bias. The techniques of keeping diaries and life course reconstruction have been used to improve recall of significant events to enhance the reliability of outcome data (Davies, 1989).

In addition to denial, participant bias in self-report may be caused by item refusal, over- and underreporting, and test–retest reliability. If there are high item refusal rates on some areas, such as sexual behavior, there may be insufficient data to analyze that question. This is a critical problem because if there is an under- or overestimate of the amount of high-risk behaviors, persons at risk may be misidentified, which may consequently undermine prevention efforts. The stability of people's self-report may present another confound. A change score on a self-report measure may index actual change or be an artifact of poor test–retest reliability of the instrument. An essential area of AIDS research is to develop multimethod, multimodal ways to assess outcome in behavioral studies.

13. DATA ANALYSIS

Some innovative data analysis methods may be needed to tease out what is happening in AIDS research. Because of the high attrition rates in AIDS research due to illness and death, survival analysis may provide a better strategy to use in analyzing the data from many studies (Ellenberg *et al.,* 1992).

In this book, an entire section is devoted to the special data analytic needs in AIDS research. James M. Robins describes some new methods to estimate the effect of treatment which may be the only available methods to adjust for the effects of additional nonrandomized treatments in randomized clinical trials.

Analytic methods are suggested by Victor De Gruttola and Marcello Pagano that are robust enough to handle differential data quality issues that are inherent in surveillance data bases. Nicholas P. Jewell and Stephen C. Shiboski discuss the design and analysis of partner studies and suggest a framework for assessing the probability of HIV transmission in modes of contact and the role cofactors play in promoting or suppressing transmission.

14. ETHICAL ISSUES

Ethical guidelines are essential in AIDS research because there is a continual balance between the need for data on which to predicate prevention efforts and the privacy of individuals about highly personal, stigmatized, and sometimes illegal behaviors. In their chapter, Howard C. Stevenson, Dorothy De Moya, and Robert F. Boruch review the historical precedents for ethical guidelines and pose five fundamental questions about the relationship between the investigator and subject and about privacy and confidentiality. These are basically issues of who, when, where, what, and how, which can determine whether the balance between good and harm to an individual can be established. They present options to increase ethical behavior in AIDS research.

15. CONCLUSIONS

In this Introduction, we have tried to describe the sociocultural milieu within which this monograph was developed and to summarize the methodological issues and concerns addressed by the individual chapters. While AIDS has indeed presented a set of new and challenging methodological problems in the design and conduct of studies, a broad and comprehensive research program has been mounted by researchers and funded by the National Institute of Mental Health (NIMH) to address the neuroscience, behavioral, and prevention research questions posed by HIV. NIMH is committed to strengthening current AIDS projects as well as mental health HIV research applications by providing state-of-the-art assessment strategies and by addressing methodological challenges in HIV behavioral research. This book is a major effort that is designed to ensure that the second decade is even more productive than the first one in confronting these pressing research issues.

REFERENCES

Catania, J. A., Gibson, D. R., Chitwood, D. D., and Coates, T. J. (1990). Methodological problems in AIDS behavioral research: Influences on measurement error and participation bias in studies of sexual behavior. *Psychol. Bull.* **108**:339–362.

Davies, P. (1989). Using personal interviews with diary keeping to provide improved measures of sexual behavior. *Joint Centre for Survey Methods Newsletter* **10**:8–9.

Dawes, R. M. (1992). How do you formulate a testable exciting hypothesis? In W. Pequegnat and E. Stover (eds.), *How to write a successful research application.* Washington, D.C.: National Technical Information Service.

Ellenberg, S. S., Finkelstein, D. M., and Schoenfeld, D. A. (1992). Statistical issues arising in AIDS clinical trials. *J. Am. Stat. Assoc.* **87**:562–569.

Gagnon, J. (1989). Sex research and sexual conduct in the era of AIDS. *J. AIDS* **1**:593–601.

Herek, G. (1992). Development of a theoretical framework and rationale for your research proposal. In W. Pequegnat and E. Stover (eds.), *How to write a successful research application.* Washington, D.C.: National Technical Information Service.

Reinisch, J. M., Sanders, S. A., and Ziemba-Davis, M. (1988). The study of sexual behavior in relation to the transmission of human immunodeficiency virus. Caveats and recommendations. *Am. Psychol.* **43**:921–927.

Remien, R. H. (1992). Instrumentation: Off the shelf or on your own. In W. Pequegnat and E. Stover (eds.), *How to write a successful research application.* Washington, D.C.: National Technical Information Service.

Taylor, H. G. (1992). Developing the analytic plan. In W. Pequegnat and E. Stover (eds.), *How to write a successful research application.* Washington, D.C.: National Technical Information Service.

Turner, C. F., Miller, H., and Moses, L. E. (1989). *AIDS, sexual behavior, and intravenous drug use.* Washington, D.C.: National Academy Press.

Design and Sampling Issues

Ethical Issues and Approaches in AIDS Research

HOWARD C. STEVENSON,
DOROTHY DE MOYA, and
ROBERT F. BORUCH

1. INTRODUCTION

Mark Twain once said, "Always do right. This will gratify some people and astonish the rest." Doing the right thing is what the public expects of scientists who conduct research to improve the quality of life. AIDS researchers are faced with a unique challenge in uncovering the mysteries of AIDS transmission and gathering data on the private behaviors of individuals that contribute to its spread. Researchers are responsible for knowing the possible negative effects of their research procedures and for balancing the need for research information with the protection of the participant's rights. Many issues of distrust and stigmatization affect AIDS research programs and set the stage for difficult data gathering ventures.

  Our task for this chapter is to outline ethical issues facing AIDS researchers. We will examine briefly the history of scientific impropriety, identify various ethical principles and guidelines, discuss the propriety of randomized field experiments, explore options to increase confidentiality and privacy in AIDS research, note specific examples of ethical and confidentiality dilemmas, and make suggestions about where research seems warranted.

HOWARD C. STEVENSON and ROBERT F. BORUCH • Graduate School of Education, University of Pennsylvania, Philadelphia, Pennsylvania 19104-6216.   *DOROTHY DE MOYA* • Correctional Health Solutions, Chalfont, Pennsylvania 18914.

Methodological Issues in AIDS Behavioral Research, edited by David G. Ostrow and Ronald C. Kessler. Plenum Press, New York, 1993.

1.1. Basic Definitions

Clarifying the definitions of terms can avoid needless confusion. The definitions of privacy, confidentiality, and security are multidimensional and reiterated here (Boruch, 1990).

Privacy. Privacy refers to an individual's right to control personal information, such as beliefs, attitudes, and behaviors. It also includes the participant's control over his/her bodily integrity as well as personal space (Melton, 1983). Privacy of the institution is not the concern of this chapter. To the extent that an individual divulges information about him- or herself, privacy is diminished. While there are statistical and procedural ways to reduce the compromise of privacy, AIDS researchers are expected to design methods that do not appeciably reduce privacy while still yielding socially meaningful information.

Confidentiality. Confidentiality is the protection against the unauthorized disclosure of personal information. Once disclosed, it is incumbent on the AIDS researcher to prevent the redisclosure of the information and to ensure its use for research purposes only. To the extent that a participant's disclosed information is held to be confidential and protected by law against appropriation by agencies outside of the research institution (e. g., police and human services agencies), privacy is also protected.

Security. Security protects against accessing the system that stores, tabulates, and manages research information. It is usually a function of the mechanical and electronic capabilities of that system. While not a focus of this discussion, there can be general public fear regarding how personal information in a computer is less protected than when filed away in a locked drawer.

Privacy work involves further distinctions between administrative or clinical records and research or statistical records. Administrative or clinical records involve personal information about a participant and are referred to when decisions about that individual are made. Statistical or research records are designed solely for the promulgation of research and identification is necessary only to the extent a researcher can continue tracking or measuring on some variable. Privacy as defined from the participant's perspective must also be recognized given the concerns regarding the integrity of scientific ventures.

The examination of ethical guidelines for AIDS research has been subjected to serious critique (Gray and Melton, 1985; Melton and Gray, 1988; Melton *et al.,* 1988). The emotionally charged and difficult questions of ethics have challenged AIDS researchers in ways similar to other stigmatizing social dilemmas. In their summary statement, Bayer *et al.* (1984) state clearly the rationale for the development of ethical research guidelines:

> The identification of Acquired Immune Deficiency Syndrome (AIDS) three years ago has created a crisis of confidence. Persons with AIDS and others who might be research subjects recognize that research is essential to understand, treat and prevent this devastating disease, yet they are concerned that information divulged for research purposes might be used in ways detrimental to their interest. Unless they have confidence in the system designed to protect their privacy and in the people to whom personal information is entrusted they may provide invalid or incomplete data. The problem then is: What procedures and policies will both protect the privacy interests of research subjects and enable research to proceed expeditiously? [p. 5]

Three broad categories of approaches have been designed to protect the privacy and confidentiality of participants in AIDS research. They include procedural approaches, statistical approaches, and legal approaches (Boruch and Cecil, 1979, 1983). Since the discussion of privacy and confidentiality relates primarily to the reduction or avoidance of adverse effects on participants/respondents, it may prove worthwhile to develop models of understanding the practice of ethics and confidentiality from the participant's perspective. Historical examples of the misuse of personal information or the lack of protection of privacy are important for any discussion of research ethics. Before addressing the question of privacy protection, a historical look at ethical guidelines is warranted.

2. HISTORICAL ANTECEDENTS OF CONTEMPORARY ETHICAL GUIDELINES

To say that recent history has generated doubts about the integrity of scientific endeavors understates the matter (Zuckerman, 1990). Developing research agendas on highly sensitive topics requires entry into communities that are often hostile to the tenets of research. It requires more than a research track record, university clout, and political savvy. In fact, lessons of drug regimen sharing between control and experimental group participants from AIDS clinical trials have led some researchers to suggest that research apart from a community/scientist partnership may suffer from an overabundance of unhelpful solutions (Melton *et al.,* 1988). Concern has arisen about the integrity of science and the value-laden decisions of scientists.

> Historians, sociologists, and other students of science have shown that social and personal values unrelated to epistemological criteria—including philosophical, religious, cultural, political, and economic values—can shape scientific judgment in

fundamental ways. . . . The obvious question is whether holding such values can harm a person's science. In many cases the answer has to be yes. The history of science offers many episodes in which social or personal values led to the promulgation of wrong-headed ideas. For instance, past investigators produced "scientific" evidence for overtly racist views, evidence that we now know to be wholly erroneous. Yet at the time the evidence was widely accepted and contributed to repressive social policies. [Committee on the Conduct of Science, 1990, pp. 215–216]

For example, the Tuskeegee Syphilis Study conducted by the Public Health Service from 1932 to 1972 was the longest nontherapeutic study conducted in the history of the United States. It involved the withholding of medical treatment from 400 black men in the South with the expressed purpose of tracking syphilis into the tertiary stages (Jones, 1981). This was an unethical experiment not only because the men were not treated for syphilis, but also because they were led to believe that they were receiving treatment. Attempts to keep these men from receiving treatment were prompted by optimism and application of the longitudinal research principle of controlling for variables (i. e., any form of medical intervention) that might interfere with legitimate results. Medical science's desire to eradicate a major health problem, its wrongful assumptions of black sexuality, and its deception of available but vulnerable research participants all contributed to a neglectful stance toward this research (Jones, 1981).

The Nuremberg Code of 1947, which addressed problems in human experimentation by establishing the protection of human subjects, had been developed long before the Tuskeegee episode was concluded. The World Medical Association in 1964 drafted a more explicit set of ethical guidelines called the Declaration of Helsinki that enunciated the following principles: (1) Clinical research should be based on scientific principles and committee-proved research design; (2) the researchers should be scientifically qualified; (3) the research objectives should be in proportion to the inherent risk to subjects; and (4) the right of the patient to privacy and dignity must be safeguarded. One of the major contributions of the Helsinki Declaration was the fundamental distinction between therapeutic research aimed at the diagnosis and treatment of patients, and nontherapeutic research aimed at purely scientific knowledge without treatment value to the individual research participant. The guidelines for this dichotomy were:

1. Subjects should be protected from unnecessary harm in nontherapeutic research.
2. Investigators should have a strong justification for exposing a healthy volunteer to a substantial risk of harm simply for increasing scientific knowledge.

3. Investigators are responsible for protecting the life and health of research participants.
4. Each participant must be adequately informed of the nature of the study and must give free consent.

The authors stated: "The concern for the interest of the subject must always prevail over the interests of science and society" (Levine, 1986, p. 288). These and other examples justify the development of ethical codes for professionals of various disciplines and the invention of methods to facilitate their use.

3. ETHICAL PRINCIPLES THAT APPLY TO AIDS RESEARCH

Various ethical guidelines and principles have been proposed to help establish an ethic toward conducting research for AIDS patients (Ankrah, 1989; Bayer *et al.,* 1984; Committee for the Protection of Human Participants, 1986; Fineberg, 1990; National Commission for the Protection of Human Subjects in Biomedical and Behavioral Research, 1978).

Fineberg (1990) identifies four ethical principles: bodily integrity, balancing good and harm to an individual, preventing harm to others, and striving toward justice. The first principle suggests that researchers develop public policy around HIV infection screening that protects the autonomy of the individual's interest over and above the interests of society. Second, balancing the conflict between societal and individual interests implies that where harm does occur, either as expected or unintentionally, a "net effect of good" must result. Third, researchers and clinicians are expected to engage in harm prevention activities as they establish the strategies to conduct HIV infection screening. Finally, Fineberg argues for a commitment to justice that implies a "fair distribution across individuals, of the burdens as well as the benefits associated with our social interventions" (p. 30). Fineberg's counsel is focused on operational programs (i. e., screening) rather than research. Insofar as research on such programs is sensible the counsel is pertinent here also.

The fear of intrusiveness from government and other large societal institutions has been a driving force behind the preponderance of ethical mandates. These calls have centered around the principles of respect for personal autonomy, beneficence or good will toward participant, justice, avoidance of maleficence, and fidelity (Committee for the Protection of Human Participants, 1986; Melton *et al.*, 1988).* Another related principle is that of equipoise. Equipoise has been defined by Freedman (1987) as a state of genuine uncertainty on the part of a scientist regarding the imperative therapeutic merits of a specific intervention. It has also been interpreted to mean the ambivalence that may exist within the entire medical community toward a preferred treatment regimen (Freedman, 1987).

A Hastings Center group of behavioral research experts developed a set of specific ethical guidelines and recommendations for AIDS researchers, public health officials, institutional review boards (IRBs), legislators, and community organizations (Bayer *et al.*, 1984). These recommendations address the following: when identifiers are needed and when they are not; who should and who should not have access to personally identifiable information obtained during research or surveillance; explanation of experimental design and procedures, confidentiality procedures, the need to remove identifiable personal information as soon as research purposes have been achieved, and rationale for the study; when research information can be redisclosed to other researchers; enhancing legal protections available to research subjects; and the role of IRBs.

IRBs were created under federal law to review the ethical propriety of experiments in biomedical and behavioral research. The criteria used by IRBs to judge the ethical propriety of research are based on intensive work by, among others, the National Commission for the Protection of Human Subjects in Biomedical Research (1978). Put plainly, the IRB criteria include determining for a given survey or experiment that:

1. Risks to participants are reasonable in relation to benefits.
2. Risks are minimized.
3. Selection of participants is equitable.
4. The individual's consent to participate in the experiment is informed.
5. Privacy of the individual and confidentiality of information are assured.
6. Data are monitored continuously.

---

* Definitions for these principles are taken from Melton *et al.* (1988). *Beneficence* relates to the researcher maximizing social good toward and high degree of concern for the social welfare of research participants. *Nonmaleficence* is the avoidance of doing harm to research participants. *Respect for personal autonomy* is ensuring, as is possible, that participants have the freedom to refuse involvement in research through the use of informed consent regarding all risks and benefits. *Justice* refers to the researcher's mandate to ensure fairness toward participants and that risks and benefits have been equally distributed. The duty of *fidelity* is a good faith commitment by the researcher to uphold all implicit and explicit agreements with the participant.

These criteria accord well with ethical principles enunciated by the American Psychological Association (1990). These and other criteria often justify *and* raise concerns about the use of randomized, controlled, and natural experiments to protect the rights of the participants.

With regard to regulation of unethical behavior of psychologists, Hess (1980) has outlined five sources of control: general criminal law, peer ethics committees, profession-specific legal controls (e. g., state licensing boards), civil litigation of malpractice complaints, and federal laws and regulations. These controls may not be known to the general public so there is some skepticism as to how they may be accessed by, say, persons with AIDS, who feel victimized by their participation in a control group or in an alternative treatment that resulted in no demonstrable improvement in health or access to health care.

Federal Judicial Center Guidelines

Despite the scientific importance of randomized experiments, they are rarely given great publicity. As a consequence, the rationale for randomized experiments is not a matter of common knowledge. For the public, at least, this raises the question: Why conduct a randomized experiment? Under what conditions is an experiment ethically acceptable or desirable or fair?

The question of whether to use random assignment looms large given the controversy likely to boil once the randomized experiment is undertaken. Borrowing from the Federal Judicial Center's (1981) book on experimentation in the courts, there are five threshold conditions that must be considered if randomized experiments are to be used in the judicial system. These conditions are also applicable, within limits, to determining the ethical propriety of research on AIDS and to work in biomedicine, and elsewhere. Cast into question form, the threshold conditions are:

1. Does present practice or policy need improvement?
2. Is there "significant uncertainty" about the value of the proposed regimen?
3. Is there any practical means other than randomized control to determine the value of the proposed regimen?
4. Will the results of the experiment be used to improve practice or policy?
5. Is there a mandatory component to participation in the experiment?

4. THE EMPIRICAL STUDY OF RESEARCH ETHICS

The empirical study of research ethics and of ways to better meet ethical standards is a relatively recent social science endeavor. Work described by

Boruch and Cecil (1979), for instance, helped to clarify some of the perplexities raised by various forms of sensitive data gathering. Questions raised by this area of inquiry include: Can one assure individual privacy and protect the confidentiality of individual records? What factors influence researchers' perceptions of the risks of their research? What strategies or guidelines are likely to increase researchers' sensitivity to privacy, intrusiveness, and unique ethical issues endemic to their research? What are the differential responses by participants to informed consent procedures? All of these questions are important and can influence how AIDS research is conducted (Stanley *et al.,* 1987).

4.1. Intrusion, Anxiety, and Informed Consent

Exploiting data collected prior to the research effort offsets the intrusive quality of AIDS research. Educating the participants about the study's purpose, scope, and possible outcome fulfills the research requirement of informed consent. It may also serve to allay the fears of the unknown, remove false assumptions, and encourage the participant's control over the situation.

Preliminary studies suggest that anxiety reactions to consent information do not necessarily lead to individuals refusing to participate in studies on diagnostic angiography (Alfidi, 1971). Other studies argue that the more target individuals comprehend the procedures and consequences of participating in a research endeavor, the more likely they are to agree to participate (Epstein and Lasagna, 1969; Stuart, 1978). Others have found that the amount of information and assurance of confidentiality that is given to respondents in survey research does not appreciably influence their willingness to cooperate in answering sensitive questions (Singer, 1978, 1979, 1983).

Other informed consent dilemmas have been explored but have not been investigated rigorously. While Stanley *et al.* (1987) argue that under no circumstances is the relinquishing of informed consent an option for researchers, Wan (1990) claims that ethical guidelines stipulated by the Belmont Report (45 Code of Federal Regulations 46.) allows for the waiving of informed consent in situations of unlinked anonymous HIV seroprevalence screening.

Distress lies in the nature of AIDS research, namely, examining intimate and illegal behaviors. Added to this is the threat of morbidity and mortality associated with an AIDS diagnosis. Examples of distressing contacts include receiving a letter requesting participation in an AIDS research study or being asked to answer questions after or during one's visit to a public health clinic. Even the initiation of contact from an AIDS researcher or clinic worker can raise questions in the minds of participants about their seropositivity.

4.2. Cultural and Gender Issues in AIDS Research

Researchers are challenged to view research and ethical concerns from the participants' position(s). Ankrah (1989), for instance, discusses two significant points regarding the analysis of cultural differences. One is the research views of local persons who are asked to be participants in the study. Second, their beliefs about disease, sickness, and death are related to their view of AIDS. She goes on further to state that researcher sensitivity to these sociocultural dimensions is crucial in understanding ethical conduct. AIDS research is plagued by situational ethics and cultural differences between populations (Ankrah, 1989). African protest at the use of the terms "prostitute" and "promiscuity" by Western scientists was centered around the underlying moral implications of the terms and ignored certain economic realities and sometimes respectful perceptions of "working women" held by members of some African communities. This was considered disrespectful and made data gathering especially difficult because potential participants doubted the ability of the researchers to investigate personal issues fairly and in good faith (Brokensha, 1988).

Ethnographic techniques in AIDS research include the "discovery of culturally sensitive categories of HIV knowledge, attitudes, and behavior in presentation of HIV infection, and by enabling more effective service provision" (Herdt and Boxer, 1991, p. 171) and can be useful in gathering sensitive information (Miller et al., 1990). Ethnographic research is not without its public relations problems either (Ankrah, 1989). People who are asked to contribute to research may work hard to present a favorable image to researchers and give less than accurate information.

The distrust between the investigators of the sexual behaviors of African-Americans and the African-American community can be a major stumbling block for AIDS researchers and service providers [Fullilove and Fullilove, this volume; Stevenson (in press); Williams, 1972]. Moreover, research that does not account for the history of distrust that exists in certain ethnic communities may be vulnerable. University researchers who seek to complete a research agenda in a community with which they are unfamiliar would do well to avoid research strategies that increase research participant anxiety and suspicion (e. g., by getting endorsement from respected African-American leaders before initiating research).

Ethnographic research can be used to construct more ethical randomized field experiments (Coyle et al., 1991; Herdt and Boxer, 1991). First and foremost, selecting suitable informants experienced with the population to be studied is a must. An example may include the decision to use key informants such as AIDS outreach case managers who have developed relationships with i.v. drug users through the passing out of bleach and sterile needles. Carrier and Magana (1991) describe the use of STD clinic patients as informants in locating the meeting places for prostitutes. This led to the systematic field observation and interviewing of prostitutes serving a Mexican-American population. Key informants are helpful in gathering the basic information but may be even more useful in the selection and development of questions to be asked and how to ask them. There are implicit rules and practices that are not ascertainable through means other than those experienced by workers who are daily involved in the community. Appropriate behavior is situationally and culturally defined and the ethical behaviors of i.v. drug users and the rules for disclosure of information about their i.v. drug use need to be understood before AIDS research is initiated.

The characteristics of the investigator such as age, gender, sexual orientation, and race are also important in increasing trust and decreasing fears of intrusiveness when information about at-risk behaviors are asked. In an ethnographic study of a Chicago Women and Children With AIDS Project, Herdt and Boxer (1991) defend their use of former women i.v. drug users, mothers of children with AIDS, prostitutes, and adolescents with AIDS who act as paid outreach workers. The use of investigators or key informants who fit the sexual orientation of the respondents has been a concern for many gay and lesbian youth. In a study that is part of the National AIDS Demonstration Research Project, Johnson *et al.* (1990) through ethnographic strategies identified reactive and proactive outreach worker styles that were effective in distributing AIDS materials, information, and prevention education to various ethnic and sexual minority communities. They found differences between black, Hispanic, and gay multiethnic outreach workers with blacks adopting more of a direct, proactive style and Hispanic and gay multiethnic workers adopting more of a reactive style. Proactive efforts involved initiating conversations with clients with the explicit objective of providing HIV prevention information. A reactive style is characterized by a passive presentation to clients by "hanging out" and making oneself available should a client care to ask about HIV prevention. This difference in how outreach is conducted can inform AIDS researchers about how to increase cultural fit by interviewing respondents in a cultural style that maximizes disclosure.

Different ethical guidelines have been proposed depending on the target population of the participants and the design of the research. Protest over the exclusion of women from the AIDS clinical trials for reasons that drug regimens may prove in the future to impair child-bearing abilities has been raised (Merton, 1990). This is especially interesting since AIDS is now the number one killer of young women in New York City. Moreover, issues of ethics and confidentiality can vary because different risks are incurred when different groups of participants are involved.

There are two other ethical issues that are related to the initiation of research in ethnic minority communities. One is the researcher's need to demonstrate competent culture-specific knowledge of the values behind the attitudes and behaviors of the particular ethnic group to be studied. The difference between racial groups (e. g., Blacks, Latinos) and ethnic groups within race (e. g., Central Americans, Mexican Americans, Puerto Ricans, etc.) is an important distinction. This knowledge can be communicated through informed consent discussions with participants (without compromising experimental integrity) or when discussing the research and getting permission from key community leaders prior to the study's initiation. A second related issue is the conscious exercise or use of that knowledge in the research design (e. g., measures or sampling selection procedures). Knowing ethnic differences within racial groupings can help to decrease unethical decisions, such as considering a particular racial group to be homogeneous, when it is not.

Suppose a researcher wants to include a representative group of Hispanics in the clinical trials of research or in a survey investigating intravenous drug use. Investigating at-risk behaviors is not an easy task. The incidence of at-risk behaviors varies from one Latino ethnic group to another, as in the case of the intravenous drug use sharing of needles (Selik *et al.*, 1989). Puerto Rican–born persons showed a cumulative incidence of AIDS in heterosexual intravenous drug abusers seven times greater than that of other Latin American–born individuals (e. g., Cubans, Mexicans, etc.). Sensitive scrutiny and interpretation, replication of findings, and review of results with key informants are necessary to understand and substantiate this phenomenon across the course of the AIDS epidemic, but not to consider this type of difference in research design would constitute a breach of ethics.

Improving ethics policy and research practice must include the diversity as well as the uniqueness of the AIDS populations. Within- and between-group cultural, gender, and geographic differences may alter the administration of AIDS survey research. Increased knowledge of human sexual behavior and its different expressions across sexual, societal, and ethnic minority groups will inform public policymakers about potential research issues. In contrast, despite the cultural and social diversity of the AIDS population, this remarkably disparate group is intensely tied together by the common denominator of uncertainty regarding their care and cure. Threats of imminent death, social ostracism, financial imperatives, and public disclosures of intimate behaviors require remarkable sensitivity by AIDS researchers to the privacy needs of a vulnerable research population.

4.3. Investigator/Respondent Interaction

The ethical issues of privacy and confidentiality in AIDS research pose five fundamental questions regarding the AIDS investigator/respondent interaction.

1. *Who are the research respondents and who are the investigators?* Interviewers indigenous to the research community have practical knowledge and sensitivity about AIDS issues but may or may not be viewed as trustworthy by the respondents. The importance lies in the ethnic community's support or sanction of the investigator despite his or her ethnic or cultural background. For instance, a white female investigator may interview black male respondents if she is endorsed by an African-American community based organization that serves black gay men. However, a black male investigator not endorsed by the agency may be denied access to the research population (personal communication, Dr. Stephen Thomas, Director of Minority Research Health Laboratory, 1991).

2. *Where is the research conducted?* Ensuring privacy may include changing the location of the research interview to a private and protected area to minimize the respondent's vulnerability to exposure. Access to AIDS research participants may be easier in the field where the respondents live, seek health care, or recreate. One researcher having completed a detailed interview with an AIDS respondent at a men's health clinic avoided greeting him at a nearby restaurant. She was cautious to avoid disclosure of his HIV-positive status through association with her (personal communication, Dr. Mary Elizabeth O'Brien, Catholic University of America, 1991).

3. *When is the research conducted?* Patients suffering from AIDS often exhibit signs of AIDS dementia early in the disease process. Obtaining informed consent from such patients creates an ethical dilemma. For short-term dementia, the patient's capacity to receive information and give informed consent may be compromised. If no next of kin is available, questions of the patient's lover serving as the patient's legal guardian must be considered (personal communication, Dr. Denise Korniewicz, Johns Hopkins University School of Medicine, 1991).

4. *What can occur between the investigator and respondent that may trigger an ethical dilemma?* The investigator's status of authority can lead to misuse of power or control over the respondent. Viewing the investigator/respondent relationship as a scientific alliance rather than an unequal or subjective relationship neutralizes the power the investigator has over the respondent. A researcher in a debriefing session discovered that one of his interviewers felt a sexual attraction toward one of his respondents and wished to date him. By not knowing more about the interviewer's personal agenda,

the respondent was vulnerable to manipulation. By using the information for his own needs, the interviewer creates an ethical dilemma.

5. *How does the investigator present the purpose of the study to prospective respondents in the least threatening way?* How does the investigator encourage the respondent to communicate the necessary information with the least amount of discomfort and inaccuracy? Knowing the different types of language associated with sexual behavior assists the researcher in clearly eliciting and reporting information. For instance, heterosexual intercourse may be described in ordinary language as sexual intercourse, in clinical language as coitus, in romantic language as making love, and in street language as fucking. An example of miscommunication in language is when a participant responds "No" to having problems with ejaculation and reveals later that he has difficulty coming. Knowledge and comfort with the respondent's unique expression of sexual language increases the options that investigators have of obtaining accurate information while minimizing discomfort.

5. APPROACHES TO REDUCE THE DIMINISHING OF PRIVACY AND CONFIDENTIALITY

The options discussed in this section are procedures that ensure confidentiality of an individual's response to questions in legitimate research and evaluation studies, and permit statistical analysis by legitimate researchers and analysts outside the original data collection agency.

In particular, the following question is raised: "Which ethical dilemmas or research approaches impact on or are more likely to increase respondent trust in the researcher or to decrease fears of his or her unethical misuse of private information?" Figure 1 is an attempt to map various options to combat the diminishing of privacy along two dimensions: one is a control dimension and relates to the amount of control the participant or researcher has or is perceived to have in the engagement of that option; the second dimension is study duration, from prestudy to poststudy periods so that one might examine when various options are best applied. It is noted that there are fewer options available to participants to protect the privacy of shared information. The options are also categorized according to whether they are procedural, statistical, or legal approaches.

5.1. Procedural Approaches

Building participant trust in researcher competence is an important step toward protecting the confidentiality of participants in behavioral research.

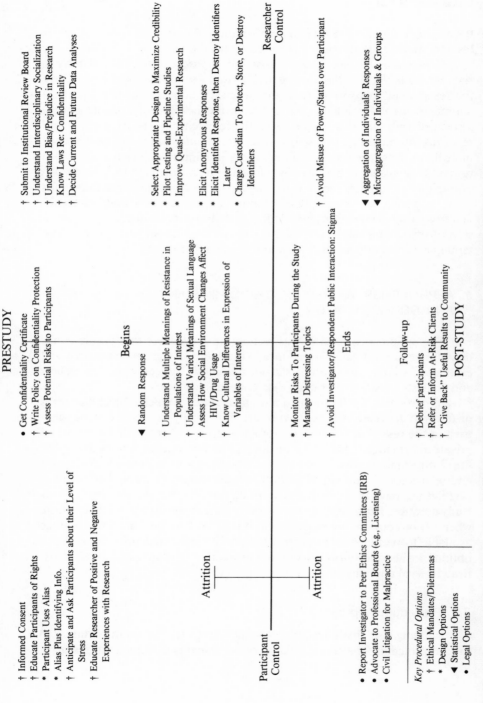

Figure 1. Options to increase ethical behavior in AIDS research.

Resistance includes a set of behaviors under the control of participants who may mistrust the research process. Fantuzzo & Stevenson (1993) have discussed the importance of understanding and facing the resistance of various research participant populations. To do so is to increase the trust of those populations such that the research endeavor will be perceived as a scientist–participant partnership rather than an autocracy. Facing the resistance can include understanding the multiple and empowering meanings behind one's resistance (e. g., as reflected in participants who say "no" or who refuse to participate or who participate reluctantly because they feel to do so is to protect one's community from excessively negative interpretations), giving informed consent, and receiving education from the participants about the history of researcher abuses within the specific community to be investigated.

Asking for anonymous responses to a mailed questionnaire is a simple example of a procedural approach to confidentiality assurance. This approach, and others, are more vulnerable to subversion than one might expect. All such approaches must be tailored to the research design.

The following covers options in three kinds of research designs commonly used in educational and social research, including studies of sensitive topics such as AIDS: cross-sectional, longitudinal, and multisource linkage. The vulnerability of the options is considered in the special context of deductive disclosure.

5.1.1. Deductive Disclosure

Friedson's (1978) assertion that the only way of "absolutely assuring confidentiality of sources is to destroy all record of their identities" is wrong. Deductive disclosure is possible despite destruction of identifiers. Witness, for instance, Kruskal's (1975) suggestion that, in Carroll's case study of government attempts to appropriate research data, the "Chicago studies of live juries in the 1950's [are] . . . not identified as such but are clearly recognizable." Gibbons (1975) penetrated the "Prairie City" research on criminal justice to show that the city was Decatur by purusing the U.S. Census Bureau's statistical reports on cities.

The strategies developed to ensure confidentiality in educational and social research are vulnerable in varying degrees to deductive disclosure. For instance, it would be easy for the counterfeit researcher to elicit information from respondents that would be in effect unique identification, ensuring that deductive disclosure is possible. Similarly, it would not be difficult to deduce identification for certain target populations or institutions.

A social scientist's record on an anonymous i.v. drug user, for example, composed of entries from police records and the researcher's record, might be easily penetrated by a hostile interrogator simply because parts of police records are public information. If sufficiently unique, this public information is a device for identifying the individual who was the respondent in the research. To remedy such a problem, the archive supplying records to the inquiring agency may use one or more of a variety of techniques normally used to impede deductive disclosure with public use data tapes or to present redisclosure.

5.1.2. Cross-sectional Studies

Consider a research design in which an independent sample of individuals is surveyed each year to estimate the incidence of drug use. The methods invented to protect privacy of respondents or to ensure confidentiality of their response in such cross-sectional studies include (1) eliciting anonymous responses directly from the respondent, (2) eliciting identified response in the interest of ensuring sampling validity, then destroying identifiers, (3) using the custodian of a list of individuals (e. g., a clinic) as an intermediary where even the identification (of, say, pregnant teenagers) is sensitive, and obtaining anonymous responses directly from the respondent, and (4) using the list custodian as intermediary in both eliciting information and as an interim recipient of responses where identification is sensitive and the custodian is capable of deleting identifying information or summarizing records.

For instance, some of the Centers for Disease Control's seroprevalence surveys involve eliciting no identifying information from individuals who provided blood samples (Ladine Newton, CDC, personal communication, 1988). The State of New York's (1988) surveys of school students' knowledge of AIDS-related behavior, undertaken in grades 9–12, asked respondents to refrain from putting any identification on questionnaires answered in classroom settings, for example.

Methods that involve not eliciting the identity of an individual are simpler than other methods discussed later. They have the merit of not diminishing an individual's privacy with respect even to the honest researcher. The methods have notable disadvantages. For instance, securing an anonymous response from a person to a questionnaire usually engenders the problem that some individuals do not respond and respondents to a survey often differ from nonrespondents. When nonresponse rate is high, the trustworthiness of a survey based on such methods will be debatable. The respondent sample characteristics may not match the populations. The problem is especially acute in research on sensitive topics, such as AIDS, where the cooperation rate in surveys of young men, for instance, often does not exceed 50% (Miller, Turner, and Moses, 1991). To reduce the problem of nonresponse in mail surveys, the researcher may ask respondents to return postcards to independently verify that they did indeed respond to a questionnaire returned anonymously and under separate cover. This tactic permits the researcher to follow-up on nonrespondents and, if population data are available, permits a statistical comparison of the respondent and nonrespondent groups.

The methods can be subverted. A marketing research firm, for instance, announced that responses to its survey of *National Observer* subscribers would be anonymous. The commercial firm identified questionnaires covertly, an act that was not understood clearly by the sponsor of the survey. One need not use invisible identifiers as the commercial firm did to identify survey respondents. Collateral information on an individual or an institution known to have responded, for example, can sometimes be used to deduce their identification from a nominally anonymous questionnaire (i. e., deductive disclosure).

5.1.3. Longitudinal Studies

Longitudinal studies require that the researcher link records obtained from individuals at one point in time to information obtained from the same individuals at other times. For instance, one may repeatedly survey a sample of high school students and dropouts in the interest of understanding changes in high-risk behavior related to drug or other substance abuse. In legitimate research, the individual's identification serves only as a vehicle for linkage among reports collected at different times.

To accomplish the linkage, but avoid diminishing privacy or threats to confidentiality, a variety of methods have been field-tested. One of the simplest is to ask that respondents use an alias. Nominal aliases have been tried out with some success in short-term studies. Rossi *et al.* (1971), for example, used numerical aliases constructed by respondents on the basis of an arithmetical algorithm in their studies of students' drug abuse. The algorithm depended on the respondent's knowing his or her parents' birth dates, a flawed assumption it appears. The CDC's surveys of prostitutes ask respondents to use an alias in conjunction with a code number to ensure that respondents can be appraised of HIV test results without risk (Ladine Newton, CDC, personal communication, 1988).

Alternatives have been developed for situations in which aliases are not satisfactory. Consider, for example, the link file system used at the American Council on Education during the early 1970s in research on political protests on U.S. campuses (Astin and Boruch, 1970). The process involved using a code dictionary of researcher-created aliases, kept outside the United States, as a device for linking information collected periodically from a sample of college students. The use of the code dictionary reduced the need to hold identified records, and because the dictionary was kept outside the country, it lowered the likelihood that a prosecutorial agency would appropriate data for use against the individuals who responded to the longitudinal surveys. Variations on the strategy include (1) providing numerical aliases to respondents, eliminating clear identifiers in response entirely, (2) using intermediaries in transmitting inquiry and response or analyses, and (3) using several principals to construct parts of a given numerical alias.

Such methods have clear disadvantages (Boruch and Cecil, 1979). They impede the quality control of sampling and investigation of response validity unless special measures are taken. They may be objectionable on other grounds. For instance, in a study of assaults on police, Oklahoma police refused to use aliases because they believed "only criminals used aliases." The possibility of deductive disclosure or covert identification is no different from that in the strategies described earlier that rely on anonymous questionnaires. Finally, the procedures impede linkage with other independent sources of information, making validation studies difficult or impossible.

5.1.4. Linking Records from Different Sources Including Follow-up

Records from independent archives must occasionally be linked in the interest of assessing the relative accuracy of records, reducing respondent burden in surveys, or for other reasons. For instance, in estimating the effects of a program designed to reduce the risk of AIDS among adolescents, one might link welfare records, medical records, and independent survey data on the same individuals.

5.2. Statistical Approaches

Personal interviews with identified respondents, rather than mail surveys, for instance, are sometimes essential. If the inquiry concerns sensitive topics such as illegal behavior, the respondent may be discomfited whether the exchange is voluntary or not and despite assurances to the contrary. Statistical approaches involve the sophisticated use of demographic characteristics rather than participant personal identification information. These approaches require much time and effort and have limits to their use (Boruch and Cecil, 1979) but they do serve the purpose of reducing discomfort, protecting against being subpoenaed for legal proceedings against a respondent, and protecting against disruption of the research. Three statistical techniques identified here are randomized response, aggregation of an individual's response, and microaggregation of individuals, groups, or organizations.

In one variant of the randomized response method, the target respondents are divided randomly into Sample A and Sample B. Each individual in Sample A is presented with two questions, an innocuous one, such as "Did you have two or more meals yesterday?," and a sensitive one that is of interest to the researcher, such as "Have you used marijuana in the last two days?" Each respondent is asked *not* to respond directly but instead to roll a die, choosing the first question if "one" turns up on the die and the second if "two," "three," etc. turn up. The respondent does not disclose which question is chosen, but merely provides a truthful "yes" or "no" response. In Sample B, only the innocuous question is asked. With the known odds on choosing each question in Sample A, the proportion estimated from Sample B, and the overall proportion of "yes" responses in Sample A, one can exploit elementary probability theory to estimate the proportion of substance users. The process and its symbolic representation are given in Table 1; full calculations and variants are given in Boruch and Cecil (1979) and references therein, in Soeken (1987), and in Tracey and Fox (1986). Three limitations to the use of this technique involve the larger number of subjects necessary to make adequate judgments, the problem of determining how truthful respondents will be regardless of which question they answer, and that the power of the technique is much related to the ability to estimate accurately the probability of response to the nonsensitive question (Soeken, 1987). Field experiments that have utilized randomized response methods are given in Boruch and Cecil (1979).

The major benefit of the approach is that it permits the researcher to elicit and obtain information on sensitive behaviors of individuals without knowing the behavior of the particular individual. That is, even in personal interviews, the interviewer cannot know from a "yes" response whether the respondent has engaged in risky behavior.

Table 1. Simple Variation on Randomized Response

Sample A

   1/6:   Have you used marijuana in the last two days?

   5/6:   Did you have two or more meals yesterday?

Sample B

Did you have two or more meals yesterday?

$P_A(Y)$ = Proportion of YES responses observed in Sample A

P_C = Unknown proportion of people who have used marijuana

P_T = Fraction of two or more meal eaters in Sample A, estimated using Sample

   B

$P_A(Y) = 1/6 P_C + 5/6 P_T$

$P_C = [P_A(Y) - 5/6 P_T] 6$

Aggregation of an individual's response constitutes the second statistical method for ensuring that there is no direct link between a response to the researcher's sensitive questions and the individual. A respondent is presented with a set of questions, some sensitive and most not, to which simple responses are expected. Instead of answering each question in the set, the respondent is asked to give an aggregate answer for the entire set. Through statistical technique and a little algebra, it is possible to estimate the proportions of respondents who have a certain combination of statistical properties. For references of the statistical properties of the estimate, see Boruch and Cecil (1979). This technique has received very little field testing and is useless if the respondent cannot do simple arithmetic.

A final statistical method for ensuring confidentiality is microaggregation and requires no collection of individually identified data. Small clusters of individuals are carefully constructed from which information is obtained. Each cluster is considered to be a synthetic person, a composite of the properties of the small set of individuals it comprises. Individual privacy is ensured to the extent that no relationship between the cluster and a particular individual is derived. Although examples of its use can be found in economic research on banks and commercial organizations, construction and statistical analysis of the clusters presents considerable technical difficulties, making this method unpopular.

5.3. Statutory Approaches

A great many educational and social research studies rely on information provided by anonymous respondents. The work includes surveys of what adolescents know about AIDS and the transmission of the virus, surveys that focus on incidence of infants born of adolescents in selected metropolitan areas, and surveys directed at high-risk behavior of adolescents. These efforts to produce reliable statistical descriptions of the scope of problems are important.

Other efforts, no less important to science and policy, attempt to understand how individuals change or how prevention programs designed to reduce high-risk behavior alter individuals' behavior. These efforts usually require that the research participants be identified and asked to provide information periodically. The need to retain identification in such work can put the individual at risk for legal or social sanctions.

A number of federal laws prevent the government's using research information on identifiable respondents for nonresearch purposes including sanction or harassment. The laws facilitate the researchers' adherence to a promise of confidentiality in research on AIDS and other sensitive topics.

They make explicit the researcher's legal responsibility to ensure confidentiality and provide legal support for it. To the extent that prospective research participants regard such statutory protection as necessary, these laws may also enhance individuals' cooperation rates in the research.

Two relevant statutes are described briefly here and along with other statutes, their provisions are summarized in Table 2. Boruch and Cecil's earlier treatment (1979) suggested ways to evaluate these laws and their guidelines are used in what follows. In particular, the following evaluative questions are addressed to assay the quality of the statute:

- Is immunity automatic rather than authorized separately for each research project?

Table 2. Statutes Providing Grants of Qualified Immunity for Research Information and Their Provisions[a]

Statute	1	2	3	4	5	6	7
Public Health Services Act Sections 303 (a) and 308 (d). Pub.L. 91-513, 42 U.S.C.A. & 242a (a)	Y	N	N	Y	Y	Y	Y
Crime Control Act of 1973. Pub.L. 93-83, 42 U.S.C.A. & 3771	Y	Y	Y	Y	Y	N	Y
Juvenile Justice and Delinquency Prevention Act of 1977. Pub.L. 95-115	Y	Y	Y	Y	Y	N	Y
Controlled Substances Act Section 502 (c). Pub.L. 91-513, 21 U.S.C.A. & 872c	Y	N	N	Y	Y	Y	N
Drug Abuse Office & Treatment Act. Pub.L. 92-225, Amended, Section 408. Pub.L. 93-282, 21 U.S.C.A. & 1175a	Y	Y	Y	YC	N	YC	Y
Alcohol Abuse Act. Pub.L. 93-282, 45 U.S.C.A. & 4582a	Y	Y	Y	YC	N	YC	Y
Privacy of Research Records Act	Y	Y	Y	Y	Y	Y	Y
Hawkins–Stafford Act, Pub.L. 100-297	Y	Y	Y	Y	Y	N	Y

[a] Definitions of provisions: 1 = protects identification; 2 = protects identifiable information; 3 = automatic, rather than authorized; 4 = immunity from administrative inquiry; 5 = immunity from judicial inquiry; 6 = immunity from legislative inquiry; 7 = provisions for secondary analysis, in regulations or law. Field key: Y = yes, covered explicitly; N = no, not covered explicitly; YC = court order required for disclosure.

- Does immunity refer to administrative and/or judicial, and/or legislative agencies seeking to appropriate records?
- Is all information or just the identification of respondents covered?
- Are there provisions that permit independent reanalysis of the data by
  researchers?

5.3.1. Public Health Services Act

Two sections of the Public Health Services Act provide legal mechanisms
to protect the disclosure of the research participant and to prevent any use of
the disclosure against the participant. They differ in character and target of
attention. In the first of the two sections, the Secretary of the U.S. Department
of Health and Human Services may:

> Authorize persons engaged in biomedical, behavioral, clinical, or other research
> (including research on mental health, including research on the use and effect of
> alcohol and other psychoactive drugs); to protect the privacy of individuals who
> are the subject of such research by withholding from all persons not connected with
> the conduct of such research the names or other identifying characteristics of such
> individuals. Persons so authorized to protect the privacy of such individuals may
> not be compelled in any Federal, State, or local civil, criminal, administrative,
> legislative, or other proceedings to identify such individuals. [Section 301(d) of the
> Public Health Services Act]

This section of the Act (42 USC s.242a, 1982) can be important to health
researchers in that the identity of the research participants can be protected
legally. Moreover, the reference to "other identifying characteristics" ensures
that the researcher can even prevent deductive disclosure or the ability to
determine who or where the identifying characteristics refer to by knowing
other facts.

The law's requirement that researchers be engaged in mental health research comports with what *some* AIDS researchers and evaluators do. Trying
to understand predictors of suicide or depression, or relationships with friends
and families, social support systems, risk reduction behavior, and other topics
are relevant to mental health. Projects with these aims arguably fall in the
ambit of the Act.

Three limitations of the statute are important. First, if a government
agency already knows the identity of a survey respondent, then the researcher
can be compelled to disclose the research record on that respondent. The
privilege arguably covers only the discovery of the individual's identification,
if unknown. Gray and Melton (1985) remind us that at the time of their
writing, this limitation "has not been confronted by the courts" (p. 670).

Second, the privilege must be conferred by the Secretary; it does not
automatically accrue to the researcher. Consequently, educational researchers

who investigate politically controversial topics, such as the effect of students' sexual behavior related to the transmission of AIDS, may be at risk for not obtaining the grant of immunity or of having it rescinded. No information is available of the Secretary's refusal of grant applications. Third, there are no provisions for disclosure of research records to independent researchers for reanalysis.

A second major class of protection of respondents in research is given in Section 308(d) of the Public Health Services Act. Put simply, 308(d) bears on research undertaken by the National Center for Health Services Research and Health Care Technology Assessment, the National Center for Health Statistics, and the research grantees or contractors of each. Recently, NCHS was reorganized under the Centers for Disease Control and CDC legal counsel have argued that the relevant protection applies to CDC more generally (Ladine Newton, personal communication, 1988). The AIDS-related work of these agencies is substantial, such as NCHS (1988) surveys of the public's knowledge about AIDS. Consequently, the protection is important.

5.3.2. Hawkins–Stafford Act

The Hawkins–Stafford Act (PL 100-297) is the most recent privacy protection law enacted by the federal government. It covers research data obtained by the U.S. Department of Education's National Center for Education Statistics. Part of the merit of the statute lies in the fact that it is automatic. A Commissioner of Education Statistics could not withhold such protection from a project in the field that covered topics that were controversial (cancellation of the entire project is possible at any stage, however). The merit of the statute lies also in covering all information collected on individuals, not just their identity. The statute requires that none of the information can be divulged without the consent of the individual concerned. Data not collected under the provision of the Act, under the Department of Education, are not covered.

6. THE CASE OF RANDOMIZED EXPERIMENTS

One may identify a pool of AIDS victims who are eligible and willing to participate in a test of a new drug, then randomly allocate the individuals either to the new drug or to conventional treatment. The object is to estimate the effectiveness of the new drug relative to the convention. Or, one may assign entire cities to one of two or more prevention programs to understand which, if any, reduce i.v. needle sharing.

Analogous experiments are undertaken in surgical research, education, welfare, law and criminal justice, health therapy, and other fields to judge the effectiveness of innovations. They have been important to policy in that they can inform decisions about initiating, operating, or terminating programs. They are scientifically important insofar as they yield durable understanding about the effects of interventions.

But randomized experiments can engender ethical and legal problems. The random assignment may appear to put some individuals at risk or to deprive them of their rights. Randomization may also present some individuals with an opportunity they might not otherwise have, putting others at an ostensible or artificially induced disadvantage. Our purpose here is to explore the ethical propriety of randomized experiments relative to recent guidelines on ethics in research. The special context is AIDS-related work.

6.1. Federal Judicial Center Guidelines Applied

The Federal Judicial Center's guidelines were developed to assist judges in determining when randomized tests are appropriate, relative to ethical standards, in settings where the target individuals may be vulnerable, notably to unwarranted social or legal pressure. The fundamental questions implied by the guidelines are also likely to be helpful in enhancing the ethical propriety of controlled tests for planning and evaluating HIV/AIDS-related programs. The questions are not always easy to address much less to reach agreement on, to be sure. But they are important to judge from what follows.

1. Does present practice or policy need improvement?

In a general view of AIDS research, answering this question will always result in the affirmative. With the limited knowledge we have on IVDU and sexual behavior in general and specifically the underlying factors which motivate persons to engage in high risk behaviors despite the relative certainty of AIDS transmission, researchers are always needing to develop new ways of collating the latest information into some coherent policy and practice. Brown, DiClemente, and Reynolds (1991) have criticized research on the effectiveness of adolescent HIV prevention programs for being too descriptive and for not following any clear theoretical model to guide the research. They argue for the development of "innovative theoretical perspectives" in order to more clearly understand HIV-related risk taking, and to predict the effectiveness of prevention programs on risk taking behavior. Such is the mandate for most of AIDS research, a continual commitment to build upon the last finding because the field is so new.

The amount of time and effort necessary to conduct randomized experiments is not justified without some reasonable logic that the study will contribute significantly to the existing body of knowledge. Moreover, randomized research on populations not at-risk are unnecessary. For instance, mounting randomized trials on drugs designed to impede AIDS in heterosexual relationships among non-IV drug users are unlikely simply because the risk in this group is relatively low so far. How "risk" is defined more finely is important, as it is often based on untestable assumptions. In fact, in advocating for improvement in the conduct of AIDS research, many researchers have argued for less investigation of "high risk groups" and encouraged that AIDS research should focus on individual factors and the determinants of at-risk behaviors to avoid needless stigmatization and to confront the denial on the part of persons who engage in risky behaviors but who do not fall into any of those stigmatized groups (Martin, 1986; O'Reilly, 1988).

2. Is there "significant uncertainty about the value of the proposed regimen"?

Whether there is "significant uncertainty" about the proposed innovation is often a matter of such debate. That AZT, for example, has toxic effects as well as possibly beneficial ones lies at the heart of uncertainty about it and related drugs. Adding to uncertainty is plausible wishful thinking, even among experts. Getting independent evidence of an effective drug becomes crucial in an atmosphere, say, where drug companies have strong financial reasons to declare that their particular drug is effective. The enormous difficulties uncovered in evaluations of drugs in the past justify great care in this respect and similarly justify an empirical research strategy that tries to understand whether, and how well, the innovation worked. Clearly there are differences of opinion between scientists and the public regarding the possibility of finding innovative techniques effective.

3. Is there any practical means other than randomized control to determine the value of the proposed regimen?

A National Academy of Sciences report on evaluation of AIDS prevention programs addressed the question in considerable detail (Coyle et al., 1991). Put far too simply, the conclusions are as follows. Recall that the random assignment produces equivalent groups and, therefore, fair comparisons among treatment alternatives. Groups that are constituted in ways *other* than through randomization usually differ in known and unknown ways. The differences among them are inextricably tangled with the effects of program variations. This may make poor treatment variations look good, good variations appear worthless, and can make harmful variations appear merely worthless.

Two technologies of research methods, quasiexperimentation and econometric modeling, have been developed to understand how good estimates of a program's effect can be produced without random assignment. The technologies are quite sophisticated and demanding.

Both depend heavily on prior data or strong theory or both. Data and theory are often absent, or at least imperfect, for "new" target groups and for new programs. Individuals who have been exposed to the AIDS virus, for example, are properly classifiable as a "new" target group in the sense that good data or theory on responsiveness to certain chemicals and treatment regimens are imperfect. The sparseness of data and good theory helps to justify a randomized field test of the proposed intervention.

4. Will the experimental results be used?

Certainly bad evidence has been used in the past. This is no reason to discontinue conducting sound research. The U.S. General Accounting Office, for instance, publicly distinguishes between trustworthy and untrustworthy studies in some of its reports, e. g., on teenage pregnancy, and recognizes randomized versus other tests. The National Academy of Sciences and the National Research Council take quality of evidence seriously and consider it in their reports (e. g., on youth employment programs and the evaluation of AIDS intervention programs). These organizations inform the Congress. They are vehicles for encouraging the use of high-quality research.

5. Is the participation in randomized experiments mandatory?

The implication is that special attention should be paid to the mandatory character of the criminal justice system, in contrast to the "voluntary" character of social and biomedical systems. This qualification is important but ambiguous. The freedom to choose to or not to participate in AIDS research is a fundamental right. It is a freedom that puts individuals at an advantage relative to those who have no opportunity to engage in such programs or are *required* to participate in certain programs.

6.2. Social Concerns about Randomized Experiments

Asking certain questions of AIDS victims or their relatives, for instance, may be legal. But the act of questioning may be "unfair" insofar as the question causes grave discomfort to a victim or because responses cannot be protected from uses that harm the victim or relatives. The same is true of survey respondents who do not have AIDS but whose sexual behavior is important in understanding the epidemic. The evidence for discomfort may be strong or weak.

The recent concern regarding the involvement of participants in the clinical trials of AIDS drug testing has run into conflict, at times, with the basic rationale for certain experimental research rules (e. g., selection of subjects; randomization of subjects into control and experimental groups). The uncertainty of the effectiveness of a drug has not been enough to dissuade persons at risk for AIDS or who have contracted the disease from wanting to be selected for experiments that test new medications.

Considerable research attention is dedicated to those groups of persons who are at highest risk of AIDS. This reflects the desire to demonstrate potential effectiveness of the given drug on the most difficult at-risk group.

Defining risk is difficult and relative depending on whether you are the scientist or the population at risk for AIDS. Those who are at earlier stages of AIDS may argue that their participation in AIDS research clinical trials is just as scientifically important as for populations at later stages of the disease. One is challenged ethically as to how to justify the exclusion of certain "at-risk" groups even though they may suffer from early symptoms of the disease. A problem with these concerns is the lack of information regarding how AIDS is best arrested and the lack of a clear solution. Issues raised by these concerns ignore the other ethical dilemma of experimentation on persons who are not at risk, nor would be helped by the medication anyway.

Several options have been proposed for ameliorating the social criticism of randomized experiments. Criticism and options are considered next.

1. *Control group members are perceived to be deprived.* During the early clinical trials of AZT, accounts of attempts of experimental participants to give the experimental drug to participants in control groups only heightened the serious challenge that AIDS raises for experimental research conditions (Melton *et al.,* 1988). The uncertainty about the drug's effectiveness was a concern secondary to the possibility that one might not otherwise have had the opportunity to receive the drug.

One option for handling this social concern is to give something to everybody, including the control group. A second option is to use the rationale that resources are limited and therefore must be spent wisely. A third option involves the communication by the researcher that sacrifice now for a short period of time can lead to long-term benefits. A fourth option and the one strongly recommended by the National Research Council (Coyle *et al.,* 1991) is to use an alternative treatment situation instead of a no-treatment control group which is considered unethical. A fifth option involves changing the unit of analysis from individuals to institutions or geographic areas where, for example, cities are randomized. Each option assumes that the researchers are taking reasonable steps to ensure that the innovation introduced for testing or intervention is one that will have a desired effect. This is not easy given the low rate of effects that new programs tend to produce, yet it can avoid unethical treatment for those participating in the intervention condition.

2. *Ineligible clients have needs that some view as absolutely critical.* Eligibility criteria for randomized experiments or the need to have homogeneous groups may lead some worthwhile and needy candidates to be excluded. In addition, there is the difficulty in determining an appropriate at-risk group. The research questions entangled with this concern are: What types or levels of interventions work best with persons with AIDS at various stages of the disease? Who is likely to respond the most from a given intervention?

In AIDS research and other high-quality experiments, the eligibility for an individual's participating in the experiment is usually defined in some detail. This detail can be said to define the eligibility "narrowly," i. e., to include only those with a particular disease or form of disease, age range, gender, physical condition.

There are two major *technical* reasons for narrowness in eligibility requirements. Narrowness produces a more homogeneous group. With a group of similar people, it is far easier (1) to detect a promising effect of treatment if it is there and (2) to interpret the results. The first of these technical reasons, producing homogeneous groups for comparison, has some ethical justification. In particular, if the experiment is technically unlikely to detect an effect, it should not be run.

The first option to address this concern includes the holding open of slots for the most needy, a number of whom are not included in the randomized test. The second option is to educate others about how narrowing of the eligibility criteria helps to limit the number of participants who may not benefit from ineffective alternative or control conditions. Reducing the number of people exposed to potentially burdensome standards can ultimately reduce participant costs.

3. *Participants may suffer from misperception and lack of knowledge of experimentation.* The difficulty of explaining random assignment to persons unfamiliar with experimental design results in objections to its use. Random assignment is not an easy principle to understand or explain. Options to offset this concern include having the researchers explain repeatedly the meaning and benefit of random assignment with the goal that eventually community-based organization administrators or key public health officials will understand. Several meetings with community leaders may be necessary to resolve conflicts

over random assignment and the rumors that may spread as a function of the misperception. A second option may involve the direct training of basic experimental principles to nonresearchers with the hope that they will become educators of others. This has been accomplished in other areas [e. g., the Rockefeller Foundation's experiments on the Minority Female Single Parent Program (Boruch *et al.*, 1988)].

4. *How informed is informed consent?* Getting reasonable and substantial information to participants is not easy. Some research suggests that one-third to two-thirds of the information given at the beginning of the study is lost by the participants by the end of the study. Problems of misinterpretation and miscommunication can abound. Also, some participants may doubt that they are being told the truth.

The object of ensuring "informed consent" is to avoid involuntary involvement in experiments that could have damaging effects. In behavioral ameliorative programs, on the other hand, consent may or may not be required, advisable, or informed, depending on the program. For example, providing information to the effect that the individual is in a short-term experiment may subvert attempts to understand behavior. Telling a woman that she may be assigned to a control group or program group (randomly) may, for instance, induce an attitude of "I'll wait and see if I can get into the program next year" among the control group women.

This, in effect, could cause harm to the control group women if ultimately the program does not continue because they will have delayed seeking treatment for their illnesses. For control group members not to access other treatment alternatives could artificially inflate the benefits of the experimental program and make the control group appear artificially weak. Experimental tests of new regimens *sound* exciting to some, but the regimens may be far less effective than they seem to be. One of the reasons the federal government requires review from IRBs is because it is not clear how "informed" the informed consent can be. Particular relevance of these issues to AIDS research is where misinterpretation or harmful behavior may result from receiving additional information.

Approaches to this concern include the conduct of research on research ethics, e. g., whether participants like or dislike random assignment; determining the severity of distress reactions to a variety of sensitive questions; repeating informed consent procedures throughout the experiment (where this does not disrupt the intervention regimen); and conducting assessments of participants' understanding after informed consent has been given. Lessons from this type of research suggest that it would enhance the ethical propriety of an experiment to ask respondents how they reacted to their participation in the AIDS research.

About attitudes, we know little. But evidence is accumulating. In Australia, for instance, J. M. Innes has studied how individuals view random assignment to new family therapy programs when various justifications for such assignments are stressed to the eligible families. The justifications include the scientific need for evidence on the program's effect, the equity of randomization when resources are scarce, and the possible negative effects of innovative treatment. The results suggest that the appeals to scientific or equity arguments do not appreciably affect a favorable attitude toward randomization but that the possibility of negative program effects on participation does.

7. SUMMARY

Ethical dilemmas in AIDS research are substantial and there are historical research examples that demonstrate the necessity for universal codes of ethics. The AIDS epidemic has exposed weaknesses in science's ability to protect the human rights of research participants. Where possible, researchers should develop a clear set of ethical principles and policies for each research endeavor that will guide the investigation and identify potential issues that might interfere with the protection of research participants. To be sure, the need for extensive empirical study of research ethics is critical. Moreover, one must not forget the unique ethical and research dilemmas presented by cultural, gender, and geographic differences. A strong collaborative relationship between investigators and the community of interest will contribute to contextually meaningful and ethical research.

Procedural, statistical, and statutory approaches have been proposed to protect the privacy and confidentiality of persons who agree to participate in research. There is an inherent conflict between the amount of control and freedom at the disposal of the participant toward protection of rights versus the control at the disposal of the researcher.

Randomized experiments can augment the knowledge of which drug regimens or prevention strategies work best. Their use is not without controversy. Taking into consideration social concerns regarding the use of randomized experimental designs and the potential ethical challenges is a wise step. As the war against the spread of AIDS continues and research on the private and intimate behaviors of people is initiated, a call for ethical propriety will need to be sounded.

ACKNOWLEDGMENTS. Research on this topic has been supported partly by grants from the U. S. Department of Health and Human Services, U.S. Department of Education, and the National Science Foundation.

REFERENCES

Alfidi, R. J. (1971). Informed consent: A study of patient reaction. *J. Am. Med. Assoc.* **216**:1325–1329.

American Psychological Association (1992). Ethical principles of psychologists and code of conduct. *Am. Psychol.* **47**(12):597–1611.

Ankrah, E. M. (1989). AIDS: Methodological problems in studying its prevention and spread. *Soc. Sci. Med.* **29**(3):265–276.

Astin, A. W., and Boruch, R. F. (1970). A "link file system" for assuring confidentiality of research data in longitudinal studies. *Am. Educ. Res. J.* **7**:142–143.

Bayer, R., Levine, C., and Murray, T. H. (1984). Guidelines for confidentiality in research on AIDS. *IRB Rev. Hum. Subj. Res.* **6**(6):1–7.

Boruch, R. F. (1990). *Resolving confidentiality and data sharing problems in educational and social research.* Background research supported by National Institute of Justice. Prepared for the National Center for Education Statistics, April 25.

Boruch, R. F., and Cecil, J. S. (1979). *Assuring the confidentiality of social research data.* Philadelphia: University of Pennsylvania Press.

Boruch, R. F., and Cecil, J. S. (eds.). (1983). *Solutions to ethical and legal problems in social research.* New York: Academic Press.

Boruch, R. F., Dennis, M., and Carter-Greer, K. (1988). Lessons from the Rockefeller Foundation's experiments on the Minority Female Single Parent Program. *Eval. Rev.* **12**(4):396–426.

Brokensha, D. (1988). A report. *Seminar on the anthropological perspectives on AIDS research in Africa.* Washington, D.C., January 7–8.

Carrier, J. M., and Magana, J. R. (1991). The use of sexual data on men of Mexican origin: HIV/AIDS prevention program. *J. Sex Res.* **28**(2):171–187.

Committee for the Protection of Human Participants. (1986). Ethical issues in psychological research on AIDS. *J. Homosexuality* **13**:109–116.

Committee on the Conduct of Science. (1990). *On being a scientist.* Washington, D.C.: National Academy Press, pp. 215–216.

Cook, J., Camarigg, V., and Boxer, A. (1990). Educating low-income minority women at risk of AIDS: Evaluating effectiveness and cultural relevance. Paper presented at the annual meetings of the Midwest Sociological Association, Chicago.

Coyle, S., Boruch, R. F., and Turner, C. (1991). *Evaluation of AIDS prevention programs.* Washington, D.C.: National Academy Press.

Darrow, W. W. (1988). Behavioral research and AIDS prevention. *Science* **239**:1477.

Dawson, D. A., Cynamon, M., and Fitti, J. E. (1988). AIDS knowledge and attitudes for September 1987: Provisional data from the National Health Interview Survey. *Vital Health Stat. Natl. Cent. Health Stat.* **148**.

Epstein, L., and Lasagna, L. (1969). Obtaining informed consent: Form or substance? *Arch. Intern. Med.* **123**:682–685.

Fantuzzo, J. W., and Stevenson, H. C. (1993). Understanding the multiple meanings of "NO" or informed dissent in ethnic minority research (unpublished).

Federal Justice Center. (1981). Advisory committee on experimentation in the law. *Experimentation in the law.* Washington, D.C.: FJC.

Fineberg, H. V. (1990). Screening for HIV infection and public health policy. *Law Med. Health Care* **18**(1–2, Spring/Summer):29–40.

Fox, J. A., and Tracy, P. E. (1986). *Randomized Response.* Newbury Park, California: Sage.

Freedman, B. (1987). Equipoise and the ethics of clinical research. *N. Engl. J. Med.* **317**:141–145.

Friedson, E. (1978). Commentary. *Am. Sociol.* **3**:159.

Gibbons, D. C. (1975). Unidentified research sites and fictitious names. *Am. Sociol.* **10**:32–36.

Gray, J. N., and Melton, G. B. (1985). The law and ethics of psychosocial research on AIDS. *Nebr. Law Rev.* **64**:637–688.

Herdt, G., and Boxer, A. M. (1991). Ethnographic issues in the study of AIDS. *J. Sex Res.* **28**(2): 171–187.

Hess, H. F. (1980). Enforcement: Procedures, problems, and prospects. *Prof. Pract. Psychol.* **1**: 1–10.

Johnson, J., Williams, M. L., and Kotarba, J. A. (1990). Proactive and reactive strategies for delivering community-based HIV prevention services: An ethnographic analysis. *AIDS Educ. Prevention,* **2**(3):191–200.

Jones, J. (1981). *Bad blood: The Tuskeegee syphilis experiment.* New York: The Free Press.

Kruskal, W. H. (1975, June 13). Letter to Margaret Martin. Department of Statistics, University of Chicago.

Levine, R. J. (1986). *Ethics and regulation of clinical research.* Munich: Urban & Schwarzenberg.

Martin, J. (1986). Sociomedical research priorities in AIDS. In M. Witt and W. Stockpole (eds.), *AIDS and patient management. Part III. Issues in social science research.* Owing Mills, Md.: National Health Publishing, pp. 177–181.

Melton, G. B. (1983). Minors and privacy: Are legal and psychological concepts compatible? *Neb. Law Rev.* **62**(455):458–460.

Melton, G. B. (1989). Ethical and legal issues in research and intervention. *J. Adolesc. Health Care* **10**:36S–44S.

Melton, G. B., and Gray, J. N. (1988). Ethical dilemmas in AIDS research: Individual policy and public health. *Am. Psychol.* **43**:60–64.

Melton, G. B., Levine, R. J., Koocher, G. P., Rosenthal, R., and Thompson, W. C. (1988). Community consultation in socially sensitive research: Lessons from clinical trials of treatments for AIDS. *Am. Psychol.* **43**:573–581.

Merton, V. (1990). Community-based AIDS research. *Eval. Rev.* **14**:502–537.

Miller, H. G., Turner, C. F., and Moses, L. E. (1990). *AIDS: The second decade.* Washington, D.C.: National Academy Press.

National Commission for the Protection of Human Subjects of Biomedical and Behavioral Research. (1978). *The Belmont report: Ethical principles and guidelines for the protection of human subjects of research.* (DHEW Publication No. [OS] 78-0012.) Washington, D.C.: Department of Health, Education and Welfare.

New York State Department of Health. (1988). *AIDS in New York State: Through 1987.* Albany.

O'Reilly, K. R. (1988). Determinants of AIDS risky behaviors. Paper presented at the Annual Meeting of the American Academy of the Advancement of Science. Boston, February.

Rossi, P. H., Groves, W. E., and Grafstein, D. (1971). *Lifestyles and campus communities* (pamphlet questionnaire). Baltimore: Johns Hopkins University, Department of Social Relations.

Selik, R. M., Castro, K. G., Pappaionou, M., and Buehler, J. W. (1989). Birthplace and the risk of AIDS in Hispanics in the United States. *Am. J. Public Health* **79**(7):836–839.

Singer, E. (1978). Informed consent: Consequences for response rate and response quality in social surveys. *Am. Sociol. Rev.* **43**:144–162.

Singer, E. (1983). Informed consent procedures in surveys: Some reasons for minimal effects on response. In R. F. Boruch and J. S. Cecil (eds.), *Solutions to ethical and legal problems in social research.* New York: Academic Press.

Singer, E. (1979). Informed consent procedures in surveys: Some reasons for minimal effects on response. In M. L. Wax and J. Cassell (eds.), *Federal Regulations: Ethical issues and social research.* Washington, D.C.: American Association for the Advancement of Science.

Soeken, K. L. (1987). Randomized response methodology in health research. *Eval. Health Prof.* **10**(1):58–66.

Stanley, B., Sieber, J. E., and Melton, G. B. (1987). Empirical studies of ethical issues in research: A research agenda. *Am. Psychol.* **42**(7):735–741.

Stevenson, H. C. (in press). The psychology of sexual racism and AIDS: The ongoing saga of distrust and the "sexual other." *J. Black Studies.*

Stevenson, H. C., and White, J. (1990). *Barriers to AIDS education and prevention services in minority communities: Making the best of a "grave" situation.* Unpublished manuscript. Philadelphia Refugee Service Center.

Stuart, R. B. (1978). Protection of the right to informed consent to participate in research. *Behav. Ther.* **9**:73–82.

Turner, C. F., Miller, H. G., and Moses, L. E. (1989). *AIDS: Sexual behavior and intravenous drug use.* Committee on AIDS Research and the Behavioral, Social, and Statistical Sciences. National Research Council. Washington, D.C.: National Academy Press.

Wan, L. (1990). The legality of unlinked anonymous screening for HIV infection: The U.S. approach. *Health Policy* **14**:29–35.

Williams, R. (1972). The death of the white researcher in the black community. In R. Jones (ed.), *Black psychology.* New York: Harper & Row, pp. 403–417.

Zuckerman, D. M. (1990). Conflicts of interest and the public interest. *Sci. Agenda* **2**:10–11.

2

Sampling Considerations in Research on HIV Risk and Illness

GRAHAM KALTON

1. INTRODUCTION

This chapter deals with sampling issues for surveys related to HIV risk and illness. Surveys are used to study a wide variety of issues related to the AIDS epidemic, for example:

1. General population surveys provide information about the public's knowledge of AIDS and its modes of transmission, about attitudes toward persons with AIDS, about behaviors that put persons at risk of contracting AIDS, and about the effectiveness of public media campaigns relating to AIDS.
2. Client surveys of users of AIDS counseling and testing services provide information about the characteristics and behaviors of these persons and about the types and effectiveness of the services provided.
3. Surveys of members of high-risk groups, such as gay men, bisexuals, i.v. drug users, and prostitutes, provide information on the members' risk behaviors, knowledge about AIDS, attitudes to changing risk behaviors, and contacts, if any, with counseling and testing services.

The sampling methods that may be employed for general population surveys are well established. Depending on whether a general population survey is to be conducted by face-to-face or telephone interviewing, standard area or random digit dialing (RDD) sampling methods may be used. Area sampling

GRAHAM KALTON • Westat, Inc., Rockville, Maryland 20850-3129.

Methodological Issues in AIDS Behavioral Research, edited by David G. Ostrow and Ronald C. Kessler. Plenum Press, New York, 1993.

methods are described in sampling texts such as that by Kish (1965a) and telephone sampling methods are described in Groves *et al.* (1988). When lists of clients for counseling and testing services are available, the samples for client surveys may be drawn in a straightforward way. When such lists are unavailable, as occurs for instance when clients are treated anonymously, clients may be sampled by sampling contacts with the services. In this case, it needs to be recognized that an equal probability sample of contacts does not yield an equal probability sample of clients; rather, clients who use the services frequently have greater probabilities of being selected. Adjustments are needed in the analysis to compensate for these unequal selection probabilities if the unit of analysis is to be clients rather than contacts (see Section 9). Apart from this latter complication, special concerns about nonresponse arising from the sensitivity of the survey subject-matter, and concerns about confidentiality in client-based surveys, the sampling issues for surveys in categories 1 and 2 in general present no unique problems. Sampling issues for surveys in these categories will therefore not be treated further here.

Sample design for the third category of surveys listed above—surveys of high-risk groups—poses severe challenges. These groups constitute what are termed rare populations in the survey sampling literature. The main challenge in sampling a rare population is to find economic methods for obtaining the sample, a challenge that is made more difficult in the present context by the social stigma associated with membership in these high-risk groups. The groups are not only rare but, because of this stigma, they also tend to be hidden, so that their members will not be readily identified by other people. This chapter considers the application of general approaches for sampling rare populations (Kish, 1965b; Kalton and Anderson, 1986; Sudman and Kalton, 1986; Sudman *et al.,* 1988; Kalton, 1993) to sampling groups at high risk of contracting AIDS. For illustrative purposes, the specific example of selecting a sample of gay men in a single city will be used. However, the general issues raised are equally applicable for other high-risk groups.

The chapter emphasizes probability sampling, the importance of which is discussed in the next section. Subsequent sections describe the range of techniques that may be used for sampling rare populations and consider their applicability for surveys of gay men. For ease of exposition, the techniques are discussed separately, although in practice several of them may be used together. The various techniques are:

1. Screening
2. Disproportionate stratification
3. Multistage sampling
4. Multiple frames
5. Multiplicity sampling

6. Two-phase screening
7. Location sampling
8. Snowballing

After reviewing each of these techniques, the chapter finishes with some concluding remarks.

2. PROBABILITY SAMPLING

As noted by the National Research Council's Committee on AIDS Research and the Behavioral, Social and Statistical Sciences, "much of what is now known about the epidemiology of AIDS has come from small-scale, local studies among subgroups thought to be at high risk for infection" (Miller *et al.,* 1990, p. 365). These studies have generally relied on convenience samples of the high-risk groups, obtained from clinics or treatment centers, newspaper advertisements, membership lists of local organizations, friendship networks, or recruitment in bars or on the streets. While these studies have often provided valuable information, they suffer the limitation that their samples may be severely biased as a result of the manner in which they were generated. Harry (1990), for instance, has noted that the usual convenience samples of gay men appear to underrepresent those over 50, probably those in their late teens and early twenties, and to be made up of highly educated and mainly white respondents (see also Harry, 1986). The great advantage of rigorously executed probability sampling is that it guards against the potential biases that may seriously distort the findings from convenience and other forms of nonprobability sampling.

The development and execution of a probability sample have to be conducted with considerable care if the full benefits of probability sampling are to be derived. First, the target population for the survey needs to be precisely defined: for a survey of gay men in a certain city, the meaning of "gay" needs to be clearly specified to meet the survey's objectives (for instance, is it to be based on behaviors, on affect, on self-identification, and what precise definition is to be used?), the boundaries of the city need to be clearly identified, decisions about whether to include men in institutions need to be made, and the time of the survey needs to be specified. Second, ideally the sample design should provide every gay man in the target population with a known, nonzero, probability of being selected for the sample. In practice, often certain subgroups of the target population are excluded from the frame from which the sample is drawn because those subgroups are difficult and expensive to survey. The proportion of the population in these noncovered subgroups needs to be kept small, however, if the risk of serious bias is to be avoided. Third, data should be collected from all of the gay men who are selected for the sample. There are two considerations here: one is that all of the sampled men who fit the survey definition of "gay" are identified as members of the population of interest, and that none of the other sampled men is falsely classified as "gay"; and the other is that all of the sampled gay men respond to the survey. Both of these considerations present severe practical difficulties. Some gay men may not be willing to tell the survey interviewer that they are gay, and nonresponse may present a serious problem because of the sensitive nature of the survey content. However, it is only when the initial sample is drawn from almost the total target population and when valid responses are obtained from a high proportion of the sampled individuals that the secure inferences of probability sampling can be realized.

As will become clear in what follows, obtaining a good probability sample of the gay men in a city is likely to be an expensive operation, even when the various techniques discussed in later sections are employed. Rather than incur the high costs involved in sampling gay men throughout the city, the sample may be restricted to a part of the gay population, such as those who live in areas with high concentrations of gay men, men who are members of gay organizations, or men who visit gay bars. In terms of the original target population of all gay men in the city, such restrictions may give rise to serious noncoverage problems. The survey findings from the restricted sample will provide biased estimates for the original target population to the extent that those included differ from those excluded from the restricted sampling frame. Since those included on the frame are often likely to be more overtly and actively gay, and hence to be more knowledgeable about AIDS, and have different sexual behaviors, etc., the biases may well be substantial. When the sampling frame is restricted to only a part of the gay population, the statistical inferences are valid only for the part of the population from which the sample is drawn. This limitation should be borne in mind in interpreting the survey results and assessing their utility.

3. SCREENING

A common component of many designs for sampling rare populations is some form of screening. If a large enough sample of the general population is screened to identify members of the rare population, a sample of the rare population of sufficient size can be obtained. The limitation of screening is the high costs associated with its use. If gay men, as defined for the survey, constitute 10% of the adult male population of a city, then a sample of 10,000 adult males, or about the same number of households, needs to be screened to generate a sample of 1000 gay men. If under the survey definition gay men constitute only 5% or 1% of the adult male population, then the corresponding screening sample sizes are 20,000 or 100,000, respectively. As these numbers illustrate, the screening sample size increases dramatically as the prevalence of the rare population declines.

A major concern when large-scale screening is employed is the minimization of the screening costs. One widely used method of screening is by telephone. The telephone interview may be used simply to identify the rare population, with subsequent follow-up of members of the rare population by face-to-face interviewing, or the full interview may be conducted by telephone. The main requirements for the appropriate use of telephone screening for gay men are that a high proportion of gay men live in housing units accessible by telephone, that a high response rate can be achieved, and that valid responses can be obtained to the screener questions over the telephone.

In general it is important to obtain a high response rate when screening for a rare population. The need for a high response rate is particularly acute in this case because even a high overall response rate to the screener questionnaire may mask a low response rate for the rare population. For instance, an overall screener response rate of 95% is not inconsistent with a response rate of only 30% in a rare population that comprises 5% of the total population.

Even though individuals agree to participate in a screening interview, this does not necessarily imply that they will respond accurately to the screener questions. The screener questionnaire needs to be carefully developed to minimize the risk of misreporting of rare membership status. In particular, some gay men may not be willing to report that they are gay in a screener interview. The development of an effective screener questionnaire involves not only the wording and ordering of the questions asked, but also such issues as making confidentiality commitments that are trusted by respondents, securing sponsorship for the survey from gay organizations, obtaining advance publicity for the authenticity of the survey, and the use of interviewers who are more likely to obtain valid responses. Extensive pilot work is needed to determine appropriate strategies for obtaining sample members' initial cooperation and then persuading them to respond accurately to the screener questions.

When face-to-face interviewing is used for screening, it is usually economical to employ a cluster sample design, and to screen large clusters. Thus, for instance, a sample of blocks in the city might be selected, and all of the households in selected blocks could be screened to identify gay men. For surveys of the general population, the selection of large samples in sampled clusters is statistically inefficient, but this does not apply for sampling rare populations because the number of rare population members in the clusters is relatively small. Further discussion of cluster sampling is given in Section 5.

Another widely used method for economic screening is to allow the screening information to be obtained from persons other than the sampled individuals. Thus, for instance, another member of the household may answer the screening questions on behalf of an absent sampled person in a telephone survey, and a next-door neighbor may provide the screening information for the members of an absent household in a face-to-face survey. The collection of screening information from proxy informants can work well for straight-forward, obvious, characteristics such as race and gender, but it is unlikely to be useful for identifying gay men. At most, its utility seems confined to determining the gender and age components in the identification of gay men.

4. DISPROPORTIONATE STRATIFICATION

Sometimes the general population can be divided into a set of strata with different prevalence rates of the rare population. Thus, the city may be divided into districts, with some districts having higher concentrations of gay men. The strata (districts) with higher concentrations may, for example, be identified as areas where the census shows that there are high proportions of unmarried adult males and/or as areas where there are sizable numbers of deaths recorded from AIDS. When such strata can be identified, it can be efficient to sample the strata where the gay men are concentrated at higher rates. With such a disproportionate stratified sample design, weighting adjustments are needed in the analysis of the survey data in order to compensate for the unequal selection probabilities assigned to members of the different strata.

Disproportionate stratification of the type described above is a useful technique to employ in sampling rare populations. However, the gains in the precision of the survey estimates that it generates are frequently not as great as might be imagined. Substantial gains accrue only when two conditions both apply: the prevalences of the rare population in the strata where it is concentrated need to be much greater than in other strata *and* the proportion of the rare population in the strata where it is concentrated needs to be large. The fulfillment of only one of these conditions is not sufficient to produce marked gains in precision (Kalton and Anderson, 1986; Waksberg, 1973; Kalton, 1993). Frequently, there may be a fairly high concentration of the rare population in certain strata, but nevertheless a sizable proportion of the rare population is to be found in other strata. In such cases, the gains from disproportionate stratification are modest. This situation seems generally likely to apply to concentrations of gay men in a city, so that only moderate gains in precision can be expected from the use of disproportionate stratification. These gains may be well worth securing, but the use of disproportionate stratification will often not produce major savings (say, 50% or more) in survey fieldwork costs.

To illustrate this point, consider a simple sample design with only two strata, one with a high proportion of the rare population and the other with a low proportion. We assume that the purpose of the survey is to estimate the mean of variable y for the rare population, that the element variances of y are the same in the two strata, that simple random samples are selected in each stratum, that the finite population correction factors can be ignored, that the per element data collection costs in the two strata are the same, and that the per element data collection costs are the same for sampled members from the rare and from the nonrare populations. Under these assumptions, the optimum choice of the sampling fraction to use in stratum 1, where the rare population is concentrated, relative to that in stratum 2 is

$$\phi = \sqrt{P_1/P_2}$$

where P_1 and P_2 are the prevalences of the rare population in strata 1 and 2, respectively (Kalton and Anderson, 1986).

The proportionate reduction in the variance of the sample mean from using this optimum allocation compared with a proportionate stratified sample that uses the same sampling fraction in the two strata and has the same sample size is

$$R = \frac{(W_1\sqrt{P_1} + W_2\sqrt{P_2})^2}{P}$$

where W_1 and W_2 are the proportions of the total population in strata 1 and 2, respectively, and P is the overall prevalence of the rare population. An alternative interpretation of R can be obtained by considering the sample sizes needed to give the same level of precision for the sample mean under the proportionate and disproportionate designs. Then R represents the multiplier to be applied to the sample size for the proportionate design to give the sample size needed for the disproportionate design. For example, if $R = 0.8$, then the disproportionate stratified design requires a sample only 80% as large as that of the proportionate stratified design to provide an estimate of the same precision.

Consider now the application of these results to sampling a rare population that has an overall prevalence of 5%. Table 1 presents the values of ϕ and R for various combinations of P_1 and θ, where θ is the proportion of the rare population in stratum 1. Table 1 also gives the values of W_1 and P_2. Values of P_1, θ, W_1 and P_2 are given in percentages.

The first row of Table 1 shows that, if the prevalence of the rare population in stratum 1 is $P_1 = 10\%$, and if that stratum covers $\theta = 20\%$ of all of the rare population, the stratum covers $W_1 = 10\%$ of the total population and the proportion of the rare population in stratum 2 is $P_2 = 4.4\%$. The stratified

Table 1.   Values of ϕ, R, W_1, and P_2 for Various Combinations of P_1 and θ, with $P = 5\%$

P_1	θ	W_1	P_2	ϕ	R
10	20	10.0	4.4	1.5	0.98
	40	20.0	3.7	1.6	0.95
	60	30.0	2.9	1.9	0.91
	80	40.0	1.7	2.4	0.83
	100	50.0	0.0	∞	0.50
20	20	5.0	4.2	2.2	0.94
	40	10.0	3.3	2.4	0.87
	60	15.0	2.4	2.9	0.78
	80	20.0	1.2	4.0	0.64
	100	25.0	0.0	∞	0.25
40	20	2.5	4.1	3.1	0.91
	40	5.0	3.2	3.6	0.80
	60	7.5	2.2	4.3	0.67
	80	10.0	1.1	6.0	0.50
	100	12.5	0.0	∞	0.13
80	20	1.2	4.1	4.4	0.88
	40	2.5	3.1	5.1	0.75
	60	3.7	2.1	6.2	0.59
	80	5.0	1.1	8.7	0.40
	100	6.2	0.0	∞	0.06
100	20	1.0	4.0	5.0	0.87
	40	2.0	3.1	5.7	0.73
	60	3.0	2.1	7.0	0.57
	80	4.0	1.0	9.8	0.38
	100	5.0	0.0	∞	0.05

design with the optimum allocation will sample from stratum 1 at a rate $\phi =$ 1.5 times that of stratum 2, and this oversampling will yield a small decrease of 2% in the variance of the sample mean (i. e., $R = 0.98$), or equivalently the same level of precision can be obtained with a 2% smaller sample by using the optimum allocation.

The following rows of Table 1 show that the rate of oversampling and the gains from the optimum allocation increase as θ increases. When $\theta =$ 100%, stratum 2 has no members of the rare population, so that no sampling is needed from that stratum. When $P_1 = 10\%$, this occurs when $W_1 = 50\%$ and hence $R = 0.50$. When P_1 is larger than 10%, the gains in precision are larger for a given level of θ, as can be seen in the lower part of Table 1. The results for R in Table 1 show that major gains in precision, or reductions in sample size, occur only when both P_1 and θ are large.

The results in Table 1 apply only for the simple sample design described above. They nevertheless also serve as useful approximations for other designs.

One assumption made in deriving the formula for R is that the costs of data collection for members of the rare population and the screening costs for members of the nonrare population are equal. Often in practice the rare population data collection costs will be larger than the screening costs, sometimes appreciably so. When this is the case, the gains from using the disproportionate allocation are less than those indicated in Table 1.

It should also be noted that the results in Table 1 are based on the assumption that the optimum sampling fractions are used in the two strata. These sampling fractions require knowledge of P_1 and P_2. Estimates of these quantities are usually based on out-of-date information, and are therefore likely to be somewhat inaccurate. The use of inaccurate estimates of P_1 and P_2 in determining the sampling fractions will also result in smaller gains than indicated in Table 1.

5. MULTISTAGE SAMPLING

When a household survey is to be conducted by face-to-face interviewing in a large city, some form of multistage sampling is almost certain to be used. In many cases a two-stage sample will serve well. Often, a sample of city blocks (the primary sampling units, or PSUs) is selected at the first stage, and then a sample of households is selected within the sampled blocks at the second stage. This section will review some special considerations that apply when this basic design is applied to sampling a rare population such as gay men.

First, as noted in Section 2, it is efficient to select much larger subsamples in selected PSUs when sampling a rare population than when sampling the general population. As a rule, clustering the sample in a two-stage design leads to some loss of precision in the survey estimates. This loss in precision, which derives from the fact that individuals within PSUs almost always exhibit some degree of similarity to one another, may be measured by the design effect, defined as the multiplier to be applied to the variance of a survey estimate under simple random sampling to take account of the complex sample design. In the case of a two-stage sample of the general population, the design effect for a sample mean, $\bar{y}$, can be represented by

$$D^2(\bar{y}) = 1 + (\bar{b} - 1)roh$$

where $\bar{b}$ is the average subsample size per selected PSU and roh is a synthetic measure of homogeneity of the y variable within the PSUs (Kish, 1965a). Since roh is virtually always positive, $D^2(\bar{y})$ exceeds 1, and hence the two-stage sample produces less precise estimates than a simple random sample of the same size. The larger the value of $\bar{b}$, the larger is $D^2(\bar{y})$. For example, with $roh = 0.05$, $D^2(\bar{y}) = 1.5$ if $\bar{b} = 11$ and $D^2(\bar{y}) = 2.5$ if $\bar{b} = 31$. The choice of $\bar{b}$ to use in a particular survey is determined by considering both the increase in variance that arises through increasing the value of $\bar{b}$, and the economies to be obtained by restricting the number of PSUs sampled. See Kish (1965a, Section 8.3B) for a formula for the optimum value of $\bar{b}$.

We now turn to consider the optimum value of $\bar{b}$ for sampling the rare population of gay men. Assuming that gay men are fairly evenly spread throughout the PSUs, then the above formula for $D^2(\bar{y})$ can be applied for the mean of variable y for gay men, but with $\bar{b}_0$ replacing $\bar{b}$, where $\bar{b}_0$ denotes the average number of gay men sampled per PSU, and where roh now measures the homogeneity of the y variable for gay men in the PSUs. The replacement of $\bar{b}$ by $\bar{b}_0$ implies that a large value of $\bar{b}$ can be tolerated, since with a rare population it will result in a small value for $\bar{b}_0$. For example, with a 5% prevalence rate for gay men, a value of $\bar{b} = 50$ gives $\bar{b}_0 = 2.5$, and a value of $\bar{b} = 100$ gives $\bar{b}_0 = 5$.

Another factor to be taken into account when designing a two-stage sample for a rare population is that the cost components differ from those for a general population survey. In particular, a substantial proportion of the survey budget is expended on screening out nonmembers of the rare population. This factor argues for $\bar{b}_0$ to be smaller than the $\bar{b}$ value that would be chosen for a general population survey with a similar value of roh and an otherwise similar cost structure. Suppose, for instance, that a value of $\bar{b} = 10$ is considered optimum for a general population survey. Then, for a rare population with a prevalence of 5% and for a survey where the per element screening costs are one-third of the per element data collection costs, the corresponding optimum value of $\bar{b}_0$ is about 3.7 rather than 10 (Kalton, 1993). Nevertheless, the number of individuals to screen to generate this number of members of the rare population remains large at $\bar{b} = 3.7/0.05 = 74$.

The second issue to be discussed in this section is that rare populations are often not evenly distributed across the PSUs. Thus, for example, gay men are likely to be more heavily concentrated in certain city blocks. When this occurs, disproportionate stratification, as discussed in Section 4, may be used. This involves separating the blocks into strata according to their estimated prevalences of gay men, and sampling at higher rates in strata where gay men are more prevalent. The form of the two-stage sample design can be varied between strata to give efficient sample designs in each stratum. For instance, the choice of $\bar{b}$ may be varied across strata to reflect the differing prevalences of gay men.

When PSUs have variable numbers of members of the rare population, it can be efficient to sample them with probabilities proportional to their numbers of members of the rare population. When PSUs are selected in this way, then the selection of the same number of rare population members from each selected PSU produces a sample in which every member of the rare population has an equal probability of selection. A limitation to the use of this design is that in general the numbers of rare population members in each PSU are unknown. Sudman (1985) describes an adaptation of the widely used Waksberg–Mitofsky random digit dialing sampling method in telephone surveys (Waksberg, 1978) that can be used to deal with this situation (see also Sudman and Kalton, 1986). The process involves first selecting one PSU with probability proportional to total population, and then selecting one individual in that PSU. If the sampled individual is a member of the rare population, the PSU is accepted for the sample; if not, the PSU is rejected. This process amounts to selecting the PSU with probability proportional to its number of members of the rare population. The process is repeated until the required number of PSUs is accepted. In each selected PSU, further screening interviews are conducted until k additional members of the rare population are interviewed. This procedure can be applied in telephone surveys, where the PSUs may for instance be banks of 100 numbers (see, e. g., Blair and Czaja, 1982; Waksberg, 1983), and in face-to-face interview surveys. A disadvantage of the procedure with face-to-face interviewing is that an interviewer has to travel to a PSU to conduct the initial interview, but then will often find that the PSU is rejected. A modification of the basic procedure that attempts to address this issue is to select more than one individual initially. Then a further k interviews with members of the rare population are sought for each individual found to be a member of the rare population.

6. MULTIPLE FRAMES

An initial step in any survey of a rare population is to seek a special frame that provides complete coverage for members and that includes few nonmembers of that population. When such a frame exists, it can be used for sample selection, and the rare population sampling problem disappears. Such a list frame probably often exists, for example, for clients of AIDS counseling and testing services. When there is no such list with complete coverage, there may be lists that cover parts of the rare population. Lists with partial coverage may be used in sampling rare populations in a multiple frame design. For instance, membership lists of gay clubs and organizations may serve as partial lists of the gay men in a city for sampling purposes, provided that permission to use them for sample selection can be obtained.

The use of a multiple frame design does not obviate the general requirement that every member of the target population should have a chance of being selected for the sample. Thus, every member of the rare population needs to be on one or more of the sampling frames. Since the special lists of parts of the rare population in combination seldom provide complete coverage, a general population frame (an area or telephone frame) is often needed as part of a multiple frame design. Thus, a sample of gay men in a city may comprise samples from the lists of several gay organizations together with a sample of gay men screened from a general population survey.

When a sample of a rare population is made up of an aggregation of samples from several frames, the problem arises that population members may appear on more than one of the frames. This is the well-known sampling frame problem of duplicate listings (Kish, 1965a). There are several possible solutions to this problem.

One solution is to compare the listings and to delete all duplicates so that every member of the rare population appears only once on the merged frame. Whether this is possible depends on the ordering and size of the lists, and the identification information available. This operation might be feasible with some membership lists for gay organizations. However, names are often misspelled and addresses are changed, causing problems in matching listings across frames.

A second solution for duplicate listings is that of unique identification. The lists are not cleaned of duplicates: instead, rules are made to identify each population member with only one of his listings, with all of his other listings being treated as blanks on the sampling frame. For example, the lists of gay organizations could be placed in a specific order, and a man could be identified with only the first organization for which he is listed. The general population frame would then be taken to exclude anyone listed for one or more of the participating gay organizations. This solution in effect converts the sample design into a stratified design, the strata being those on the list of organization 1, those on the list for organization 2 but not on the list for organization 1, etc., with the final stratum being gay men who are not members of any participating gay organization. Following the discussion in Section 3, the strata with higher concentrations of gay men (i. e., the gay organizations) are then sampled at higher rates than other strata (the general population frame). In general, the conclusions reached in Section 3 apply here also: the gains from disproportionate stratification are relatively modest unless both the proportion of those on the membership lists who are gay men according to the survey definition (P_1) is large, *and* the membership lists cover a high proportion of such men (θ). While the first of these conditions probably applies (with P_1 being perhaps 80% or higher, depending on the definition of "gay" adopted for the survey), the second may well not.

The unique identification solution works well when the unique listing can be determined from the frames as the sample is being selected. If, however, sampled individuals have to be contacted to determine whether the sampled listings are their unique listings, then the solution is generally less useful. If contact is made with the individuals, then it is usually better to complete the interviews. In this case, the probability that an individual is selected for the sample depends on the number of listings he has. The third solution to the duplicate listing problem is then to accept sampled individuals from any of their listings, and to reweight in the analysis to compensate for unequal selection probabilities.

The use of a multiple frame design for sampling gay men in a city, using special membership lists of gay organizations and a general population frame, holds promise for increased efficiency. This design depends, however, on gaining access to the membership lists, and being able to locate sampled men from the information provided on the lists. Even if these issues are resolved satisfactorily, the gains in precision from the multiple frame approach are likely to be modest unless the lists cover a substantial proportion of all gay men in the city.

The gains in precision from a multiple frame design also depend on the relative costs of sampling from the several frames. The multiple frame design will be more beneficial the lower are the costs of surveying members sampled from lists as compared with individuals sampled from the general population frame. The general theory of multiple frames is given by Hartley (1962, 1974), Cochran (1964), Lund (1968), and Fuller and Burmeister (1972). Groves and Lepkowski (1985) describe an application of a dual frame design with an area frame and a telephone frame.

7. MULTIPLICITY SAMPLING

The basic idea of multiplicity, or network, sampling is to reduce the amount of screening that is needed to identify members of a rare population by collecting more information in the screening interviews. With conventional survey procedures, respondents report only about themselves (although sometimes they are also asked to act as proxy informants for other household members). With multiplicity sampling, they are asked to report for themselves and also for others linked to them in clearly specified ways. Commonly used linkages are to certain relatives, perhaps siblings only, siblings and parents, or siblings, parents, aunts, uncles, and children. Linkages to neighbors have also been used.

By expanding the reporting of membership of the rare population from the sampled individuals alone to those linked with them, multiplicity sampling introduces the problem of duplicate listings. With linkage to siblings, for instance, an individual without siblings has only one route for sample selection, whereas an individual with three siblings has four routes. Provided that the linkages can be identified and counted, weighting adjustments can be applied in the analysis to compensate for the unequal selection probabilities resulting from multiplicity sampling. Clearly specified linkages are needed in order that these weighting adjustments can be made.

A key issue in deciding on the choice of linkages is whether individuals are able and willing to report the rare population statuses of those linked to them. As a rule, individuals are more able to report accurately for themselves than for others. Hence, the extension to reporting on behalf of others that multiplicity sampling entails will generally increase the level of response error. The use of multiplicity sampling for identifying gay men seems particularly problematic in this regard. It is highly questionable whether a linkage rule can be found such that nearly all of those linked to gay men will be able and willing to report the men's gay status.

Multiplicity sampling is most useful for measuring the size and prevalence of a rare population. In this case, all that respondents need report is the rare population statuses of those linked to them, perhaps together with some basic demographic and other characteristics to enable the sizes and prevalences to be estimated for some major population subgroups. When a survey aims to study a range of the characteristics of a rare population, respondents' reports with multiplicity sampling may be used to identify members of the rare population, but then the identified members need to be contacted in person to find out their characteristics, such as their behaviors and attitudes. In this case, the original respondents must be able to provide addresses or telephone numbers for the rare population members they identify. Tracing rare population members from inaccurate or out-of-date addresses can significantly add to survey costs.

There is a sizable literature on the theory of multiplicity sampling, including Birnbaum and Sirken (1965), Sirken (1970a,b, 1972a,b, 1975), Sirken and Levy (1974), Levy (1977a,b), and Nathan (1976). It has been applied in surveys or exploratory studies for such topics as drug abuse (Fishburne and Cisin, 1980), cancer patients (Czaja *et al.,* 1986), Vietnam War veterans (Rothbart *et al.,* 1982), and ethnic minorities (Brown and Ritchie, 1981).

8. TWO-PHASE SCREENING

There are occasions when accurate identification of rare population members is difficult or expensive, yet a cheap, easily administered, but imperfect, method of identification is available. For instance, expensive medical tests may be needed for a firm diagnosis of an illness, but responses to an inventory of symptoms relating to the illness may provide a good guide as to whether an individual has the illness. Two-phase, or double, sampling can be useful in such situations. At the first phase of data collection, the cheap but fallible test is administered to a large sample of individuals. On the basis of the results, these individuals are separated into strata according to the likelihood that they are members of the rare population (i. e., in the above example, that they have the illness). Often only two strata are created, one comprising those thought to be members and the other of those thought not to be members of the rare population. A disproportionate stratified sample is then selected for the second phase of the survey, sampling those thought likely to be members of the rare population at higher rates. The accurate method of identifying members of the rare population is applied to the second-phase sample, and the survey questionnaire is then administered to those identified to be members of the rare population.

When only two strata are formed after the first phase, the strata may be considered to be an initial fallible classification of rare population status. There are two types of misclassification that may be made from the first-phase screening: some nonmembers of the rare population may be misclassified as members (the false positives) and some members may be misclassified as nonmembers (the false negatives). As Deming (1977) points out, for two-phase screening to be effective, the number of false negatives should be kept small. The number of false positives is not so critical. It may be noted that this finding is in line with the discussion in Section 3 of the need to have the stratum with the high concentration of the rare population contain a large proportion of the rare population.

In some cases it is safe to assume that there are no false negatives, or that at most there is only a negligible number of them. When this holds, no sampling is needed in the stratum of initial negatives, and this can result in a great saving if that stratum is large. However, the decision not to sample in the stratum of initial negatives needs to be made with care, because if even only a small proportion of the members of that stratum is false negatives, but that stratum is large, then the false negatives may comprise a substantial proportion of the rare population.

In considering the use of two-phase sampling, the cost-effectiveness of the design needs to be carefully assessed. Some of the survey resources are expended on the first-phase sample, thus reducing the size of the sample on which the accurate determination can be made. The two-phase approach is beneficial only when the first-phase fallible screening costs are much lower than the second-phase costs. Deming (1977) shows that the ratio of the second- to first-phase per element data collection costs needs to be at least 6:1, and preferably much larger. Otherwise, a single-phase sample, using all of the survey resources for accurate testing, will generally be more effective.

The application of two-phase sampling for sampling gay men does not appear promising. One possible application would be to collect only nonsensitive information that is predictive of being gay at the first phase, such as being unmarried and living in a household without females. However, since such information would fail to satisfy the requirement of yielding a classification that produces few false negatives, this approach seems unlikely to be useful. Although two-phase sampling may not hold much promise for sampling gay men, it may prove useful for sampling other rare populations of interest in AIDS-related surveys.

9. LOCATION SAMPLING

A common method of generating a sample of gay men is to recruit the men at such places as gay bars, bathhouses, and bookstores. These samples are generally obtained as convenience samples, with the recruiting being conducted at times when the numbers of gay men at the locations are high. A more rigorous method of sampling is to use a time/space location sampling design.

Time/space sample designs are widely used to sample flows of human populations, such as international travelers, voters at polling booths, and visitors to museums and hospitals (Kalton, 1991). The essence of such designs involves first constructing a sampling frame of PSUs that consist of time period/location combinations during which and where the flow takes place. A sample of PSUs is drawn and a sample of visitors is then selected, often by systematic sampling, in the selected PSUs.

As an illustration, consider a sample of visits to the four AIDS testing clinics in a given area in a given 13-week period. Suppose that three of the clinics are open from 8 a.m. until 5 p.m. each weekday, and that the fourth is open on Mondays, Wednesdays, and Fridays from 10 a.m. until 6 p.m. and on Saturdays from 9 a.m. until noon. The PSUs for the time/space sample design could be formed as, say, half-day shifts at each clinic when it is open. There are then ten PSUs per week for each of the first three clinics, 8 a.m.–12.30 p.m. and 12.30 p.m.–5 p.m. for the five weekdays, and seven PSUs per week for the fourth clinic, 10 a.m.–2 p.m. and 2 p.m.–6 p.m. on Monday, Wednesday, and Friday and 9 a.m.–noon on Saturday. For the 13 weeks, there are thus 481 PSUs in total. A sample of these PSUs is selected, and fieldwork data collection is conducted in the sampled PSUs. A simple scheme is to count clients as they enter (or leave) a sampled clinic during the sampled shift, selecting every kth one for interview.

A time/space sample is a simple two-stage design, and the usual considerations in two-stage sampling apply. The PSUs may be sampled with probability proportional to estimated sizes (i. e., their predicted numbers of clients) to handle the unequal flows across times and clinics, and stratification may be applied to ensure that the selected PSUs cover the different clinics, times of day, days of weeks, and weeks of the study period in the desired way. Further details of time/space sampling are given by Kalton (1991).

An important feature of time/space sampling is that it produces a probability sample, often an equal probability sample, of *visits* not *visitors*. In many surveys of flows of human populations, the visit is the appropriate unit of analysis. If, however, the visitor is to be the unit of analysis, then the problem of duplicate listings arises, since visitors who make several visits to the locations in the survey period have multiple chances of selection. When the purpose of the time/space sample design is to sample visitors rather than visits, the sampling scheme may be termed location sampling.

As discussed earlier, one solution to duplicate listings is unique identification. With location sampling, unique identification can be achieved by identifying each visitor with his first visit during the survey period, and treating subsequent visits as blanks. The implementation involves asking each sampled visitor if this visit is his first visit in the survey period. If the answer is "Yes," then the full survey interview is conducted; if "No," then the interview is terminated. A disadvantage of this procedure is that it can create an uneven work load for the interviewers. Nearly all visitors selected early in the survey period will be making their first visits, and hence are eligible for the survey. However, many of those selected near the end of the survey period will have made previous visits, and will therefore be ineligible. A way to address this problem is to sample the time period/location PSUs with probabilities proportional to their estimated numbers of *eligible* visitors, rather than *total* visitors. For a sample design that gives all visitors in the fieldwork period equal probabilities of selection, this modification results in higher subsampling fractions being applied in selected PSUs that are later in the fieldwork period (where the numbers of eligible visitors are small). It will, of course, usually be difficult to estimate the numbers of eligible (i. e., first-time) visitors to a PSU. However, to the extent that the estimated numbers of eligible visitors used in the PSUs' selection probabilities are reasonably accurate, this procedure will tend to equalize the interviewers' work loads in each sampled PSU.

Another solution to duplicate listings is to employ weighting in the analysis to compensate for the unequal selection probabilities. The difficulty with this solution in the present case is that the true extent of duplication is not known. Even if a visitor sampled at a particular time can report accurately how many previous visits he has made since the start of the survey period, he will generally not be able to predict well how many visits he is going to make between the time of interview and the end of the survey period. If weighting adjustments are to be used, they must generally be based on only an estimate of the number of visits each visitor makes during the survey period. When visit patterns are fairly regular, such estimates may be based on reports of the numbers of visits made in a previous comparable time period. For instance, the sampled visitors to the clinics could be asked about the numbers of visits they made in the 13 weeks preceding the interview, and the weights could be made inversely proportional to these numbers.

Despite the problems created by duplicate listings, location sampling may be a cost-effective way to sample gay men who frequent gay bars and other gay establishments for which no membership lists exist. If the survey period is made sufficiently long to ensure that nearly all gay men who frequent these establishments will do so at least once during the period, the coverage rate for the population of gay men frequenting the establishments on the sampling frame will be high. However, this population does not cover all gay men. If the survey's target population is all gay men in the city, then location sampling alone is inadequate. It may, however, serve as a useful component of a multiple frame design (see Section 6 on the qualities that an incomplete frame requires to be an effective part of a multiple frame design).

An application of location sampling for sampling street prostitutes is described by Berry *et al.* (1989).

10. SNOWBALLING

The key idea behind the technique of snowballing is that members of some rare populations know each other. The technique is applicable only for rare populations for which this condition holds. Snowballing works by first identifying some members of the rare population, asking these members to identify others, asking those so identified to identify yet others, and so on. There are two different ways in which snowballing can be used in sampling a rare population: one use is for the direct generation of the sample, and the other is for constructing a sampling frame for the rare population from which a sample is then selected. It is the former use that is generally meant by the term *snowball sampling,* or alternatively *chain referral sampling.* In this case, the chain referral process is continued until a sample of the desired size has been achieved. Snowball sampling has been widely used in sociological studies of deviant behavior, and in particular in studies of drug use and addiction (e. g., Biernacki and Waldorf, 1981; Kaplan *et al.,* 1987).

Snowball sampling provides a relatively inexpensive way of generating a sample of a very rare population provided that the members of that population know and are willing to identify each other. It would appear to be potentially applicable for a number of the populations that are at high risk of contracting AIDS (e. g., male prostitutes). Snowball sampling is, however, a nonprobability sampling procedure, and is therefore subject to the inherent weaknesses of this form of sampling. With snowball sampling, members of the rare population who have many contacts with other members of that population have greater chances of being selected for the sample than those with few contacts, and those who are socially isolated from other members of the rare population have minimal chances of selection. Although attempts may be made to reweight the sample to compensate for this effect, there is no dependable way of doing so. Estimates obtained from snowball samples are potentially subject to serious biases, and need to be interpreted with due caution. Consequently, snowball sampling should be reserved for use as a last resort, when all forms of probability sampling have been ruled out as impractical.

The use of snowballing for sampling frame construction does not have the same limitations as snowball sampling. For frame construction, snowballing may be applied, along with other procedures, to create a list of members of the rare population. The snowballing process is continued until no additional members of the rare population can be found. Then a standard probability sample design can be employed to produce a sample of cases for study in the survey. The key issue with this use of snowballing is the completeness of the resulting sampling frame. Provided that the frame has a high coverage for the rare population, then a good probability sample can be produced. The risk with snowballing for frame construction is that socially isolated members of the rare population are more likely to be missing from the frame. If many socially isolated members are missing, and if they differ appreciably from other members of the rare population in terms of the characteristics studied in the survey, then the survey estimates could be seriously biased.

11. CONCLUDING REMARKS

Obtaining a high-quality, reasonably priced, probability sample of a specific population group at high risk of HIV infection is a challenging problem. The battery of techniques for sampling rare populations reviewed in this chapter can be helpful in addressing this problem, but generally there are no simple solutions. Rather, the sample design for a population group at high risk of HIV infection is likely to require an imaginative use of a combination of sampling techniques, almost certainly including a large-scale screening operation as one component. A sample of gay men in a city could, for instance, include the use of multiple frames (lists of memberships of gay organizations), disproportionate stratification and multistage sampling (oversampling in areas of the city with high proportions of unmarried males), and perhaps location sampling (time/space sampling at gay bars). In planning a survey of such a high-risk population, adequate allowance needs to be made for the developmental work needed to construct the sample design. Before an efficient probability sample can be selected, considerable research efforts need to be devoted to investigating the quality and availability of various frames, and to fashioning a design that meets the survey's objectives in a cost-efficient manner.

The quality of a sample depends not only on efficient design but also on effective implementation. Nonresponse is a serious threat to the quality of all samples, and especially so to surveys in AIDS research because of the sensitivity of the subject matter (see the discussion in Chapter 6 in Miller *et al.,* 1990, on participation in sex surveys). High response rates are essential if the benefits of probability sample selection are to be realized. The achievement of high response rates requires intensive efforts to minimize both noncontacts and refusals, and especially the latter. Methods that may be applied to increase response rates include mass media campaigns, the use of proxy informants, the use of alternative modes of data collection for reluctant respondents, providing payments or other forms of incentive to respondents, training interviewers in persuasion techniques, and the use of highly skilled interviewers for refusal conversion (Groves, 1989). Sufficient resources should be allocated to the fieldwork to enable high response rates to be obtained, and often substantial resources will be required. Without a high response rate, the efforts to design a good probability sample of a high-risk population will be largely wasted.

REFERENCES

Berry, S. H., Duan, N., and Kanouse, D. E. (1989). Developing a probability sample of prostitutes: Sample design for the RAND study of HIV infection and risk behaviors in prostitutes. In *Proceedings of the Fifth Conference on Health Survey Research Methods.* U.S. Department of Health and Human Services, pp. 195–198.

Biernacki, P., and Waldorf, D. (1981). Snowball sampling. Problems and techniques of chain referral sampling. *Sociol. Methods Res.* **10**:141–163.

Birnbaum, Z. W., and Sirken, M. G. (1965). *Design of sample surveys to estimate the prevalence of rare diseases: Three unbiased estimates.* Vital and Health Statistics, Series 2, No. 11. Washington, D.C.: U.S. Government Printing Office.

Blair, J., and Czaja, R. (1982). Locating a special population using random digit dialing. *Public Opinion Q.* **46**:585–590.

Brown, C., and Ritchie, J. (1981). *Focussed enumeration. The development of a method for sampling ethnic minority groups.* London: Policy Studies Institute and Social and Community Planning Research.

Cochran, R. S. (1964). Multiple frame sample surveys. *Proceedings of the Social Statistics Section, American Statistical Association,* pp. 16–19.

Czaja, R. F., Snowden, C. B., and Casady, R. J. (1986). Reporting bias and sampling errors in a survey of a rare population using multiplicity counting rules. *J. Am. Stat. Assoc.* **81**:411–419.

Deming, W. E. (1977). An essay on screening, or on two-phase sampling, applied to surveys of a community. *Int. Stat. Rev.* **45**:29–37.

Fishburne, P. M., and Cisin, I. (1980). *National survey of drug abuse: Main findings.* No. 108. Washington, D.C.: National Institute of Drug Abuse.

Fuller, W. A., and Burmeister, L. F. (1972). Estimators for samples selected from two overlapping frames. *Proceedings of the Social Statistics Section, American Statistical Association,* pp. 245–249.

Groves, R. M. (1989). *Survey errors and survey costs.* New York: Wiley.

Groves, R. M., and Lepkowski, J. M. (1985). Dual frame, mixed mode survey designs. *J. Off. Stat.* **1**:263–286.

Groves, R. M., Biemer, P. P., Lyberg, L. E., Massey, J. T., Nicholls, W. L., and Waksberg, J. (eds.). (1988). *Telephone survey methodology.* New York: Wiley.

Harry, J. (1986). Sampling gay men. *J. Sex Res.* **22**:21–34.

Harry, J. (1990). A probability sample of gay males. *J. Homosexuality* **19**:89–104.

Hartley, H. O. (1962). Multiple frame surveys. *Proceedings of the Social Statistics Section, American Statistical Association,* pp. 203–206.

Hartley, H. O. (1974). Multiple frame methodology and selected applications. *Sankhya C* **36**:99–118.

Kalton, G. (1991). Sampling flows of mobile human populations. *Surv. Methodol.* **17**:183–194.

Kalton, G. (1993). *Sampling rare and elusive populations.* United Nations Statistical Division, National Household Survey Capability Programme. Technical Studies Series. New York: United Nations.

Kalton, G., and Anderson, D. W. (1986). Sampling rare populations. *J. R. Stat. Soc. A* **149**:65–82.

Kaplan, C. D., Korf, D., and Sterk, C. (1987). Temporal and social contexts of heroin-using populations: An illustration of the snowball sampling technique. *J. Nerv. Ment. Dis.* **175**:566–574.

Kish, L. (1965a). *Survey sampling.* New York: Wiley.

Kish, L. (1965b). Selection techniques for rare traits. *Genetics and the epidemiology of chronic diseases.* Public Health Service Publication 1163, pp. 165–175.

Levy, P. S. (1977a). Optimum allocation in stratified random network sampling for estimating the prevalence of attributes in rare populations. *J. Am. Stat. Assoc.* **72**:758–763.

Levy, P. S. (1977b). Estimation of rare events by simple cluster sampling with multiplicity. *Proceedings of the Social Statistics Section, American Statistical Association,* pp. 963–966.

Lund, R. E. (1968). Estimators in multiple frame surveys. *Proceedings of the Social Statistics Section, American Statistical Association,* pp. 282–288.

Miller, H. G., Turner, C. F., and Moses, L. E. (eds.). (1990). *AIDS: The second decade.* Washington, D.C.: National Academy Press.

Nathan, G. (1976). An empirical study of response and sampling errors for multiplicity estimates with different counting rules. *J. Am. Stat. Assoc.* **71**:808–815.

Rothbart, G. S., Fine, M., and Sudman, S. (1982). On finding and interviewing the needles in the haystack: The use of multiplicity sampling. *Public Opinion Q.* **46**:408–421.

Sirken, M. G. (1970a). Household surveys with multiplicity. *J. Am. Stat. Assoc.* **65**:257–266.

Sirken, M. G. (1970b). Survey strategies for estimating rare health attributes. In *Proceedings of the Sixth Berkeley Symposium on Mathematical Statistics and Probability.* Berkeley: University of California Press, pp. 135–144.

Sirken, M. G. (1972a). Stratified sample surveys with multiplicity. *J. Am. Stat. Assoc.* **67**:224–227.

Sirken, M. G. (1972b). Variance components of multiplicity estimators. *Biometrics* **28**:869–873.

Sirken, M. G. (1975). Network surveys. *Bull. Int. Stat. Inst.* **46**(4):332–342.

Sirken, M. G., and Levy, P. S. (1974). Multiplicity estimation of proportions based on ratios of random variables. *J. Am. Stat. Assoc.* **69**:68–73.

Sudman, S. (1985). Efficient screening methods for the sampling of geographically clustered special populations. *J. Market. Res.* **22**:20–29.

Sudman, S., and Kalton, G. (1986). New developments in the sampling of special populations. *Ann. Rev. Sociol.* **12**:401–429.

Sudman, S., Sirken, M. G., and Cowan, C. D. (1988). Sampling rare and elusive populations. *Science* **240**:991–996.

Waksberg, J. (1973). The effect of stratification with differential sampling rates on attributes of subsets of the population. *Proceedings of the Social Statistics Section, American Statistical Association,* pp. 429–434.

Waksberg, J. (1978). Sampling methods for random digit dialing. *J. Am. Stat. Assoc.* **73**:40–46.

Waksberg, J. (1983). A note on "Locating a special population using random digit dialing." *Public Opinion Q.* **47**:576–578.

3

Quasiexperimental Designs in AIDS Psychosocial Research

RONALD C. KESSLER

Psychosocial AIDS surveys are designed to study risk behaviors for HIV transmission and, increasingly, the determinants of these risk behaviors. Some psychosocial AIDS surveys, like the AIDS supplement to the ongoing U.S. National Health Interview Survey, have the limited goal of providing descriptive data on trends in risk behaviors (e. g., Marcus and CDC, 1988; Kelley *et al.*, 1990) or in knowledge and attitudes related to these behaviors (e. g., Blendon and Donelan, 1988; Keeter and Bradford, 1988). The vast majority of psychosocial AIDS surveys, however, have the more ambitious goal of documenting causal relationships of variables that influence risk behaviors, such as individual differences in knowledge, attitudes, and group norms (Joseph *et al.*, 1987; Valdisseri *et al.*, 1988) and critical events like learning one's HIV antibody test results (McCusker *et al.*, 1988; Ostrow *et al.*, 1989). The hypotheses underlying these causal analyses are often poorly specified and the goal of assessing causality is often implicit rather than explicit, but this is the goal nonetheless in much of the research published from psychosocial AIDS surveys. The broad aim of this work is characteristically described as increasing knowledge of causal processes in such a way as to help design preventive interventions (Coates *et al.*, 1987; Kelley *et al.*, 1989).

This chapter discusses the problems and prospects associated with using nonexperimental psychosocial AIDS research to make causal inferences of this type, with an emphasis on seeking control through research *design* rather than through the use of special statistical analysis procedures. The chapter by Robins in Part III of this volume discusses the use of statistical analysis pro-

RONALD C. KESSLER • Institute for Social Research, University of Michigan, Ann Arbor, Michigan 48106-1248.

Methodological Issues in AIDS Behavioral Research, edited by David G. Ostrow and Ronald C. Kessler. Plenum Press, New York, 1993.

cedures to make valid causal inferences from nonexperimental data. This chapter begins by reviewing the basic problem of causal inference in nonexperimental research. We then consider a number of quasiexperimental designs that can be used to augment conventional surveys in such a way that causal inferences can be made with more confidence. Finally, the chapter reviews other ways in which AIDS psychosocial surveys can be used to help guide the development of preventive interventions other than relying on their limited ability to support strong causal inferences. The goal throughout is to provide a review of research designs that will be helpful to workers in this area of research who are grappling with the complex problems posed by the AIDS epidemic. No attempt is made to discuss the many analysis issues that arise in implementing the designs we review, as this would place too great a burden on a single chapter and would deflect the discussion from the main goal of focusing on design decisions. However, citations are provided throughout the chapter to published works that discuss the wide range of practical analysis issues associated with the use of each design reviewed.

1. THE PROBLEM: CAUSAL INFERENCE IN NONEXPERIMENTAL RESEARCH

The least complex case to consider is one in which exposure to an experience thought to play a part in reducing risky sexual behavior occurs for reasons that are random with respect to the initial value and trajectory of that behavior. For purposes of discussion throughout the chapter such an experience will be referred to as an "intervention," recognizing that this does not imply forethought on the part of either the person exposed to the experience or the persons who might have been responsible for creating the experience. Nor is the use of the term *intervention* intended to prejudge the issue of causality or randomness of exposure. It merely indicates that the experience in question is of interest to the researcher as a subject of inquiry, the main focus of this inquiry being whether the experience did, in fact, have a causal impact on some outcome.

Random exposure to an intervention occurs by design in experiments. It also sometimes occurs in naturalistic settings in the absence of planned intervention. When this latter situation is the case, the intervention can be considered a "natural experiment" and the task of causal analysis is much simplified. The main strategy in the techniques reviewed in this chapter is to search for natural experiments in a variety of ways.

An example of a situation that might approximate the conditions of a natural experiment would occur if the local newspapers in one set of communities decided to carry a syndicated series of articles on HIV transmission while the newspapers in other adjoining communities did not, for reasons having nothing to do with the comparative risk profiles of the respective communities. In a situation of this sort, when the researcher considers it reasonable to assume that exposure is random with respect to the outcomes, it is conventional to interpret an aggregate association between exposure and subsequent change in risky sexual behavior as evidence that the intervention had an effect on risk reduction. The confidence one has in estimating the magnitude of this effect, within the constraints of the assumptions about between-community equivalence and randomness of exposure, can be formalized statistically by considering the distributions of subsequent changes and the number of communities involved in the comparison.

The practical problem in an exercise of this sort is that exposure is unlikely to be entirely random with respect to initial values or trajectories of the outcomes of interest. Even a seemingly random event, like the decision of a local newspaper to carry a syndicated series of stories on HIV infection, might occur in some communities for reasons that involve personal experiences that are related to structural determinants of the outcome variable of interest. When this is the case, an evaluation of causal influence based on the assumption of random exposure will yield a biased estimate.

2. SOME DESIGN SOLUTIONS TO THE PROBLEM

In some cases where random exposure cannot be assumed, it is possible to regain inferential power by using one of several different research designs that approximate the control provided by a true experiment. The most promising of these designs are reviewed in this section, beginning with simple cases and then progressing to more complex ones.

2.1. Regaining Inferential Power by Aggregation

It is important to recognize in the example given above that the decision of a particular individual to read a newspaper story cannot be considered random even if between-community variation in publication of the stories is random with respect to the aggregate distributions of individual risk behaviors across the communities. This means that the interpretation of causal influence would, in this particular example, be more legitimate at the community level than at the individual level. A researcher who analyzes data at the community level in order to exploit the ability to assume random exposure at this level of aggregation, even though he or she is fundamentally interested in the effect of the intervention at the individual level, is using aggregation as a design strategy.

This use of aggregation to regain inferential power is similar in some ways to what is known as the "random invitation design," a type of field experimental design where a random subsample constituting the experimental group is invited to participate in an intervention while this invitation is not extended to an equivalent control group (Caplan *et al.*, 1989). The virtue of this design is that it allows the analyst to invoke the assumption of random assignment even though only a small percent of the experimental group may actually participate in the intervention. The main weakness of this design is that the estimated experimental effect is not the effect of primary interest to the researcher (i. e., the effect of the intervention) but rather a complex product of the success of the invitation in attracting a subset of eligible participants and the success of the intervention in this subset. A powerful program could very easily be judged ineffective in a mechanical use of the random invitation design because of poor success in attracting participants.

In cases where the invitation is an integral part of the intervention one seeks to evaluate, as in the case of a program to distribute brochures about safe sex in a school setting, it is perfectly legitimate to restrict analysis to the level of aggregation where the invitation was randomized because the program would only be considered successful if it both succeeded in getting people to read the brochure and in promoting behavior change among those who did so. In cases where there is also interest in knowing whether the program was effective in the (nonrandom) subsample who were exposed to it, the aggregate effect could usually be taken as a lower bound estimate and multivariate analysis could be used to narrow the range of uncertainty about the upper bound. The success of this narrowing effort hinges centrally on whether the researcher is willing to assume that the invitation had no effect on the outcome among the subsample of experimental subjects who did not participate in the program. When this assumption is plausible, as it often is, an unbiased estimate can be obtained of the program's effect on the subsample of people who took advantage of the invitation. The logic and analysis procedures used to obtain this estimate are presented by Bloom (1984, 1985).* This estimate is useful in situations where the strategy of attracting participants to the program can be improved, in which case an estimate of the program's impact can help planners decide whether to invest in increased recruitment efforts.

---

* It is important to note that while Bloom's (1984) discussion of parameter estimation is correct and useful for the researcher who wishes to use the random invitation design, his discussion of standard errors is incorrect. The significance tests of the aggregate-level effects of the intervention are identical to those of the reparameterized effect estimates, which means that there is no increase in statistical power associated with this procedure. The main benefit is, rather, the substantive one of obtaining a more accurate estimate of the true magnitude of the intervention effect in the subsample of exposed respondents.

An estimate of treatment effect is also very useful in the more general case where the researcher is evaluating a nonexperimental intervention, like a newspaper story about AIDS risk, where exposure and motivation to read the story are likely to be nonrandom within a community. It is very important in cases of the latter sort, however, for the researcher to appreciate that the effect of the newspaper story (or other exposure) may be quite different for the subsample of people who self-selected into exposure than for the broader population. Some sense of the limits of external validity can often be obtained by estimating selection equations for nonrandom exposure at the individual level in the experimental communities and using the results of these equations to generate subsample replications of the basic evaluation among respondents who vary in probability of taking advantage of the intervention opportunity. Variation in these estimated effects can be used to assess external validity. This strategy requires the construction of quasicontrol groups in the control communities by applying the selection equations to the individual-level data in the control communities in order to locate a subsample of respondents who are "the kinds of people" who would likely have read the newspaper stories if they were available. The persuasive power of this external validity analysis will vary directly with the strength of the selection equations on which this exercise is based and, for this reason, a researcher making use of the random invitation design is usually well served by building in measures designed explicitly to predict individual-level selection into exposure (Vinokur et al., 1991).

2.2. Regaining Inferential Power by Matching

A broader strategy for regaining inferential power is to use ancillary information obtained from both exposed and unexposed subjects to match cases and controls and construct an after-the-fact comparison that might be considered random. It is unfortunate that this strategy is not used more often in nonexperimental research, because there are many cases where a persuasive case could be made for essentially random exposure to an intervention within a carefully matched subsample. Indeed, this is the real power of matching. The more typical use of matching is mechanically to construct matched samples on such variables as age, sex, and other demographic characteristics in the vague hope that this will improve the *precision* of comparison. The *validity* of comparison is seldom taken into consideration in such efforts.

It is important to recognize that a good deal of careful analysis is required to implement a persuasive matching design, one that can be analyzed as if exposure to the intervention was random. In the case of an evaluation of the effects of a series of newspaper stories on the sexual behaviors of community residents, for example, the researcher would have to investigate the reasons behind editorial decisions about publishing the series of stories on a case-by-case basis in the communities sampled. An investigation of this sort would lead to certain communities that carried the stories being excluded from the analysis (e. g., communities where interest in the stories was stimulated by the recent AIDS-related death of a prominent citizen) because of special circumstances that invalidate comparisons with communities that did not carry the stories. It would also lead to the exclusion of certain communities that did not carry the stories (e. g., communities with a strong fundamentalist citizenry who shape editorial decision-making) because of special characteristics of community composition or ethos that vary in some important ways from the broader set of communities in the investigation. If it is possible, after this careful sorting and sifting, to end up with a meaningful subsample of communities in which the determinants of publication are known and can be considered random with respect to the outcome under investigation, a good case can be made for treating the comparison as equivalent to an experimental evaluation.

The limiting condition in constructing a matched comparison sample of this sort is that the range within which exposure can legitimately be considered random will sometimes be quite narrow. Indeed, there may be no reasonable comparison group for certain important subsamples, as when virtually all communities of a particular type (like those, mentioned above, that experienced the recent AIDS death of a prominent citizen) carry stories about HIV infection in their local papers. In a case of this sort, it is impossible to ascertain the effects of the event under examination in all places it occurred. This may be the typical case. If so, it implies that an accurate assessment of the impact of the intervention is more likely to be obtained by focusing on a subset of thoughtfully compared communities that can be considered a series of "natural laboratories" than by attempting to generate a single overall estimate in a broad-based analysis of a much more diverse sample.

It is worth noting that even in cases where legitimate comparison groups can be constructed, some researchers might not find the narrow population within which exposure can be considered random an interesting one to study. This is another issue of external validity. The researcher who works with nonexperimental data should place a higher priority on establishing the conditions to support a clear causal inference in one or more subsamples than on striving for less firmly justified causal inferences about the total sample. This position is based on the view that the task of generalizing a finding beyond the subsample(s) in which it is initially documented is most effectively achieved by means of theory-guided cross-validation based on firm documentation of a causal relationship in one or more particular subsamples.

A researcher adopting the opposite approach, of using less firm arguments about causal inference in the total sample, needs to recognize that no matter what data analysis strategy or research design he uses to study the effects of naturally occurring interventions, each such case has a particular range of the population over which exposure was random. This range may not be apparent to the researcher, but it exists. It varies from one situation to another, and it plays a part in shaping estimates of the effects of the intervention even when the researcher fails to take it into consideration. The researcher will seldom be successful in making causal inferences without developing sufficient knowledge about the situations he studies to define this range of valid inference and without understanding the implications of this range for his estimates. This knowledge will often argue for the use of matching to construct subsample quasiexperimental contrasts as the most convincing strategy for making causal inferences. In cases where this is not true and the use of statistical modeling is seen to be the preferable strategy, the development and interpretation of these models will almost certainly be done more intelligently than in the absence of such information if the researcher has a firm background knowledge about the determinants of exposure.

2.3. Regaining Inferential Power by Using a Random Component

The successful use of matching to make causal inferences requires the researcher to accept assumptions about the total set of conditions leading to exposure for a subset of respondents. This kind of *total* understanding is often impossible to achieve other than in situations where exposure is known to have occurred for one specific reason that was random with respect to the outcome. A more typical situation is where the researcher knows about some of the influences on exposure, which are thought to be random with respect to the outcome, but not all influences. In a situation of this sort, the method of instrumental variables can sometimes be used to obtain an accurate estimate of the effect of an intervention. This method was developed by econometricians and has a long history of use in econometrics, where problems of nonrandom exposure and reciprocal influence are common occurrences (Fisher, 1965).

The critical feature required to use this method is that the researcher is able to measure one or more variables (the instrumental variables) that are correlated significantly with the outcome and that can plausibly be assumed to have no effect on the outcome other than through exposure to the intervention. When this assumption is true, the component of variance in exposure to the intervention that is caused by the instrumental variables can be interpreted as a random assignment component. It is possible to use either a direct variance decomposition procedure or an estimation procedure based on simultaneous equation methods to estimate the causal effect of the intervention purged of the selection bias that might influence other components of exposure. A limiting condition in using this analysis strategy is that powerful estimation of the intervention effect requires the instrumental variables to explain a substantial part of the variance in exposure (Bielby and Matsueda, 1991). It should also be noted that the resulting estimates are extremely sensitive to minor misspecifications.

Keeping with the focus of this chapter on design rather than analysis, estimation issues involved in using the method of instrumental variables will not be discussed. A detailed discussion of these issues can be found in any standard textbook on econometrics. A particularly good treatment is provided by Amemiya (1985). Instead, the fact is emphasized that the availability of this analysis strategy creates design opportunities that the researcher should consider when seeking to make causal inferences from nonexperimental data. A good example is the case considered by Robins in his chapter in this volume on the effect of nonrandomly assigned aerosolized pentamidine in a clinical trial to evaluate the effect of AZT on survival of AIDS patients. As noted by Robins, there was a confounding between assignment to the low-dose treatment arm of this clinical trial and exposure to prophylaxis therapy for PCP with aerosolized pentamidine because of the fact that men assigned to the low-dose condition developed more cases of PCP than those in the high-dose condition. The fact that men in the low-dose condition had longer average survival times than those in the high-dose condition raised the question whether the nonrandomly assigned prophylaxis therapy had a more powerful effect on survival than the experimental treatment.

The method of instrumental variables could have been used to address this question if it was possible to conceptualize and measure one or more determinants of exposure to prophylaxis therapy that influenced survival risk only through the mediating effect of exposure to prophylaxis. The practice style of the treating physician could have served as a variable of this sort. As noted by Robins, a great many physicians served as primary providers for the men in the AZT trial and these providers were allowed to use their own clinical judgment to decide on therapies other than AZT. If it was possible to assess variation in clinical judgment among these providers in a rigorous fashion and conceptualize this variation as a determinant of individual differences in exposure to aerosolized pentamidine which affected mortality risk of participants only through the mediating effect of this exposure, the method of instrumental variables could have been used to obtain a direct estimate of the effect of prophylaxis therapy on longevity.

I do not want to suggest that the use of this design-based strategy would have been superior to the model-based strategy proposed by Robins. Design-based and model-based approaches are both potentially useful, but the extent to which this is true in a particular application depends on the circumstances confronting the researcher in that instance. In the ideal case, a number of design-based and model-based strategies would all be feasible and the researcher would use all of them and see whether they converge on the same conclusion. In the more typical case, only one or none will be feasible. In the particular example considered by Robins, it turns out that the method of instrumental variables would not have worked because the question about the effect of prophylaxis therapy on survival was not raised until so late in the course of the AZT trial that the opportunity to collect data on the practice styles of providers was no longer feasible. Furthermore, it is unclear that the amount of variance in exposure to prophylaxis therapy resulting from this instrumental variable would have been large enough to provide a powerful estimate of the causal effect of prophylaxis on longevity even if it was possible to obtain the required measures.

2.4. The Regression Discontinuity Design

Although it is only rarely used, it is useful to consider a special case of the multivariate control approach known as the regression-discontinuity design before turning to the more general case. This design can be used when exposure to an intervention occurs for reasons that are *completely* determinate. The impact of an AIDS awareness education program in high schools could be evaluated by means of this approach, for example, if the funding for this program was totally determined by some formula defining need, such as a community-wide index based on combining information about the percent of teenage pregnancies and results of heelstick surveys in local hospitals.

The logic of the regression-discontinuity design is to create a synthetic comparison group with adjusted levels of the outcome variable by studying the relationship between the selection variable and the outcome in the subsample not exposed to the intervention. This relationship is imputed to the subsample with the intervention to provide an expected value of the outcome in the absence of the intervention, based on the assumption that the functional form of the relationship is the same in the two subsets. This assumption is often a more plausible one than the assumption required in more conventional linear regression analyses that all relevant common causes have been controlled. Based on the assumption of constant functional form, the expected value of the outcome is compared with the observed value to estimate the impact of the intervention. The regression-discontinuity design is discussed in greater detail by Trochim (1984). A variant on the regression-discontinuity design known as the regression-point-displacement design is discussed by Cook and Campbell (1979) and, with examples relevant to psychosocial AIDS research, by Coyle *et al.* (1991).

2.5. The Multivariate Control Approach

Although the designs reviewed above all offer advantages over uncontrolled comparisons of nonexperimental data, they are not used very often in nonexperimental research. The far more common situation is for the researcher to use control variables in a multivariate analysis to approximate matching. This approach can yield valid inferences of causal impact if certain restrictive conditions are met by the data. However, neither the nature of these restrictions nor their low likelihood of being fulfilled is widely appreciated by practicing researchers.

The multivariate control approach uses the logic of multivariate analysis to estimate the causal impact of an event or behavior in cases where exposure is assumed to be nonrandom with respect to the outcome variable. The main practical problem in using this approach is that we seldom understand the determinants of the outcome sufficiently to include all relevant control variables in the prediction equation and, in the absence of relatively complete controls, it is unclear whether estimates of causal influence are improved compared with the situation where no controls are added (Marini and Singer, 1988). The chapter in this volume by Robins provides a very elegant extension of the conventional use of multivariate controls that is effective in sorting out causal influences in nonexperimental data, but this approach is similar to the more general use of multivariate controls in that it requires the researcher to assume that he has accurately measured *all* of the joint determinants of the critical predictor variable and the outcome variable. The necessity of having to make this unrealistic assumption is a serious limiting factor in strategies using multivariate controls, particularly as no statement can be made about the direction or magnitude of bias introduced into the estimate of causal influence by the omission of relevant control variables unless the researcher has more understanding about the omitted variables than is typically the case. For thoughtful critiques of the multivariate control approach, see Lieberson (1985) and Freedman (1991).

2.6. The Panel Design

A popular strategy for correcting this problem is to use data collected on a panel of respondents over multiple points in time to measure the outcome variable prior to the time when the intervention occurs. In this approach, the assumption is made that by controlling the earlier value of the outcome variable one can successfully adjust for initial differences between subjects who were subsequently exposed and not exposed to the intervention, thus yielding an unbiased estimate of causal influence (Plewis, 1985).

This assumption is seldom based on a clear consideration of the ways in which bias is produced. Use of a time 1 measure of the outcome as a control variable will correct missing variable bias only in a restrictive set of situations, the most plausible of these being when the only source of bias is due to earlier values of the outcome affecting exposure to the intervention. This could occur, for example, in an individual-level evaluation of the effect of newspaper stories on change in risky behavior, if the individual's involvement in risky sex motivated him to read the series. (An unbiased estimate would not be obtained, however, if a subset of the determinants of risky behavior, rather than the behavior itself, were the motivating factors.) It is important to note that even in the narrow class of situations in which this simple type of selection process is the only source of nonrandom exposure, the use of a lagged measure of sexual behavior as a control variable will remove this bias in the estimated effect of the intervention only if the lagged variable is measured accurately and is assessed at the correct time lag and at the correct level of aggregation (Kessler and Greenberg, 1981).

2.7. The Interrupted Time Series Design

A more persuasive approach to the estimation of causal effects is available when a time series of observations on a dependent variable is available both before and after a nonexperimental intervention. As a practical matter, this situation most often occurs when there are (or can be set up) time series of informative administrative records, although it is also possible (but much more expensive) to use a long series of tracking surveys for the same purpose. A case in point might be the use of data on the number of people calling the National AIDS Hotline by month across a series of several years to evaluate the effects of major societal interventions. Visual inspection of a time series such as this one, with a particular focus on the existence of a sharp change in the level or slope of the series at the time of intervention, can sometimes be used to make inferences about the influence of a particular intervention. There was a dramatic increase in the number of calls to the National AIDS Hotline, for example, shortly after the popular sports figure Magic Johnson announced that he was HIV seropositive in October, 1991. Tests of significance for changes of this sort are available (Box and Tiao, 1975) and occasionally can be used to document significant effects on slopes even in cases where visual inspection fails to recognize them. The statistical power of these tests depends importantly on the number of data points in the time series and the stability of the series prior to the time of intervention. A number of examples along these lines are reported by Campbell (1976).

As in all designs that lack random assignment to the intervention, the researcher who uses the interrupted time series design to evaluate naturally occurring interventions should search for plausible alternative explanations of any change in the series that occurs near the time of the intervention. This should not be merely a superficial part of the data analysis, but a serious effort that might use such things as interviews with key witnesses and searches through local media records to investigate the possibility of important confounding events that occurred close in time to the intervention. There are times when it is difficult to envision any plausible alternative of this sort, as in the case of the increase in AIDS hotline calls following Magic Johnson's press conference. In cases of this sort, the interrupted time series design can be a very persuasive way of arguing for cause-and-effect relationships without carrying out a true experiment. Indeed, assuming that stable baseline time series exist, this approach could prove to be the most practical way of evaluating the effects of individual-level interventions—either novel approaches aimed at changing a long-standing pattern of risky sexual behavior or innovative therapies aimed at changing the progression of HIV-related symptoms—without the enormous costs, logistic difficulties, and ethical dilemmas associated with randomized clinical trials (Campbell, 1985). There are times, of course, when randomized clinical trials are absolutely necessary, but evidence for consistent and dramatic change from a stable baseline or reversal of a stable pattern of decline across a broad range of subjects assessed at diverse time points can sometimes be equally compelling. Even when the results of such an analysis are not definitive, they can provide a practical way of screening across multiple rival interventions in search of a subset that should be submitted to a randomized clinical trial.

There are other cases where plausible alternative explanations exist. For example, it often happens that nonrandom exposure to an intervention occurs as a result of a change in a time series, as when a school district initiates a program of AIDS education in response to an extreme recent increase in the rate of teenage pregnancies in the community. This sort of situation could lead to serious confounding and the appearance of what seem to be positive effects of the intervention on subsequent changes in that same time series that are, in fact, due to a regression artifact (Campbell, in press). McCleary and Hays (1980) discuss a number of general-purpose strategies that can be used to search for rival explanations of this sort.

A particularly appealing general-purpose strategy along these lines involves the disaggregation of the time series into meaningful subsamples that can be used to search for a dose–response relationship (thus providing additional support for the effect of the intervention) and for specifications that would argue for alternative interpretations. There has been some discussion of using this strategy to evaluate the effects of CDC's America Responds to AIDS national public service announcement campaign, applying the strategy to a disaggregated monthly multiple time series of the number of calls received by the National AIDS Hotline across separate television markets throughout the country. As noted by Flay et al. (1991), even though the volume of calls handled by this hotline increased from roughly 70,000 per month in 1987 to over 200,000 per month in 1989, it is difficult to attribute this aggregate increase to the CDC campaign both because the hotline's 800 number is available through means other than exposure to the CDC public service announcements (e. g., directory assistance, AIDS support groups) and because changes in the hotline itself (e. g., changes in the number of lines, which shorted the amount of time callers were put on hold, and changes in the use of live operators rather than taped phone answering machines) as well as events external to the hotline that occurred at the same time as increased use of AIDS public service announcements (e. g., broader media coverage) could have created fluctuations in the series in ways that make it appear to be associated with the introduction of public service announcements. Flay and his colleagues argue that a more powerful evaluation could be carried out by disaggregating the national time series to the market level where the America Responds to AIDS campaign is carried out. Market-level data on variation in the airing of America Responds to AIDS public service announcements could then be used in conjunction with this disaggregated time series to provide information on dose–response relationships and to sort out otherwise plausible alternative hypotheses about causes of variation in the volume of hotline calls.*

3. USING NONEXPERIMENTAL RESEARCH TO DEVELOP INTERVENTIONS

It was noted earlier that one of the main goals of nonexperimental research on AIDS risk is to provide information that can be used to help target intervention opportunities. Yet few of the investigators who are involved in designing and analyzing psychosocial AIDS surveys have gone on to develop preventive interventions based on the results of their survey research. Indeed, few of these survey researchers have any experience designing or evaluating interventions of any kind. Nor have most of these researchers worked closely with intervention specialists in developing research questions to be used in their surveys. As a result, the AIDS risk surveys carried out up to now have been less useful than they could have been in guiding the development of preventive interventions. This same state of affairs, it should be noted, is true for many other areas of research, where survey researchers and intervention specialists live in two largely separate intellectual worlds. While survey re-

---

* Incoming phone numbers can be readily captured and stored on a computer data file with readily available hardware. However, the CDC has up to now not collected this type of data based on concerns about confidentiality of information and disincentives for using the Hotline if such a master file was known to exist. This is very unfortunate from the perspective of the researcher, particularly as the interests of the researcher would require data to be collected only on the area code and central office code of each call, not on the full number.

searchers make frequent reference to the goal of studying causal processes as a means to the larger end of designing interventions, the reality of the situation is that they typically carry out their surveys without any serious input from an intervention specialist and without any real appreciation of what information an intervention specialist would find useful.

The irony of this situation is that when intervention specialists have an opportunity to influence the research questions posed in surveys, their questions usually turn out to be easier to answer than the questions posed by survey researchers. The reason for this, broadly speaking, is that intervention specialists place the burden of demonstrating causal connections on their experimental interventions rather than on the surveys that precede them. Surveys are seen as most useful in providing descriptive information and hunches about causal influences that can be tested more rigorously in subsequent field experiments (Gersten et al., 1991). Intervention specialists also rely on surveys carried out in the course of evaluating interventions to provide nonexperimental data that can be used to diagnose problems and pinpoint opportunities for increased effectiveness in subsequent generations of the intervention program (West et al., 1991).

A wide range of statistical techniques can be used in this type of insight-generating work, including causal modeling procedures aimed at tracing out pathways by which high risk status is associated with adverse health outcomes (Umberson et al., 1992) and at evaluating the importance of potential intervention targets as either mediators or modifiers of these pathways (e. g., Turner et al., 1991). These techniques have all of the problems of causal inference reviewed above, but they can nonetheless be useful when the analyst sees them as generating plausible hunches for further experimental testing rather than as providing definitive tests of causality. Once this more modest goal is accepted, a broader range of strategies for survey data collection and analysis present themselves.

One such strategy is to obtain testimonial data about the dynamics of naturalistic interventions. We suspect that systematic focused interviews (Merton et al., 1990) with relevant samples aimed at obtaining this type of data would generate important insights about the structural forces that impede efforts to reduce risky sexual behavior in particular sectors of society. This kind of insight-generating research has, in recent years, been associated most closely with qualitative research techniques of the sort discussed by Mindy and Robert Fullilove and by Richard Zeller in their chapters in this volume. However, it is important to recognize that there is no reason why sensitive quantitative surveys that include semistructured components could not be equally effective in generating insights of this sort. Indeed, given the concerns that have been raised about the representativeness of the small samples used in focus group research, a good case could be made that surveys of representative samples designed to build rapport and elicit insights about causality could yield more valuable data than standard methods of qualitative research.

Although surveys of the sort needed to achieve these ends are not common, a number of examples exist in the recent literature. Lehman *et al.* (1986), for example, carried out a survey to study social support for people who experienced the death of a loved one, an event that has been a tragically common feature of life in the gay community since the beginning of the AIDS epidemic. The researchers found that much of the support received by the bereaved was experienced as unhelpful, largely because of support providers offering "comforting" words that inappropriately minimized the subjective sense of loss that the bereaved were experiencing. Lehman and his colleagues carried out a parallel survey with support providers to investigate why minimization was such a common strategy with the bereaved. The researchers concluded that most support providers are unprepared to deal with the intense emotions associated with death and use minimization as a way of coping with their own distress. This result provided a useful insight that has important implications for the kinds of support strategies that should be used in interventions for the bereaved.

4. SUMMARY AND CONCLUSIONS

This chapter has considered a number of nonexperimental designs that can be used to make causal inferences in the absence of random assignment to treatment and control groups. All of the strategies reviewed rely on the assumption that exposure to some naturalistic intervention can be considered random with respect to earlier values of that outcome within a certain range. This assumption is plausible in a far wider variety of situations than most researchers realize. The foregoing exposition was presented in the hope that it may motivate nonexperimental researchers working in this area to think more carefully and creatively about ways in which this is true for their particular research questions and to exploit the existence of random exposure within a range to strengthen the plausibility of their causal inferences. Of course, the fact that all of these designs require the researcher to base causal inferences on usually untested and often untestable assumptions makes them much less attractive than true randomized field experiments. However, quasi-experimental designs can be extremely helpful when the assumptions on which they are based are plausible and particularly so when multiple strategies can be used to generate several different estimates of a single effect across designs that make different assumptions. In cases of this sort, the use of nonexperimental data to make causal inferences can be a serviceable substitute for an experiment or can be used as a powerful preliminary step before launching a true experiment aimed at sorting through and possibly disconfirming otherwise plausible hypotheses and, in this way, preventing the development of ineffective interventions based on disconfirmed hypotheses.

It is important to emphasize that all of the designs reviewed in this chapter have reduced statistical power relative to true experiments of comparable size and scope. This means that the use of these designs will usually require much larger samples than one would require with a true experiment. Another caution is that the designs that require special modeling procedures, particularly models to infer individual-level effects from random invitation designs and models to separate selection from causation by the method of instrumental variables, are extremely sensitive. This means that minor misspecifications or changes in the specification of these models can sometimes lead to substantial changes in the parameter estimates. This sensitivity is not reflected in the standard errors of the parameters, which are based on the assumption that the specification is correct, and so must be investigated by means of sensitivity analysis. Sensitivity analysis should consequently be a routine part of the investigation of results when these designs are used. Useful discussions of sensitivity analysis are provided by Belsley *et al.* (1980) and by Leamer (1978).

While the main theme in Section 2 was that survey researchers should pay more attention to design issues in their efforts to make causal inferences from nonexperimental data, the main theme in Section 3 was that surveys can do more than this. They can help guide the direction interventions will take by disconfirming otherwise plausible hypotheses and by providing insights into the processes involved in successful intervention effects. It is important that survey researchers not lose sight of this important guidance function in their zeal to make causal inferences. To this end, surveys carried out to study psychosocial variables involved in AIDS risk should increase their emphasis on intervening processes and modifying influences that could be potentially useful intervention targets. They should also build in more opportunities for discovery than they have up to now. They should, finally, more closely link their efforts with the work of interventionists and come to see their work as part of a series of research activities that sorely need greater coordination than they have had up to now.

ACKNOWLEDGMENTS. Preparation of this chapter was supported, in part, by grants K02-MH00507 and T32-MH16806 from the National Institute of Mental Health. I am indebted to Donald T. Campbell for motivating me to prepare this paper and for discussing the content with me on several occasions. Campbell's unpublished paper "Quasi-Experimental Designs in AIDS Prevention Research," which was initially prepared for the NRC Conference on Nonexperimental Approaches to Evaluating AIDS Prevention Programs (Washington, D.C., January 12–13, 1990), and later revised for the NIMH

AIDS Survey Research Methodology Conference (Rockville, Maryland, July 11–12, 1991), was a particularly valuable resource in preparing my own paper. I also appreciate the helpful comments on an earlier draft provided by members of the University of Michigan Training Program in Psychosocial Factors in Mental Health and Illness.

REFERENCES

Amemiya, T. (1985). *Advanced econometrics.* Cambridge, Mass.: Harvard University Press.

Belsley, D. A., Kuh, E., and Welsch, R. E. (1980). *Regression diagnostics: Identifying influential data and sources of collinearity.* New York: Wiley.

Bielby, W. T., and Matsueda, R. L. (1991). Statistical power in nonrecursive linear models. In P. V. Marsden (ed.), *Sociological methodology.* Washington, D.C.: American Sociological Association, pp. 167–197.

Blendon, R. J., and Donelan, K. (1988). Discrimination against people with AIDS. *N. Engl. J. Med.* **319**:1022–1026.

Bloom, H. S. (1984). Accounting for no-shows in experimental evaluation designs. *Eval. Rev.* **8**:225–246.

Bloom, H. S. (1985). Using longitudinal earnings data from Social Security records to evaluate job-training programs. In L. Burstein, H. E. Freeman, and P. H. Rossi (eds.), *Collecting evaluation data: Problems and solutions.* Beverly Hills: Sage, pp. 220–246.

Box, G. E., and Tiao, G. C. (1975). Intervention analysis with applications to economic and environmental problems. *J. Am. Stat. Assoc.* **70**:70–92.

Campbell, D. T. (1976). Focal local indicators for social program evaluation. *Soc. Indic. Res.* **3**:237–256.

Campbell, D. T. (1985). Quasi-experimental approaches to therapeutic research. *Muscle Nerve* **8**:483–485.

Campbell, D. T. Systems theory and social experimentation. In W. N. Dunn (ed.), *The experimenting society: Policy essays in honor of Donald T. Campbell. Policy Studies Review Annual, Vol. 11.* (in press).

Caplan, R. D., Vinokur, A. D., Price, R. H., and van Ryn, M. (1989). Job seeking, reemployment, and mental health: A randomized field experiment in coping with job loss. *J. Appl. Psychol.* **74**:759–769.

Coates, T. J., Stall, R., Mandel, J. S., Boccellari, A., Sorenson, J. L., Morales, E. F., Morin, S. F., Wiley, J. A., and McKusick, L. (1987). AIDS: A psychosocial research agenda. *Ann. Behav. Med.* **9**:21–28.

Cook, T. D., and Campbell, D. T. (1979). *Quasi-experimentation: Design and analysis issues for field settings.* Boston: Houghton Mifflin.

Coyle, S. L., Boruch, R. F., and Turner, C. F. (1991). *Evaluating AIDS prevention programs: Expanded edition.* Washington, D.C.: National Academy Press.

Fisher, F. M. (1965). The choice of instrumental variables in the estimation of economy-wide econometric models. *Int. Econ. Rev.* **6**:245–274.

Flay, B. R., Kessler, R. C., and Utts, J. M. (1991). Evaluating media campaigns. In S. L. Coyle, R. F. Boruch, and C. F. Turner (eds.), *Evaluating AIDS prevention programs: Expanded edition.* Washington, D.C.: National Academy Press, pp. 50–82.

Freedman, D. A. (1991). Statistical models and shoe leather. In P. V. Marsden (ed.), *Sociological methodology.* Washington, D.C.: American Sociological Association.

Gersten, J. C., Beals, J., and Kallgren, C. A. (1991). Epidemiology and preventive intervention: Parental death in childhood as a case example. *Am. J. Community Psychol.* **19**:431–500.

Joseph, J. G., Montgomery, S. B., Emmons, C. A., Kessler, R. C., Ostrow, D. G., Wortman, C. B., O'Brien, K., Eller, M., and Eshleman, S. (1987). Magnitude and determinants of behavioral risk reduction: Longitudinal analysis of a cohort at risk for AIDS. *Psychol. Health* **1**:73–96.

Keeter, S., and Bradford, J. B. (1988). Knowledge of AIDS and related behavior change among unmarried adults in a low-prevalence city. *Am. J. Prev. Med.* **4**:146–152.

Kelley, J. A., St. Lawrence, J. S., Hood, H. V., and Brasfield, T. L. (1989). Behavioral interventions to reduce AIDS risk activities. *J. Consult. Clin. Psychol.* **57**:60–67.

Kelley, J. A., St. Lawrence, J. S., Brasfield, T., Stevenson, L. Y., Diaz, Y. Y., and Hauth, A. C. (1990). AIDS risk behavior patterns among gay men in small southern cities. *Am. J. Public Health* **80**:416–418.

Kessler, R. C., and Greenberg, D. F. (1981). *Linear panel analysis: Models of quantitative change.* New York: Academic Press.

Leamer, E. E. (1978). *Specification searches: Ad hoc inference with nonexperimental data.* New York: Wiley.

Lehman, D. R., Ellard, J. H., and Wortman, C. B. (1986). Social support for the bereaved: Recipients' and providers' perceptions of what is helpful. *J. Consult. Clin. Psychol.* **54**:438–446.

Lieberson, S. (1985). *Making it count: The improvement of social theory and research.* Berkeley: University of California Press.

McCleary, R., and Hays, R. A., Jr. (1980). *Applied time series analysis for the social sciences.* Beverly Hills: Sage.

McCusker, J., Stoddard, A. M., Mayer, K. H., Zapka, J., Morrison, C., and Saltzman, S. P. (1988). Effects of HIV antibody test knowledge on subsequent sexual behaviors in a cohort of homosexual men. *Am. J. Public Health* **78**:462–467.

Marcus, R., and CDC Cooperative Needlestick Surveillance Group. (1988). Surveillance of health care workers exposed to blood from patients infected with human immunodeficiency virus. *N. Engl. J. Med.* **319**:1118–1123.

Marini, M. M., and Singer, B. (1988). Causality in the social sciences. In C. C. Clogg (ed.), *Sociological methodology.* Oxford: Blackwell.

Merton, R. K., Fiske, M., and Kendall, P. L. (1990). *The focused interview: A manual of problems and procedures, second edition.* New York: The Free Press.

Ostrow, D. G., Joseph, J. G., Kessler, R. C., Soucy, J. S., Tal, M., Eller, M., Chmiel, J., and Phair, J. P. (1989). Disclosure of HIV antibody status: Behavioral and mental health correlates. *J. AIDS Educ. Prev.* **1**:1–11.

Plewis, I. (1985). *Analyzing change: Measurement and explanation using longitudinal data.* New York: Wiley.

Trochim, W. M. K. (1984). *Research design for program evaluation.* Beverly Hills: Sage.

Turner, J. B., Kessler, R. C., and House, J. S. (1991). Factors facilitating adjustment to unemployment: Implications for intervention. *Am. J. Community Psychol.* **19**:521–543.

Umberson, D., Wortman, C. B., and Kessler, R. C. (1992). Widowhood and depression: Explaining long-term gender differences in vulnerability. *J. Health Soc. Behav.* **33**:10–24.

Valdisseri, R. O., Lyter, D., Leviton, L. C., Callahan, C. M., Kingsley, L. A., and Rinaldo, C. R. (1988). Variables influencing condom use in a cohort of gay and bisexual men. *Am. J. Public Health* **78**:801–805.

Vinokur, A. D., Price, R. H., and Caplan, R. D. (1991). From field experiments to program implementation: Assessing the potential outcomes of an experimental intervention program for unemployed persons. *Am. J. Community Psychol.* **19**:543–562.

West, S. G., Sandler, I., Pillow, D. R., Baca, L., and Gersten, J. C. (1991). The use of structural equation modeling in generative research: Toward the design of a preventive intervention for bereaved children. *Am. J. Community Psychol.* **19**:459–480.

Measurement Issues

Combining Qualitative and Quantitative Techniques to Develop Culturally Sensitive Measures

RICHARD A. ZELLER

The purpose of this chapter is to propose and illustrate a strategy designed to develop valid, reliable, and culturally sensitive measures of risk perceptions, social support, and coping strategies as applied to HIV/AIDS behavior and mental health issues for special populations. The specific concern concentrates on the identification and measurement of salient social dimensions for those who face a high risk of HIV/AIDS infection. The measurement effort will address:

1. The phenomenological meanings attached to their norms, values, attitudes, and behavior patterns
2. The estimation of the incidence and prevalence of these norms, values, attitudes, and behavior patterns in the respective populations
3. The ethical issues raised by such a measurement effort

In order to accomplish these objectives, a strategy for combining quantitative and qualitative techniques will be developed. There are many different quantitative and qualitative techniques. To simplify this task, the sample survey will be used as the model quantitative technique and the focus group will be used as the model qualitative technique. Both the sample survey and the focus group encompass major opportunities for the enhancement of social knowledge. At the same time, neither technique used in isolation from the

RICHARD A. ZELLER • Department of Sociology, Bowling Green State University, Bowling Green, Ohio 43403.

Methodological Issues in AIDS Behavioral Research, edited by David G. Ostrow and Ronald C. Kessler. Plenum Press, New York, 1993.

other is immune from a substantial risk of being led astray. The value of combining these approaches into a single coherent research strategy is that the liabilities of one approach are, to a large extent, the assets of the other.

We will now turn to a description of the essential features of the quantitative sample survey and the qualitative focus group. This description will articulate the major opportunity offered by each technique. A comparison and contrast of these sample surveys and focus groups will be followed by a discussion of strategies a researcher may wish to use to combine them when developing culturally sensitive measures. Appropriate applications to research on the population of those who face a high risk of HIV/AIDS infection will be made.

1. QUANTITATIVE RESEARCH: THE SAMPLE SURVEY

The major opportunity of the sample survey is parameter estimation. For clear issues in well-defined populations, the sample survey can provide estimates of known accuracy about the opinions of hundreds of millions based upon hundreds. For vague issues in ill-defined populations across time, the sample survey can mislead, confuse, and serve vested interests. Perhaps the best illustration of the sample survey is election forecasting.*

It has been more than 40 years since any major polling agency has failed to correctly predict the winning candidate in the U.S. presidential election. Specifically, all major polling agencies correctly predicted the Bush victory over Dukakis in 1988, the Reagan victories over Mondale in 1984 and over Carter in 1980, the Nixon victory over McGovern in 1972, the Johnson victory over Goldwater in 1964, and the two Eisenhower victories over Stevenson in 1956 and 1952. These agencies declined to predict the outcomes of the close elections in 1976, 1968, and 1960.

In statistical terminology, the *population parameter* "percent of the popular vote" is the percent of the vote each candidate receives on election day. This population parameter is based on millions of voters' decisions. The size of this population has varied from 50 million to 100 million voters during the past half century. It is identifiable after an election using public records.

The *sample statistic* "percent of the popular vote" is the percentage of those interviewed, called respondents, in a sample survey who indicate that they intend to vote for each candidate. This sample statistic is based on hundreds of respondents' verbal responses to questions posed by interviewers.

* For more information about survey research, see Fowler (1988) and Lavrakas (1987).

In such a sample survey, respondents are asked questions relevant to the election. Specifically, respondents are asked whether they are registered to vote. If yes, they are asked if they intend to vote on election day. If yes, they are asked which candidate they intend to vote for. The sample percentage for each candidate derived from this procedure is then used to estimate the population parameter.

The accuracy of the sample percentage in the survey can be evaluated by comparing it to the population percentage in the election. If the sample has been selected for this study using appropriate probability criteria, statisticians can establish a confidence interval based on probability theory. The *confidence interval* indicates the range within which the population percentage can be expected to be given the observed value of the sample percentage to a certain likelihood level. For example, a 95% confidence interval of a probability sample survey of 1000 respondents who indicate their electoral preference is ±3%. That is, if candidate X was selected by 55% of the respondents in the sample survey, there is a 95% probability that candidate X will receive between 52 and 58% of the vote in the election.*

A question of substantial importance in the investigation of HIV/AIDS transmission in the gay community involves the number of different homosexual partners with whom the individual engages in homosexual intercourse. If we had perfect knowledge of who was having sexual intercourse with whom and when, we could solve for the population mean and standard deviation. However, our knowledge is far from perfect. While we suspect that this community includes millions of people, their identity is not a matter of public record. Even if we could identify them, we would still be faced with the challenge of ascertaining the number of different homosexual partners they have per month.

Operating under these handicaps, we can imagine a population parameter "mean number of gay sexual intercourse partners" per month. In order to estimate this imagined population parameter, we can conduct a sample survey from which we can derive the sample statistic "mean number of gay sexual intercourse partners" per month. In such a survey, respondents are asked questions relevant to homosexual intercourse. Specifically, respondents are asked if they are gay. If yes, they are asked if they engage in homosexual

---

* I have taken inferential liberties in this assertion. A strict constructionist statistician would argue that the 52 to 58% confidence interval applies not to the election. Rather this confidence interval applies to the population proportion of citizens who would have specified candidate X if they had been asked the questions noted above. However, the answers to such questions in an interview are not a particularly interesting population parameter; the percent who vote for a certain candidate is interesting. As noted above, this inference has been supported by comparisons with election outcomes for 40 years.

intercourse. If yes, they are asked how many different partners they have engaged in intercourse with during the past month. The sample mean derived from this procedure is then used to estimate the population mean.

Unlike election polling, the accuracy of this sample mean cannot be directly evaluated. This is because the population parameter is never produced. Hence, the inference from sample statistic to population parameter is a leap of statistical faith. The believability of this inference depends on the degree to which the circumstances governing problem definition, data gathering, and interpretation are robust. We now turn to a discussion of our representative of qualitative research, the focus group.

2. QUALITATIVE RESEARCH: THE FOCUS GROUP

The major opportunity of the focus group is the identification of the phenomenological meanings attached to their norms, values, attitudes, and behavior patterns. For vague issues in ill-defined populations across time, focus groups can provide an understanding of how people define their life-space. For clear issues in well-defined populations at one point in time, the focus group is wasteful and inaccurate and can serve vested interests. Perhaps the best illustration of the focus group is human sexuality.*

If you eliminated love, sex, commitment, intimacy, companionship, power, and interpersonal communication from the entertainment industry, little would be left. These aspects of life are fascinating and pervasive. They involve substantial connotation and emotional involvement. Many questions can be posed when examining sexual situations. Is A testing B's commitment to the relationship? Is A lying in order to convince B to engage in sexual intercourse? Is A carrying a sexually transmitted disease (STD) that threatens B's health? Is A a virgin? Is A afraid that B thinks A is ugly? From a substantive perspective, delving into the interpersonal dynamics of sexual negotiations is a challenging domain of social inquiry.

From a methodological perspective, researchers want to explore the meaning by which target individuals, called participants, define the situation. Often a focus group is useful in this situation. A *focus group* is a discussion group among 6–12 people focused on a particular topic. Led by a *moderator,* the purpose of the focus group is to create a structure within which the meaning attributed to a social event by researchers becomes isomorphic with the meaning attributed to that same social event by the participants themselves. The results of a focus group are based on the comments of a small number of

---

* For more information about focus groups, see Morgan (1988) and Krueger (1988).

participants. Within a discussion context, a moderator poses questions on the general topic of interest. As the discussion proceeds, the moderator focuses these questions more specifically on the issues under investigation by following a topic outline guide. A *topic outline guide* is a set of open-ended questions that reflect the researcher's best guess about the important dimensions of a research problem. Care must be taken to ensure that the focusing of the questions is done consistent with the participants' definition of the situation. The participants' comments are then examined for patterns and themes that the researcher hopes will provide insight concerning the participants' definition of the situation.

The validity of the results of a focus group can be evaluated in terms of the degree to which the researcher can confidently anticipate how a member of the culture under investigation would react to a given cultural situation. That is, as a discussion proceeds, situations arise in which an outsider can be asked: "What is going to happen (or be said) next?" A researcher "understands the cultural context" when he/she can accurately provide the next reaction that a member of that culture would give.

For the gay community, one question of substantial importance in the investigation of HIV/AIDS transmission involves the criteria for evaluating potential homosexual partners and the circumstances in which they will or will not engage in homosexual intercourse. When estimating the number of homosexual partners someone had per month, at least the behavior in question is relatively clear to participants and observers alike. However, when exploring the criteria for evaluating potential homosexual partners and the circumstances in which they will or will not engage in homosexual intercourse, not only are the attitudes and values not clear to observers, but they may also be unclear to the participants themselves. Before one can imagine obtaining information concerning how many people use a particular criterion, the nature, scope, and dimensions of this criterion must be established. A criterion that is salient for one individual may not be salient for another. A criterion that is defined in one way for one individual may be defined in a different way for another.

Operating in this situation, it is unreasonable to even attempt to imagine a population parameter when there is no definition for the concept of the population parameter. A step must be taken before such an "experiment of the mind." This step is to discover, at least provisionally, the issues and ideas that are in the minds of the target population.

The unique feature of the focus group over other qualitative techniques is that ideas and perspective emerge from the interaction that would not have emerged had the interaction inherent in the focus group not taken place. That is, a group dynamic occurs in focus groups that does not occur when other techniques, such as focused interviews, are used. There are advantages and disadvantages to this group dynamic feature of focus groups.

A major advantage of the focus group is the interaction process itself. One participant's comments may spark a related thought in the mind of another participant. This participant's articulation of this new thought may lead others to still other thoughts. As the discussion proceeds, aspects of the situation that participants do not usually consider come to their minds. Occasionally, focus groups are extraordinary events. Some chemistry occurs among the group that provides unusual or unimaginable insight. You get some ideas above and beyond what any individual might have provided.

For example, when crack had just appeared on the scene, Dr. Robert Fullilove* conducted research on crack use. In his survey, he asked people whether they "shoot crack." He then conducted focus groups, where he asked, "Do you shoot crack?" The participants laughed and said: "No, you don't shoot crack." They then explained how you took crack and all of the different names for it. Even though Dr. Fullilove was embedded in the community, he did not know any of these terms. The crack epidemic was evolving rapidly and the AIDS-risk relevant behaviors were totally new. Dr. Fullilove noted that these behaviors and the terms used to describe them would not have been discovered had they not used focus groups.

At the same time, the interaction process may threaten the creative juices of the participants. Often, one or two participants will be very verbal about their opinions, and this behavior will motivate the rest of the participants to be compliant. The moderator has the responsibility of managing the interaction so that verbal participants do not overwhelm the interaction. As a way of controlling the discussion, a moderator may wish to interject: "We have already heard from Bob on this question, let's hear from someone else."

The validity of an interpretation applied to the results of focus group discussions cannot be directly evaluated. This is because of the uncontrolled nature of the investigation and the variety of factors that operate within it. Hence, inference from the focus group discussion to the cultural meaning of events is a leap of exploratory faith. As with survey research, the believability of this inference depends on the degree to which the circumstances governing problem definition, data gathering, and interpretation are robust.

3. COMPARISON AND CONTRAST OF SAMPLE SURVEYS AND FOCUS GROUPS

We will now compare and contrast the sample survey and the focus group as they contribute to the inference process. Moreover, we will articulate

---

* Comments at AIDS Survey Research Methodology Conference, National Institute of Mental Health, July 11–12, 1991, Rockville, Maryland.

and illustrate the opportunities and risks associated with the integration of the sample survey and the focus group as research tools. Our goal is to establish research design criteria that result in both rigorous and vigorous inference. The assets of sample surveys and focus groups are summarized in Table 1.

First, how clear are the issues under investigation? The sample survey is appropriate for clear issues; the focus group is appropriate for vague issues. An election is a relatively clear issue. Those running for the office of president are candidates; they are seeking votes; the winner becomes president while the loser becomes a private citizen; etc. The success of electoral polling is based, in part, on this clarity.

Many issues are vague. When respondents do not understand the terms used to define an issue, sample survey results lose credibility. Frequently, when issues are controversial, competing groups seek to define the "issue" in their own terms. For example, there is a substantial difference between the wording of survey items defined by "prolife" versus "prochoice" terminology. For example, a "prolife" Likert item might read: "A mother has a right to kill her unborn baby"; a "prochoice" Likert item might read: "The government has a right to dictate to a woman what happens to her body." Substantial proportions of disagreement could be expected to both items in a national survey. Each political persuasion then claims that majorities support their respective position on the abortion question.

The connotation attached to a word can substantially alter the reaction that respondents have to the assertion. Respondents are more likely to agree with the assertion "Gays deserve equal rights" than they are to agree with the assertion "Faggots deserve equal rights." When dealing with HIV/AIDS questions, many terms carry connotative baggage that can reasonably be expected to taint the estimation process. In order for a survey to effectively estimate important population parameters, the connotations attributed to terms must be established for the target population. Focus groups can be effectively used to establish those connotations. Thus, the value of survey research is that it effectively estimates parameters for clear issues; the value of focus group research is that it clarifies vague issues.

Table 1. Assets of Sample Surveys and Focus Groups

	Sample survey	Focus group
Issue clarity	Clear	Vague
Respondents understand questions	Yes	No
Respondents know the answers to the questions	Yes	No
Standardization of format	Maximum	Minimum
Sampling	Heterogeneous	Homogeneous

Second, do respondents understand the questions being asked? In electoral polling, most citizens understand the questions being asked. Specifically, they understand what it means to be "registered to vote," to "intend to vote on election day," and to "vote for candidate X or Y." Respondents who do not understand these situational definers of an election will be unable to intelligibly respond to the interviewer's queries. These same respondents are also unlikely to vote on election day. If they do vote, they are likely to vote in a random fashion.

Reasonable research procedure in election forecasting, therefore, suggests that the elimination of such respondents from the sample data will not harm the accuracy of the prediction of electoral victory. In statistical terms, the accuracy of the sample statistic as an estimator of the population parameter in election forecasting is robust to respondent misunderstanding of the situation.

However, such respondent misunderstanding does influence the parameter estimation robustness when conducting research on HIV/AIDS. This is because a person can, indeed, become infected with HIV even though that person does not understand the situational definers of HIV transmission.

Consider Fred, an intravenous drug user. Fred may not know what a "sterilized hypodermic needle" is. All he knows is that after sticking a pin in his arm, he "gets high." Fred has no basis for answering the question: "When you inject drugs into your arm, do you use a sterilized hypodermic needle?" However, his behavior with respect to the use of sterilized hypodermic needles has a substantial impact on his risk of contracting HIV. The elimination of Fred from the sample data will harm the accuracy of the prediction of HIV transmission. Hence, the accuracy of the sample statistic as an estimator of the population parameter is not robust to respondent misunderstanding in this situation.

The value of focus group research is that it establishes what the respondents' understanding of the topic is. The value of survey research is that when the researcher is aware of the respondents' understanding of the topic, the researcher can properly word questions so that parameter estimates are robust.

Third, do respondents know the answers to the questions being asked? In a sample survey designed to forecast the outcome of an election, most respondents know the answers to the questions being asked. They know if they are registered, if they intend to vote, and which candidate they intend to vote for.

Fred, our intravenous drug user, may know what a "sterilized hypodermic needle" is but not know whether the needle he is currently using is sterilized or not. Moreover, he may use a sterilized needle today and reuse it tomorrow. He may believe in this situation that he is using a sterilized needle.

A common way to establish "knowledge" among respondents is to ask "knowledge questions" and treat those who "know" the answers differently than those who do not. Care must be taken to ensure that "current conventional wisdom" does not substitute for "knowledge." As a researcher dedicated to "the willing suspension of belief" (Greer, 1989), there are many current conventional wisdoms in our culture today that do not pass the rigorous criteria of "knowledge" that science espouses. Indeed, credentialed scientists occasionally abandon scientific criteria rather than challenge conventional wisdoms when the conventional wisdoms challenge their ideological persuasions (Zeller, 1982).

Alternatively, a researcher may ask questions in such a way that a lack of knowledge will not hamper the respondent in answering the question. For example, consider the following items:

1. When injecting substances into yourself, do you use a sterilized hypodermic needle?
2. When injecting substances into yourself, do you use a needle that has not touched anything outside of its wrapper before you use it?
3. When injecting substances into yourself, do you use a needle that has not been used before?

Question 1 requires knowledge of sterilization; question 2 establishes sterilization by procedure without using the term "sterilized hypodermic needle"; and question 3 establishes prior use. Each of these items makes different assumptions about what the respondent understands about the question and knows about the answer.

By exploring the participant's definition of the situation, focus group research can establish how the participant thinks about the question. For example, what is the current term used to describe the injection of substances into yourself for the purpose of getting a "high"? Is it a "high" that is sought? Members of the drug-user subculture may have different definitions than members of the researcher subculture of what is going on. The focus group provides a tool by which the researcher can come to appreciate how the members of the drug-user subculture see themselves in their situation.

Thus, survey research establishes "knowledge" from the researcher's perspective; focus group research establishes "knowledge" from the target population's perspective.

Fourth, do respondents give socially desirable answers to questions being asked? There is no guarantee that what respondents say is isomorphic with what they think or what they do. *Social desirability* describes a situation in which respondents say what they think the researcher wants to hear rather than what they believe. Social desirability insidiously attacks the inference process. This often unintended attack is both subtle and alluring. The result of this attack is that researchers draw unwarranted inferences.

Both survey research and focus group research are vulnerable to social desirability. Each method employs techniques designed to minimize the effects of social desirability; neither method can claim unequivocal success at mitigating these effects. Moreover, efforts to measure the degree to which social desirability has undermined the inference process are unconvincing.

In addressing the question of social desirability, both focus group and survey research seek to put the participant/respondent at ease. Both wish to create a trusting, supportive environment in which the participant/respondent can relax and provide the relevant data to the researcher. The emphases of these two approaches differ.

Survey research seeks maximum standardization of format. The goal of this approach is the maximization of the degree to which each respondent comes to believe that all of the questionnaire responses are acceptable responses. Ideally, none of the responses on a closed-ended questionnaire is any more socially desirable than any other. Often, respondents impose such differential desirability on questionnaire response categories based on their social and cultural definitions of the situation.

For example, suppose a survey researcher wishes to find out if someone intends to vote. If voting is socially desirable among the citizenry, a reasonable hypothesis is that the percentage of citizens who reported that they voted will be higher than the percentage of citizens who actually voted. Whether a citizen votes is a matter of public record. Though I am unaware of this study having been done, a researcher could obtain lists of registered voters containing their voting records, call a probability sample of these registered voters, and ask them if they voted in the most recent election. A comparison of their responses with the data contained in the voter registration records will reveal the degree to which respondents report behavior that is more socially desirable than how they behaved.

Survey researchers attempt to mitigate the effects of social desirability by creating items that legitimate all item responses. For example, consider the following questionnaire items:

1. A municipal primary election was held last month? Did you vote in this election?
2. A municipal primary election was held last month? Some citizens voted in this election. Others who had conflicts, were too busy, or could not get to the polls, did not vote in this election. What about you? Did you vote in this election?

Item #2 provides rationalizations for the socially undesirable behavior of not voting; item #1 provides no such rationalizations. The difference between the percent who report that they voted item #1 and actual voting behavior estimates the "social desirability" effect on reported voting behavior. The difference between the percent who report that they voted item #2 and actual voting behavior estimates the "social desirability" effect on reported voting behavior *when rationalizations for socially undesirable behavior are included in the item.* The difference between the percent who report that they voted item #1 compared with item #2 represents the mitigating effect of including the rationalizations for socially undesirable behavior in the item. The American National Election Studies consistently use the latter style of items in their panel research.

Focus group research seeks minimum standardization of format. The goal of this approach is to minimize the degree to which each participant comes to believe that interpretation of the cultural setting is preferable to another. There are a variety of techniques that focus group researchers use to implement this approach. Exploration and codification of these techniques has captured much attention recently (Morgan, 1990).

For example, suppose a focus group is designed to explore the conditions under which drug users inject drugs into themselves. If use of a sterilized needle is socially desirable among drug users, a reasonable hypothesis is that drug users will report use of sterilized needles when they actually share needles. While the actual use of such needles is not a matter of public record, it is important to discover whether the needles that are being used are shared and what rationalizations and justifications are used to enable this high-risk behavior. In my view, an effective focus group moderator should engage in discussion tactics designed to legitimate reporting the use of shared needles!

Imagine a focus group among drug users concerning the use of hypodermic needles. As the discussion proceeds, questions concerning the use of needles will arise.* As these questions are explored, participants are likely to make socially desirable comments. Often, these socially desirable comments are made early in the focus group session. Once the participants come to see that comments that are usually undesirable are acceptable in this setting, they alter what they have said. It is the responsibility of the moderator to provide a context within which comments seen as socially undesirable in the outside world are acceptable in the focus group setting.

Different moderators use different techniques to establish this acceptability of socially undesirable comments. Some seek to place constraints on the repertoire of actions appropriate for moderators. Krueger (1988), for ex-

---

* I have argued elsewhere (Zeller, 1990) that in the most effective focus group, the participants will talk to one another about the topics on the moderator's topic outline guide. Such a discussion goes beyond the purposes of the current discussion.

ample, argues that substantial direction is appropriate in the training and evaluation of moderators. Such a philosophy, in my view, implicitly uses the criteria of quantitative research for the evaluation of qualitative research.

Others, such as myself, argue that the posing of rhetorical questions, argumentativeness, "leading the witness," and various other devices that are clearly prohibited in quantitative research are appropriate in focus group research. This violates the traditional criteria of "disinterested outsider" that are ordinarily used to evaluate researchers. Instead, it acknowledges the differences between quantitative and qualitative research in terms of both means and goals. Because quantitative research seeks parameter estimates, it is appropriate to demand the minimization of the influence of the researcher on the research setting. On the other hand, qualitative research uses social interaction in search of the participant's definition of the situation. Pursuing this goal with these means requires researcher involvement in the research setting.

Suppose a researcher was moderating a focus group among drug users about drug use behavior and a participant said: "When I inject cocaine into my arm, I always use a sterilized hypodermic needle." Frankly, I would suspect that this participant was patronizing me. Specifically, I doubt that drug users are in the habit of using terms like "inject" and "sterilized hypodermic needle." If my suspicion is true, I should take active, intrusive steps to "smoke out" what the participant is really thinking. Perhaps a rhetorical question would assist in this process. For example, a moderator might respond: "What the hell is a sterilized hypodermic needle?" or "You've got to be kidding me! If you are desperate for a hit and you don't have any sterilized needles around, are you going to pass up the hit?"

By traditional quantitative standards, such a moderator response introduces all kinds of biases into the data. But by qualitative standards, to allow a blatant "for public consumption" response to go unchallenged undermines the purpose of the focus group. The value of the focus group is that it can and should challenge patronization of researchers by those on whom data are being collected. I suspect that such epistemological patronization is more common than the research community has admitted. Focus groups are uniquely positioned to challenge this flaw in our inference process; sample surveys are not.

Fifth, what kind of sample capitalizes on the strength of the tool? Survey research seeks a heterogeneous sample representative of a diverse target population. Ordinarily, this is achieved by using probability sampling techniques. Focus group research seeks a homogeneous sample to reflect a common target population. Ordinarily, this is achieved by screening the participants on demographic, psychological, and behavioral characteristics.

Perhaps the best illustration of the adverse effect of nonprobability sampling on parameter estimation occurred in the famed presidential election of 1936. In that year, the respected *Literary Digest* published the results of a poll showing that Franklin D. Roosevelt would receive a paltry 40.9% of the vote and lose the election to his Republican challenger, Alfred M. Landon. When the votes were counted, Roosevelt actually received 60.2% of the vote. Gallup (1948) explains this parameter estimation error as follows:

> The *Literary Digest* sent out its ballots by mail and, for the most part, to people whose names were listed in telephone directories or to lists of automobile owners. From the point of view of cross sections this was a major error, because it limited the sample largely to the upper half of the voting population, as judged on an economic basis.

The general sampling procedure for focus groups is to have homogeneous participants. In general, it is better to have separate focus groups of officers and enlisted personnel, for married and single participants, and for men and women. To my knowledge, the best illustration of the adverse effect of an ineffectively screened set of focus group participants occurred in a focus group discussion on the use of alcoholic beverages on campus (Grabarek and Zeller, 1990). It was desirable to include in this focus group only students who drink at least occasionally. The screener questionnaire did not effectively screen out participants who abstained from drinking. This "heterogeneity" had a negative effect on the focus group. Specifically, when the discussion turned to serious drinking issues, the abstainers provided a "solution" to the "problem"—don't drink. The interjection of this comment into the focus group discussion inhibited the drinking members of the group from articulating their concerns about drinking.

A homogeneous sample renders a sample survey superfluous; a researcher need not survey lots of people if everyone thinks the same way. A heterogeneous sample renders a focus group ineffective; the purpose of a focus group is to ascertain the elements of a culture on which people agree.

A word of caution. How one interprets research data depends on that person's vested interests in the results. This statement is valid for both survey research and focus group methodologies.

Consider survey research data. Candidates who lose elections often say, prior to the election but after the polls predict their defeat, "The only poll that counts is the one that is taken on election day." The eventual loser's preelection agenda is to offset the perception that a loss is imminent, and transform the impending defeat into victory. This agenda, which usually fails to achieve its objective, is served by implying disbelief in the parameter estimate and by encouraging a volatile electorate to change their minds.

Candidates who win elections often say, prior to the election but after the polls predict their victory, "We are cautiously optimistic. However, we must guard against complacency and get out our vote." The eventual winner's preelection agenda is to reinforce the perception that victory is imminent and to assure that victory by continued attention to electoral success. This agenda, which usually succeeds in achieving its objective, is served by asserting belief in the parameter estimate and by warning about the potential that the volatility of the electorate could turn imminent victory into defeat.

Consider focus group data. The 1988 George Bush campaign based two powerful commercials on the results of focus groups.* Whether such use of focus group data elevated the campaign is debatable. What is not debatable is that the results of the focus groups were used to define political issues in graphic ways.†

A similar caveat applies to research in a sensitive research domain such as HIV/AIDS research. Some groups will have a vested interest in dramatizing the dimensions of HIV/AIDS; other groups will have a vested interest in minimizing these dimensions. In a free society, nothing can stop those who wish to reinterpret the results of research consistent with their own agendas. Social researchers are committed to resisting convenient political interpretations designed more to convince or impose one ideological perspective on society. Often, this stance leaves the social researcher vulnerable to political attack.‡

---

* One commercial presented a revolving prison door in which those who are guilty of crimes are released from prison before their sentences are fully served. The other commercial poked fun at Dukakis when he was wearing a combat helmet and rode in a tank and posed questions about Dukakis's knowledge and stature on military issues. Bush's focus groups were conducted among the homogeneous sample of "Reagan Democrats."

† In November, 1988, I was conducting a focus group on banking in a small midwestern city. After the focus group, some of the participants were asking about other uses of focus groups. I conveyed to them the Bush use of focus groups and described the two Bush commercials. Bush's focus groups were conducted among the homogeneous sample of "Reagan Democrats," voters who have traditionally supported Democrats but who voted for Reagan in the 1980s. As I was discussing this use of focus groups, one participant, who was not part of this group, overheard our conversation and joined in our discussion. She was a Reagan Democrat who was afraid of crime in the streets and wanted a strong defense. She espoused those two Bush campaign themes articulately and with much enthusiasm in our impromptu discussion. Whether one admires or detests the Bush commercials, that experience left me with little doubt that the Bush focus groups had, indeed, captured important dimensions of the political scene that were unlikely to have emerged from a survey research study.

‡ I painfully acknowledge being the target of a political repression attempt at the university on which I serve on the faculty. Radical feminists attempted to impose political correctness criteria on the curriculum of a graduate research methods course. In addition, administrators enabled this attack on unfettered investigation by simultaneously supporting the censorship efforts of the radical feminists and denying the validity of their claims. For an in-depth discussion of this event, see Zeller (1991).

4. TOWARD A NEW DEFINITION OF VALIDITY

With all of the political pushing and shoving about what is and is not known, and with all of the academic pushing and shoving about the alleged superiority of this method or that one, how is the researcher to know whether alleged "research findings" are to be taken seriously? In other words, how do we know whether our research findings are valid? The research community answers this question with a distinct flavor of multiple personality disorder.

Qualitative researchers define validity in terms of "deeper knowledge of social phenomena . . . developed in intimate relationship with data" (Strauss, 1987, p. 6). Validity from the qualitative perspective can be characterized as "pressing the flesh." Survey researchers search for statistical relationships among variables (Zeller and Carmines, 1980). Validity from the survey research perspective can be characterized as "chasing the decimal point." Experimentalists answer the validity question by appealing to the truth or falsity of causal propositions (Cook and Campbell, 1979, p. 37). Validity from the experimental perspective can be characterized as "producing the effect." In social research, I am uncomfortable with any of these approaches to validity taken in isolation from the others.

Therefore, I wish to offer a new definition of validity. This definition of validity is the criterion that I believe social research should employ. From this perspective:

> *A valid phenomenon has been established when pressing the flesh, chasing the decimal point, and producing the effect all provide the same messages about the nature of the phenomenon.*

These criteria for establishing validity are both simple and awesome. Under this definition, validity is as much a process as a product. In this view, validity requires method diversity rather than method specialization; it requires both theoretical insight and attention to detail. Validity demands a virtual obsession with the identification of argumentation and observational flaws and establishing ways that those flaws can be handled compellingly. Under these conditions, it is not surprising that efforts to conduct valid research from the perspective of a single methodological approach are unsatisfying.

Strauss does an admirable job of pressing the flesh, but his refusal to chase the decimal point or produce the effect make his work uncompelling. His strength in providing insight through rich description is not matched by an effort to explore the limits of generalizability through parameter estimation of demonstrable causation. He fails my validity test.

Joreskog (1970) is as clever and creative a data analyst as one is likely to find. But so far as I can tell, his work does not reflect any appreciation of the challenges to validity presented by data collection situations. Moreover, despite the insightfulness, elegance, and creativity of their work, it is naive for Heise and Bohrnstedt (1970) to claim to have identified a formula that differentiates reliability from validity when their formula does no more than differentiate between two kinds of reliability. They fail my test of validity.

Few experimentalists are as clever and creative as Aronson (1981). But the application of his work to actual situations leaves me unconvinced and unsatisfied. His causal propositions are demonstrated well. Moreover, he is to be commended for his noble attempt to bridge the gap between qualitative and experimental work. However, he generalizes his results well beyond what makes me comfortable, and the gap between his touchy-feely form of qualitative work and his laboratory experiments strains credulity. Thus, Aronson has clearly moved in a productive direction. At the same time, I am left with an uncomfortable sense that much remains to be done.

Cook and Campbell (1979) is a marvelous attempt to integrate experimentation and quantification. An excellent example of integrating qualitative and quantitative techniques in AIDS research is Joseph *et al.* (1984). This article is an acknowledgment of the value of making the effort to integrate diverse methodological approaches.

5. COMBINING QUALITATIVE AND QUANTITATIVE MEASUREMENT

As noted above, sample surveys and focus groups have different, compatible strengths and weaknesses. In order for research data to most powerfully speak to the question being raised by the researcher, these techniques should be used in concert. It is more difficult to be misled by the results that triangulate multiple techniques with compatible strengths than it is to be misled by a single technique that suffers from its inherent weaknesses.

Hence, the general strategy of combining qualitative and quantitative measurement is that the methods be used interactively. While such a position is easy to articulate, it is difficult to implement. This implementation challenge results, in part, from the fact that most researchers have a research method loyalty. Researchers are comfortable operating in their own area of methodological expertise; they are vulnerable operating outside that area.

At the same time, a method used in isolation from other methods does not provide compelling answers to many research problems. The reason for this is clear. Qualitative and quantitative techniques differ dramatically in their purposes, goals, objectives, tactics, strategies, strengths, and weaknesses. The original questions that prompt the research and the new questions that emerge from its results require a blending of methods. As a result, while many scholars endorse the idea of combining qualitative and quantitative measurement techniques, few actually do it. The purpose of this section is to explore ways that qualitative and quantitative measurement techniques can be blended into a coherent research strategy.

There are two basic approaches to combining qualitative and quantitative measurement. One approach seeks to guide quantitative research by the results of qualitative research; the other seeks to guide qualitative research by the results of quantitative research. In fact, an effective research program will use qualitative and quantitative research interactively. However, research projects are usually discrete entities. Hence, one approach usually precedes the other. We now turn to the advantages and disadvantages of these two approaches.

5.1. Using Focus Groups to Guide Questionnaire Construction

The results of focus groups can be effectively used to guide questionnaire construction. This is particularly valuable where the target population of the research comes from a different culture or subculture than that of the researcher. Without an infusion of cultural conventional wisdom, a researcher from one culture does not know how to create useful and meaningful questions for members of another culture. Researchers constitute a unique subculture. Often, researchers do not know how to create useful and meaningful questions for the targets of research (i. e., nonresearchers).

Focus groups can be used to enhance the degree to which the researchers appreciate the cultural conventional wisdom of a target population. Specifically, focus groups can be used to guide questionnaire construction. The usefulness and meaningfulness of questionnaire items will be enhanced when the results of focus group research guide their preparation. A transcript of a focus group discussion will provide numerous opportunities for the construction of questionnaire items in the language (i. e., slang) of the target population. A strategy for such questionnaire item construction involves the following lead-in paragraph: "The following statements have been made by others on this issue. To what degree do you agree or disagree with each of these statements." This paragraph is followed by a series of statements paired with Likert response categories.

Focus group results will provide insight concerning statements representing the same phenomenon. The validity of the categorization system inferred from the focus group results can be evaluated by applying factor analytic techniques to the battery of Likert questionnaire items. The trick of using focus group results to guide questionnaire construction is to extract from a verbatim transcript cultural conventional wisdoms that can be transformed into Likert items.

To illustrate this process, examine quotes from a recent focus group discussion (Grabarek and Zeller, 1990):

I never drank so much that I didn't know what I was doing, I mean I've always been able to remember the next day what I did the night before. I've never done anything that I wouldn't want to take responsibility for. I've never done anything really stupid and, you know, I think it's just, I know some people go out and get plowed just so they can. They go and drink a bottle of something just so they can have an excuse to beat the hell out of somebody.

I've found that . . . we use drinking not as an excuse so that you can do things, just so you can loosen up and talk more freely with your friends, you know. I just use it (alcohol) as a relaxant.

My brother is an alcoholic so I know from experience that the difference between use and abuse is that when someone thinks about getting drunk all the time or they are getting drunk all the time, I think they are abusing.

The following Likert items were written from these quotes:

1. I drink so much that I don't know what I am doing.
2. After I go drinking, I do not remember the next day what I did the night before.
3. After I drink, I don't want to take responsibility for what I do.
4. Drinking makes me do really stupid things.
5. When I get plowed, it is a good excuse to beat the hell out of somebody.
6. I use drinking as an excuse to do things.
7. I drink so that I can loosen up and talk more freely with my friends.
8. I think about getting drunk.

Using the response categories "Often," "Sometimes," "Occasionally," "Almost Never," and "Never," these items attempt to provide a quantitative measuring instrument designed to estimate the incidence and prevalence of the thoughts articulated by this focus group member. Not only do these items use cultural terms (e. g., "get plowed"), they also provide the cultural context within which alcohol consumption occurs. Perhaps a good survey researcher would have constructed these items using these terms and contexts without conducting a qualitative exploration of the attitudes, opinions, and perspectives of the target population. In my experience, however, researchers write quantitative questionnaire items more effectively after a qualitative experience.

Virtually every focus group research project ends with questions left unanswered. These questions include:

1. Did the focus groups produce sufficient cultural knowledge to achieve the sponsor's purposes?
2. How reliable and valid is this cultural knowledge?
3. How generalizable is this cultural knowledge?

Let us address these questions.

Whether focus group research produces sufficient cultural knowledge to achieve one's purposes depends on those purposes. If, for example, one is attempting to design and implement a strategy designed to reduce the risk of HIV/AIDS transmission, the results of focus groups may provide the desired emphases and accents from which persuasive communication messages can be fashioned. At a minimum, designing such a program is more informed when done with benefit of focus group results than without that input.

The validity of cultural knowledge is the degree to which an outsider can anticipate how an insider will react in a cultural situation. The reliability of cultural knowledge is the confidence that the outsider has in this anticipation. The generalizability of cultural knowledge depends on the cultural similarities and dissimilarities of the situations.

Just as quantitative criteria are used to evaluate the reliability and validity of quantitative measurement, qualitative criteria are used to evaluate the reliability and validity of qualitative measurement. A common practice for those trained in quantitative analysis who begin to use qualitative measurement is to impose quantitative criteria on the qualitative research process.

For example, I am often asked: "How many focus groups are enough?" What they really mean to ask is: "How many focus groups are enough so that the results are believable and credible?" The qualitative answer to this question is that you need to conduct enough groups so that you are confident and comfortable that when a situation arises in the groups, you know what will be said next. When they press me for a quantitative answer to this question, I say: "I am comfortable when I have heard the same thing three or four times in three or four groups." In essence, I have conveyed my believability and credibility break point.

5.2. Using Survey Results to Guide Topic Outline Guide Construction

The results of survey research often leave questions unanswered. Crosstabulations and analyses of variance often provoke these questions. For example: Why are women more likely to be concerned about X than men? Why are heterosexuals more likely to engage in Y than homosexuals? Factor analyses of items designed to measure salient attitudes and behaviors also provoke questions: Does this factor represent an important substantive dimension of attitudes, or is it merely a method artifact of the measuring instrument?*

---

* The author has addressed this question in Zeller and Carmines (1980).

Reactions to these questions vary. If the findings are consistent with the theoretical orientation that motivated the research, researchers will ordinarily claim empirical support for that theoretical orientation. If the findings are inconsistent with that theoretical orientation, researchers will frequently look for reasons why the theoretically anticipated result failed to appear. One approach to the interpretation of findings inconsistent with theoretically anticipated relationships is to engage in ad hoc theorizing. Such an approach speculates about a theoretical framework that, if it were in operation, would account for results. Another such approach is to focus on the methodological flaws of the study. From this perspective, sampling and measurement problems emerge as paramount.

One common analysis procedure is to provide special attention to participants who react differently than the majority. What operated to make this respondent different from other respondents in a similar circumstance? Why did this respondent react differently than the others? Is this individual representative of a larger group that is unrepresented in the research design? How do members of this group differ systematically from the participants in the current research?

Rather than focus on deviant cases, reasonable methodological procedure is to focus on deviant groups. More generally, reasonable methodological procedure is to focus on the differences between groups. Why did this group behave in this way while that group behaved in that way? What were members of this group thinking that led them to behave this way compared with the thoughts of the members of that group that led them to behave that way?

The differences between the behavior of groups can be efficiently and cost-effectively identified using a survey methodology. However, a survey is neither efficient nor cost-effective in an exploration of the thinking that led to those differences. Focus groups can be used to amplify and clarify these patterns.

Suppose, for example, that survey research was to reveal that knowledge of HIV transmission avenues results in a dramatic decrease in high-risk sexual behavior among gays. However, this knowledge does not decrease high-risk drug-taking behavior of narcotic addicts. What differences between these two groups led to the reduction in high-risk behavior within the one group but not the other? A focus group approach holds substantial promise of providing this insight in an efficient and cost-effective fashion. Perhaps the gays believed X while the narcotic addicts did not. Perhaps the narcotic addicts thought Y while the gays did not. Because it encourages the participants' definition of the situation to emerge as the research result, the focus group approach is uniquely qualified to provide this insight.

Once the focus groups have identified the thinking patterns that differentiate between these groups, these insights can be translated into survey items as illustrated above. A subsequent survey can confirm these differences quantitatively. In addition, a survey can show that those few gays who think like most narcotic addicts will behave in high-risk ways while those few narcotic addicts who think like most gays will behave in low-risk ways.

5.3. An Example

Perhaps the best example of the implementation of such an interactive strategy is the Portland Men's Study (O'Brien, 1989, 1991). The long-term goals of this study are to understand how personal relationships of men who have sex with men are influenced by the epidemic of AIDS—and, in turn, to understand how those relationships can help men respond to the epidemic in ways that benefit them. Focus groups and surveys were used interactively. This study has skillfully nurtured the dedication and commitment of the members of the gay community by involving those people who are ordinarily the "respondents" or "participants" in study design, sampling, analysis, and interpretation in addition to having them provide the "data" for the study. Moreover, this is a continuing study for which the commitment of members of the community enhances the prospects for genuine increases in social knowledge.

6. SUMMARY

The purpose of this chapter was to propose and illustrate a strategy designed to develop valid, reliable, and culturally sensitive measures of risk perceptions, social support, and coping strategies as applied to HIV/AIDS behavior and mental health issues for special populations. In order to accomplish these objectives, a strategy for combining quantitative and qualitative techniques was developed. The sample survey and the focus group were used as examples of quantitative and qualitative research, respectively. A comparison and contrast of the strengths and weaknesses of these two approaches was made. Then a new definition of validity was proposed. It was asserted that a valid phenomenon has been established when pressing the flesh, chasing the decimal point, and producing the effect all provide the same messages about the nature of the phenomenon. Finally, strategies for combining qualitative and quantitative measurement were suggested. An interactive research design between the sample survey and the focus group will provide the greatest increment in useful information at a minimum cost. More generally, this strategy results in a useful combining of qualitative and quantitative techniques to develop culturally sensitive measures.

REFERENCES

Aronson, E. (1981). *The social animal.* San Francisco: Freeman.

Cook, T. D., and Campbell, D. T. (1979). *Quasi-experimentation: Design & analysis issues for field settings.* Chicago: Rand McNally.

Fowler, F. J., Jr. (1988). *Survey research methods.* Beverly Hills: Sage.

Gallup, G. (1948). *A guide to public opinion polls.* Princeton, N.J.: Princeton University Press, p. 73.

Grabarek, C., and Zeller, R. (1990). *Alcohol on campus.* Prevention Center for Alcohol and Other Drug Abuse, Bowling Green State University.

Greer, G. (1989). *The logic of social inquiry.* New Brunswick, N.J.: Transaction, p. 3.

Heise, D. R., and Bohrnstedt, G. W. (1970). Validity, invalidity, and reliability. In E. F. Borgatta and G. W. Bohrnstedt (eds.), *Sociological methodology 1970.* San Francisco: Jossey Bass, pp. 104–129.

Joreskog, K. G. (1970). A general method for analysis of covariance structures. *Biometrika* **57**: 239–251.

Joseph, J. G., Emmons, C. A., Kessler, R. C., Wortman, C. B., O'Brien, K., Hocker, W. T., and Schaefer, C. (1984). Coping with the threat of AIDS. *Am. Psychol.* **39**:1297–1302.

Krueger, R. A. (1988). *Focus groups: A practical guide for applied research.* Beverly Hills: Sage.

Lavrakas, P. J. (1987). *Telephone survey methods.* Beverly Hills: Sage.

Morgan, D. L. (1988). *Focus groups as qualitative research.* Beverly Hills: Sage.

Morgan, D. L. (1990). *Focus groups and group interviews: Advancing the state of the art.* American Sociological Association Problems of the Discipline Conference, Portland, Oreg.

O'Brien, K. (1989). *The Portland Men's Study: A report to the community on progress and plans.* Department of Psychology, Portland State University, P.O. Box 751, Portland, Oreg. 97207-0751; telephone (503) 725-3900.

O'Brien, K. (1991). *The Portland Men's Study: Our second report to the community on progress and plans.* Department of Psychology, Portland State University, P.O. Box 751, Portland, Oreg. 97207-0751; telephone (503) 725-3900.

Strauss, A. L. (1987). *Qualitative analysis for social scientists.* London: Cambridge University Press.

Zeller, R. A. (1982). *Sociological myths, social realities!* Department of Sociology, University of Notre Dame, Notre Dame, Ind.

Zeller, R. A. (1990). Qualitative approaches to the study of human sexuality. In A. Chouinard and J. Albert (eds.), *Human sexuality: Research perspectives in a world facing AIDS.* Ottawa: International Development Research Centre.

Zeller, R. A. (1991). *Censoring academic freedom: Using sexual harassment regulations to impose feminist ideology.* Paper presented at the Southern Sociological Society Meetings, New Orleans.

Zeller, R. A., and Carmines, E. G. (1980). *Measurement in the social sciences.* London: Cambridge University Press.

5

Understanding Sexual Behaviors and Drug Use among African-Americans

A Case Study of Issues for Survey Research

MINDY THOMPSON FULLILOVE and
ROBERT E. FULLILOVE, III

1. OVERVIEW

The thesis of this chapter is that surveys of minority populations are attempting to describe what is, essentially, a moving target, and, as in other situations in which the target is mobile, special strategies are required in order to achieve the survey objectives. This target includes attitudes and behaviors that are being shaped and reshaped at tremendous speed; it includes constant revolutions in language, customs, and mores; and it includes changing access between sectors of the population. These problems are magnified for AIDS researchers. We want to know the most intimate, private, and even furtive details of a person's life, material the most trusting of mainstream college students (one of the most frequently surveyed groups in America) might have difficulty revealing.

In Section 2 we shall describe the conditions that have created massive social instability in the African-American and other minority communities. In Section 3 we shall discuss the problems of access in divided societies. In

MINDY THOMPSON FULLILOVE and ROBERT E. FULLILOVE, III • HIV Center for Clinical and Behavioral Studies, New York State Psychiatric Institute and Columbia University, New York, New York 10027.

Methodological Issues in AIDS Behavioral Research, edited by David G. Ostrow and Ronald C. Kessler. Plenum Press, New York, 1993.

the final section we shall review strategies used by our research team as we grapple with many of these issues. Throughout these sections we use illustrations taken from a recent research project, the "Women and Crack" project, conducted by our research group. Because we are African-Americans, and conduct our research primarily in that community, we have focused our remarks on that ethnic group. But the issues raised here are relevant for (and to) many minority groups throughout the United States.

2. CHANGING TIMES

2.1. What We Knew

A long tradition of scholars working within the black community, complemented by a small cadre of sympathetic white scientists, has accumulated knowledge of black life and culture over almost two centuries. That body of work provides the basis for several important assumptions about black life:

- Black culture in America shows important influences of African cultures, but direct ties to those cultures were lost in the process of enslavement.
- Black culture, cut off from African roots, re-formed itself in the Americas, re-creating and maintaining kinship and friendship structures, despite the pernicious, disruptive influences of slavery and post-Civil War peonage.
- Because of a traditional devotion to education, blacks have worked tirelessly to overcome the effects of long periods (lasting through the 1960s in some parts of the southern United States) during which the majority of community members were forced to be illiterate.
- Black men and women have been closer in gender role definition and gender role expectation than men and women from other cultures. For example, black women have always had to work, just as black men did.
- Racism has been an incessant and insidious part of black life in the United States for more than 300 years and has—more than any other factor—shaped the black community's mores, values, behaviors, and perceptions of itself.

Through the 1960s and 1970s, as black studies emerged as a discipline within American scholarship, these basic tenets of black studies helped to shape the important empirical work of psychologists (Reginald Williams,

Harold Neighbors), psychiatrists (Frantz Fanon, Carl Bell), feminists (Angela Davis, Bettina Aptheker), anthropologists (Leith Mullings, Niara Sudarkasa, Carol Stack), and others. The more recent work helped to elaborate both the mechanisms by which blacks survived and the social pressures that threatened that survival. An important theme of black studies in the 1970s and 1980s was that the black community, far from being a pathological creation of racism, had created unique and healthy structures that promoted group survival. The extended family/kin network, for example, was noted to be a key source of support and survival for poor, black families. The kinship networks provided emotional support and financial assistance, shared childrearing functions, and maintained social norms. Throughout that period, young black scholars examined the community and found reasons to celebrate its accomplishments.

The two great accomplishments of the scholarship of that period were (1) that the mechanisms for examining black life and culture were honed and (2) that the reframing of the black experience as a positive one allowed many to have a new perspective on old truths. The weakness of the period was that it failed to assess accurately the processes that signaled decay and destruction. This is not to say that the basic mechanisms of destruction were not apparent. Rather, the force and intensity with which they operated were serving to undermine the very strengths scholars were trying to affirm.

2.2. What Happened?

Several forces acted over time to undermine the strength of the black community. The economic structure of the United States shifted from agriculture and other unskilled labor to technology. Blacks, always "last hired/ first fired," now faced a new and more formidable challenge in the job market: that of acquiring "marketable skills." Coinciding with the national economy's increasing demands for educated workers was an absolute stagnation, and even decline, in black educational achievement that followed the Supreme Court's ruling on school desegregation. Finally, as the economic base of the older urban centers declined, the urban areas themselves began to deteriorate. The process of deterioration was accelerated in the minority areas of cities such as Newark, Detroit, Philadelphia, and New York.

The interaction and synergism between lower levels of educational achievement, loss of unskilled jobs, and urban decay resulted in massive social disintegration of minority communities. This social disintegration is characterized by the splintering of the family and the traditional kinship/friendship networks, as well as by rapid growth in anticommunity activities, such as crime and drug-taking, behaviors that were previously mitigated by—if not eliminated by—the presence of strong, proactive community organizations. It is in the context of such social disintegration that AIDS is spreading.

2.3. The Lessons of the South Bronx Burnout

The South Bronx "burnout phenomenon" as described by Wallace (1988) offers a unique glimpse of the dynamics of this disintegration as well as its role in the dissemination of HIV. This borough of New York City has suffered a tremendous loss in its housing through burnout since the mid-1970s. The process has been marked by a number of milestones: "hard social services"—e. g., fire code enforcement, fire fighting, sanitation, housing code enforcement, and housing rehabilitation—were reduced or withdrawn entirely by the City of New York in the 1970s as part of a policy to cut city spending. A sharp increase in destructive housing fires followed and as housing in the borough was lost, social networks disintegrated and members of previously stable social networks suffered forced migration. These migrants, not surprisingly, contributed to overcrowding in neighboring communities. This new overcrowding planted the seeds for further decay in the form of increases in crime, drug use, and apartment fires. As the demands for increased fire, police, and social services went unmet, the velocity of community collapse in these neighborhoods increased. By the end of the 1970s, a significant portion of the housing that was accessible to poor people had disappeared and unprecedented levels of crime, drug use, and disease became part of the pattern of borough life.

The dissemination of HIV was a major component in this downward cycle of decay. As of the end of 1990, for example, as many as one in five black men between the ages of 26 and 40 in the South Bronx were believed to be infected with HIV. The deterioration of the community forced heretofore stable drug-using networks to suffer the same migratory patterns as those of other residents of these neighborhoods. Users, already HIV-infected, became part of new drug-using/drug-works-sharing networks in the neighborhoods in which they resettled. The result was a wide-scale dissemination of the virus that, Wallace concludes, accounts for the unprecedented levels of HIV seroprevalence in this borough. This "seeding of the epidemic" would not have occurred had this pattern of fire-induced forced migration not taken place.

2.4. Patterns of Change in the Future

The direction of change in the future is influenced by the momentum of past changes, by the current worldwide recession, and by worldwide crisis between racial, ethnic, and national groups. For the moment no country appears to be free of tension between racial/ethnic groups as exemplified by recent pogroms against the Gypsies in Romania, and fighting between the Protestants and the Catholics in Ireland.

In this country, it seems inevitable that poor, predominantly black or Hispanic urban neighborhoods will undergo some variation of the South Bronx syndrome, and like the South Bronx, a predictable outcome will be a sharp increase in the numbers of new cases of HIV infection. Observing, understanding, and ultimately controlling the forces that drive the epidemic in these communities will become the major agenda item for researchers and public health officials during the 1990s. The issue, of course, is how will we gain access to communities that are perceived to be "hard-to-reach," if not closed altogether?

Coping successfully with the problem of studying the hard-to-reach— insofar as it involves conducting research with members of black communities—requires three steps: (1) gaining access to the community through knowledgeable guides and acquiring the trust of those who will participate in the study; (2) learning the language of the groups being studied; and (3) avoiding at all costs the error of taking data out of the community without leaving something of value in return for the services that community members have rendered on behalf of the research effort (Magaña, 1991; Duke and Omi, 1991; Weissman, 1991; Mays and Jackson, 1991).

3. GAINING ACCESS

The idea that any American is only six handshakes away from any other American fits well with our democratic ideals. But, in fact, our society is stratified with social barriers that have a one-way gradient, such that those in higher positions can reach those in lesser positions more easily than those in lesser positions can access those above them. Being male, white, educated, or wealthy are all associated with membership in the higher social networks. When university-based researchers use the term "hard-to-reach" to refer to poor people of color or others who are outside the sphere of the university, they are describing the largely structural barriers created by this social stratification. Yet it must be underscored that, because of their relatively privileged position in the social structure, researchers will be able to reach the poor, if they are willing to make the effort to penetrate the social barriers.

3.1. The Role of Guides

Since there are few natural connections between the black ghetto and the university, it is difficult for those within the university (the vast majority of whom are not black) to reach those on the outside. This difficulty is quite real. Because of the ways in which one spends one's time, one has access to a not unlimited set of opportunities to form associations with others in a given social network. But few of the social networks in our society cross barriers of race, sex, class, education, and geography simultaneously.

The nonblack researcher (and at times, the black researcher) who is seeking to cross the barriers created by social stratification must begin the effort by finding guides. Just as Lewis and Clark trusted Sacajawea to lead them into the wilderness, so the modern researcher must trust someone's expertise to lead the journey out of the university and into the community. Guides are community-based people who are in a bridge role. They are well known and respected in the community. They are able to engage members of the community in the processes of research. They are also able to interpret the language and concerns of the community to the outside observer. Thus, they can link the researcher with the members of the community, and can ensure that the two sides understand each other.

The critical feature of the relationship between the researcher and the guide is that the researcher is in a dependent position with respect to the guide. Researchers who have written grants, collected money, published articles, and generally "know" science can misconstrue their ability to work in the inner city, overestimating their own abilities and underestimating the contribution of the guide, who has less money, fewer degrees, and no publications. Those researchers who are most respectful and most modest will have the most success in working in the inner city. But while the guide can provide an introduction, the guide cannot make the community trust the researcher.

3.2. Gaining Trust

The distrust evinced by community members for outside researchers cannot be fully understood without reference to the real historical experiences of abuse that give rise to such feelings. The Tuskegee Syphilis Study is one of the most important examples of systematic abuse of poor people by privileged researchers, justified on the basis of "research." In 1932, the U.S. Public Health Service recruited black men infected with syphilis to participate in a study of the natural history of the disease. The men were repeatedly deceived, told they were getting treatment when they were not, and blocked from contacts outside the study that might have provided opportunities for treatment. The Public Health Service continued the study for 40 years, despite mounting evidence of the excess morbidity and mortality among those with untreated syphilis. Only when exposed in the national press did the Public Health Service end the study and reimburse those victimized in the effort. That this travesty of science was dubbed "research" has done incalculable harm to future researchers hoping to work in the black community. The legacy of this experiment has had far-reaching repercussions on black life and on the trust black Americans experience with respect to government-sponsored research (Thomas and Quinn, 1991).

Given the historical mistreatment of black people by white people—admittedly, the Tuskegee Syphilis Study is but one example—the researcher may be treated as "guilty until proven innocent." Suspicion of the white researcher may lead to feigning openness and respect while concealing one's true self. In a perceptive description of his relationship with the family maid, Howell Raines (1991) wrote,

> There is no trickier subject for a writer from the South than that of affection between a black person and a white one in the unequal world of segregation. For the dishonesty upon which such a society is founded makes every emotion suspect, makes it impossible to know whether what flowed between two people was honest feeling or pity or pragmatism. Indeed, for the black person, the feigning of an expected emotion could be the very coinage of survival. [p. 90]

It would be a serious error for a researcher to underestimate the extent to which those rules of conduct, derived from segregation, are still tools of survival.

In the context of such suspicion, it is the researcher's own conduct that will win friends and allies. The methods to accomplish this task have been well described by anthropologists and others seeking to study cultures other than their own. Margaret Mead (1969), for example, has outlined the delicate process of joining a society and of gaining the trust of its members as one that requires showing interest and respect for the group's daily life as well as its traditions. In her description, the process included the following steps:

> [The anthropologist] must live among [isolated primitive people], within sight and sound of their twenty-four-hour activities throughout a normal annual cycle (which may include periods of nomadism), if he is to give the required account of their lives. For permission to live among them and for such cooperation as he needs to obtain a house, food, and transport, he must convince them that his intentions are friendly, and the difficulties he may cause are in some way compensated for by benefits. These benefits may be material. . . . But . . . in the end the anthropologist is dependent upon enlisting intellectual curiosity that complements his own research interest. . . . [pp. 361–362]

Mead, who felt that the demonstration of respect and equality was of critical importance to the success of anthropological studies, went so far as to say, "Anthropological research does not have subjects. We work with informants in an atmosphere of trust and mutual respect" (p. 361).

Carol Stack (1974), who studied black families in a poor inner-city neighborhood in the Midwest, offered a vivid description of gaining access and trust. A fellow student, who had grown up in that area, offered to introduce her to two families. After that, Stack was on her own to win the confidence of the families. Stack relates:

> I first came by the Waters' home in the summer of 1968. Magnolia, her sixty-year old "husband" Calvin (father of six of Magnolia's children), Magnolia's oldest son

Lenny, and five of the younger children were sitting in the living room . . . folding several piles of newspapers for Lenny's five evening paper routes. . . . After a lesson from a seven-year-old on how to make the fold, I joined in on the rhythmic activity that absorbed everyone's concentration. . . . Several months later Magnolia told me that she had been surprised that I sat with them that first day to fold papers, and then came back to help again. "White folks," she told me, "don't have time, they's always in a rush, and they don't sit on black folk's furniture, at least no Whites that comes into The Flats." [p. 10]

Our own experiences provide ample support for the utility of this two-stage process. Between 1986 and 1991, our research group conducted a number of studies related to HIV disease and HIV risk behaviors within black communities in Oakland and San Francisco, California, and in New York City (Bowser, 1989; Bowser et al., 1990; Fullilove and Fullilove, 1989; R. E. Fullilove et al., 1990; M. T. Fullilove et al., 1990, 1992). These studies included examinations of crack cocaine users in three cities, as well as investigations of sexual behavior and gender roles. We have gained access to crack dealers and crack users on the streets where crack is sold and used; we have observed crack users in crack "spots" and in crack houses in East Harlem. We have discussed the dynamics of sex–drug exchanges with female crack users and asked them to give life histories that detail their involvement with drug use as well as the details of their sexual activities in pursuit of cocaine. In each of these efforts, we found colleagues who gave us an introduction to the community. Once we were inside, we had to win trust. Sometimes this involved pitching in with the work at hand. Sometimes this involved our own willingness to tell who we were. Sometimes it involved passing a test—often an unstated one—in which our willingness to "sit on the furniture" signaled that we were OK.

As an example of this process, let us describe events that occurred while we were conducting a study aimed at describing women's high-risk sexual behaviors that occurred in the context of crack use. This "Women and Crack" project began with interviews and focus groups at a drug treatment center in Harlem. We were introduced to the staff and clients at the center by a colleague who was also a member of the center staff. With his introduction, we were welcomed and allowed access to the program's clients. Our first focus group was, we thought, open and informative. The women who participated told us that they thought it had been great. One woman said, "This was the first AIDS,—well, I've taken a couple of AIDS researches and . . . all the researches I had, they give a paper like this, a book, you know. Various types, and then they mark off the questions. That's how they do it, but I find that this to be more better, right, and we can all talk. . . . I think you do a better survey this way, to be honest with you." They also promised that they would recommend the group to other women at the clinic.

Their enthusiasm was reassuring but did little to prepare us for what happened in the second focus group. Those in the first group had spread the word that not only were we OK, but also the discussion was "real." As the women arrived for the second group, we noticed that they were both tense and eager. As it turned out, it was an explosive group, in which women shared raw and painful experiences. Their openness revealed to us a fact that we had not completely understood before: many women living in the "belly" of the crack culture suffer from psychological trauma. From that hunch—that women who exchanged sex for crack were caught up in a spiral of traumatic experiences with far-ranging consequences for their addictive disorders and their prospects for recovery—came the cornerstone for one year of subsequent research. In those later studies, we were able to confirm the extent and severity of the trauma the women had experienced (Fullilove *et al.*, 1993).

This finding of widespread trauma, and trauma-related mental disorder, has important implications for HIV prevention, for recovery from crack addiction, and for mental health efforts aimed at female crack users. We did not anticipate that we would collect this information; rather, we came with our own "agenda." But the women trusted us enough to share intimate, painful details of their lives with us, taking us inside their world so that we might gain a real understanding of what had happened to them, and to some extent, why it had happened. The trust we had garnered in the first focus group was critical to our ability to reenter this and similar settings so that new findings might emerge from our further explorations.

4. LEARNING TO LISTEN

The Evolution of Language

The classic methods for conducting social science research dictate that the researcher examine the context in which behaviors occur before any attempt is made either to conduct survey research or to interpret survey data. Our experience has made it abundantly clear that understanding "context" begins with understanding language.

Our studies of crack cocaine, for example, have been marked by the development of a healthy respect for the language that crack users employ to describe every aspect of their use of the drug as well as their activities in pursuit of it. This language is not uniform and appears to vary from crack-using network to crack-using network. The same activities (e. g., exchanging sex for drugs or having sex while high on crack) have different names in the Bay Area (respectively "tossin' " and "freekin' ") than they do in New York ("skeezin' " and "parlayin' ") (Mieczkowski, 1988).

This language is also subject to tremendous evolution that is largely driven—particularly in areas like the South Bronx or Harlem—with the ever-changing patterns of life in the community. As members of user networks come and go, and as these networks re-form, grow, and change, the manner in which members speak to each other almost inevitably changes as well.

Crack users are frequently polydrug users. Since its introduction in drug-using communities, crack has been taken with other drugs. These drugs may heighten the high or mitigate its more unpleasant aftereffects. The mixing is frequently tied to the economics of the crack trade. In the summer of 1991, for example, crack users in some (but not all) sections of New York City began smoking heroin as well as crack, resulting, our informants tell us, from lower prices of heroin and shifts in the leadership of the groups dealing and distributing the two substances.

The first signal for this alteration in drug use was the appearance of a new set of terms for getting high. At the Port Authority Bus Terminal at 42nd Street, for example, dealers asked prospective buyers if they "wanna date with girlfriend?" "Girl" is a shortened form of "white girl" (a classic name for cocaine). "Girlfriend" connotes something that enhances or boosts the impact of "girl" since, to quote one of the dealers, "That's what friends are for."

At the risk of citing the obvious, attending to shifts in language is at the core of determining when, where, and how changes in the habits and behaviors of a social network have occurred. Simply put, researchers have few tools to understand what is new if they lack the means to ask about it. Moreover, the pace of social change and community disintegration that we have previously described appears to be at the core of the rapid evolution of HIV risk behaviors and, correspondingly, of the language that people use to describe their behaviors.

Our rule of thumb, therefore, has been simple: keep listening and keep talking. With each new project, we allocate time and resources to identify the emergence of new terms in the targeted community. For this purpose, we employ focus groups whose major objective is to encourage participants to speak about their day-to-day life in the language that they use among themselves.

If these groups are to be successful, four elements are necessary: (1) identifying the social networks that should be examined; (2) recruiting members of these groups for participation in a focus group; (3) carefully recording their speech as part of the set of tasks to be accomplished within the focus group; and (4) carefully decoding this speech by using the talents of someone who understands the language being spoken in the preparation of focus group transcripts.

This latter point cannot be overemphasized. Standard transcription services typically are at a loss to "hear" unfamiliar words and in the early days of our crack research, we were frequently recipients of transcripts in which 30 to 40% of the speech of participants was missing. In a recent attempt to transcribe a focus group session conducted with female crack users, members of our team spent more than 40 hours perfecting the basic transcript. This editing process attended to words that were used, the types of overlaps in speech among the participants, and the affect contained in the voices. In Table 1 we have given a brief excerpt of a transcript of a focus group (the first

Table 1. The Challenge of Transcribing: Two Versions of the Same Tape Segment

Version 1 transcribed by Standard English speaker

So that's basically it. I did crack. It's so—it takes you up so much, I started taking (inaudible). This Spanish guy used to tell me that I'm like a nervous wreck. He used to say, "Take a pill." (Inaudible) after a while when you've done so much coke, you have to take something to come down. I don't like dope, so I started taking, like, a pill, because it was convenient to take it, drink some water, and go to sleep.

Version 2 transcribed by speaker of black English vernacular

so
that's basically it
that's all I did was
I did crack
and
it's so
it takes you up so much
I starting taking
. . .
for like pills
some
this Spanish guy used to always tell me
'cause I'm like a nervous wreck
he used to say
"take a pill"
I'd always be worried he was trying to poison me
but after a while
when you do so much *coke*
you got to take something to come down
and I don't like dope
so I started taking
like
a pill
because it was so convenient
you know
just take it
drink some water
and go to sleep.

"Women and Crack" focus group referred to above). At the top we show the transcript as originally transcribed by a speaker of Standard English. In the second part we show the edited version of the transcript as produced by our research team.

We must stress again the extent to which the quality of the focus group will reflect the amount of trust that people have in the group. Groups self-monitor in many ways. Groups of people who speak black English vernacular will alter their speech when talking to someone who speaks Standard English. The monitoring of the style of speech is closely related to monitoring the content of the speech (Labov, 1972). As speakers feel constrained to speak in a manner that is socially acceptable, so too will they be constrained in the topics they feel free to discuss. The rules for social acceptability are defined by the process that occurs within the group and between the group and the research team. Therefore, trust between the researchers and the participants decreases the effect of "outsider" bias and, similarly, trust within the group will decrease the number of constraints on open communication.

We learned a great deal about group monitoring in our attempts to study women's participation in high-risk sex. We conducted several groups in San Francisco with young women who had participated in exchanging sex for drugs, the sexual behavior that carries a high risk for infection with sexually transmitted disease. Even though the young women had been willing to discuss this in one-to-one interviews, it was socially unacceptable for anybody to admit that behavior in a group setting. After the groups were over, the young women told us, "I would have said something but nobody else was talking so I kept quiet."

The focus groups that were conducted with women in recovery from crack addiction were, by contrast, unrestrained in their discussion of sex-for-drugs exchanges. In the second focus group, a heated exchange exploded because one woman contended that, as she had only had sex with friends for drugs, her behavior was different from that of the women who "did it with strangers." The others, all of whom admitted to sex-for-drugs exchanges with strangers, felt that the speaker was "in denial." In their view, that one had sex with friends was irrelevant: that this behavior occurred in an effort to get drugs was supremely important.

In these groups, the women were willing to discuss their participation in sex-for-drugs exchanges in great detail. Unlike our earlier work with teenagers engaging in this behavior, we found that these two groups of adults were far more open. The reason for the openness of one and the closed nature of the other was at first not apparent. However, another informant, when asked to help us understand why this difference existed, made it quite plain: the women in treatment were participating in a 12-step program for recovery. The first steps of this program require that participants acknowledge their status as addicts—that is, as individuals who are slaves to an addictive substance—and that they take a "fearless moral inventory" in which they acknowledge who they are and what they have done during the course of their enslavement to drugs. Our informant pointed out the obvious: our 12-step participants had both a language and a social milieu in which matters were to be discussed forthrightly and without shying away from any harsh truths that were revealed.

Our teenagers were isolated and participating in a focus group where the only bond they shared was one that they dare not acknowledge: having participated in socially scorned and despised behaviors.

5. GIVING BACK

The inner city is poor and getting poorer. It is not enough to ask a community agency for help. Researchers must be prepared to give back to the agency. Put another way, any energy devoted to the research project takes energy away from the community. To the extent that the research effort comes to the inner city, takes information, and leaves, to that extent has the effort appeared to the residents to have impoverished them. In fact, if there is no replacement—no give back—the actual resources in the community are diminished by the process of research. This must be avoided at all costs. It is critical that research understand the ways in which something must be given in exchange for what is taken.

This is difficult for many researchers to accomplish, and not solely because they lack the will or the desire to do so. Researchers must also be supported by the funding agencies. Often, in guarding the boundary between "research" and "service," funding agencies are reluctant to support the activities that "give" to the community. El-Sadr and Capps (1992) have argued that ". . . the definition of research costs should be broadened to include the funding of meals, social and outreach services, transportation, child care, and the development of educational materials." However, even without such expanded funding, much can be accomplished. For example, researchers have a great deal of knowledge about science. This knowledge is desperately needed in the community. People working in the community want to learn about science. Community workers also need some of the tools of science, such as the ability to write a simple questionnaire, and analyze the responses obtained. These tools enable community workers to conduct program evaluation activities, an increasingly critical part of surviving in the service delivery sector. Giving knowledge to the community is one highly effective manner of giving back to the community.

A second way to give back to the community is to share the results of the research. The data are important for program design, policy development, and other kinds of activities that community members are involved with. Having critical pieces of data can be powerful in the ongoing political life of the community. This kind of empowerment is a respectful way of giving something to the community. It also helps to deepen the understanding in the community of what "knowledge" is and how it can be used. Researchers are certainly concerned with using knowledge to forward their own goals: they must also be willing to use that knowledge to forward the goals of the communities they study.

Our studies of crack, for example, have suggested a number of changes in the manner in which women suffering from crack addiction are integrated into a treatment community. We have come to understand that the high prevalence of trauma and of posttraumatic stress disorder in this group amounts to comorbidity on a scale that has not been either fully understood or treated (Fullilove *et al.,* 1992). We are, at this writing, attempting to describe the necessity for altering diagnostic and treatment strategies to detect and then minister to the needs of dual diagnosed crack users. It is a small but hopefully significant way in which one uses findings from such research to improve the quality of life in the settings where research is conducted.

A third way to give back is to involve community members as coauthors of papers. All too often, the process of writing papers (which must, perforce, be left to the "lettered" researcher) never includes those other members of the team who contributed to the work. In fact, the guidelines for authorship proposed by important medical journals, which state that each author must be able to support the arguments in the paper, would work against the inclusion of those with less mastery of science. The "guides" and "interpreters" will continue to be accorded a footnote in the acknowledgments, but not coauthorship of a paper. Yet, if the contributions of the community members of the research team are recognized as indispensable ones, then their claim on coauthorship will have greater weight.

As noted earlier, in the "Women and Crack" study, we attempted to "give back" in a variety of ways. First, the identification of trauma as a problem for women in recovery was shared with staff at the treatment centers where we have conducted the research and with other treatment centers around the city and the state. This dissemination of preliminary findings, we believe, makes details of research available to the community in a timely and comprehensible fashion.

Second, women in treatment had identified the study questionnaire as a valuable resource. In cooperation with staff and clients, we adapted the instrument for use as a clinical tool. This revised "Stress Test" deleted detailed psychiatric history but expanded the inquiry into childhood problems. Staff and peer counselors worked with the research team to incorporate the "Stress Test" into the day-to-day work of the clinic. The research team also provided ongoing supervision in the use of the instrument.

6. CONCLUSION

We have suggested that minority communities are changing rapidly. Much of this change is for the worse. We need to stem the tide of epidemic disease, homelessness, illiteracy, joblessness, and other ills. Research efforts will play an important, albeit minor, role in the process of stabilizing and rebuilding these broken communities. But, in order to play this role, we must be sure that we have developed effective strategies for research in the community. The critical assumption, we have argued, is that the communities are changing rapidly. What is true today may not be true tomorrow. We must constantly search for the content and pathways of change if we wish to be on target in describing the nature of life and disease in the minority community.

ACKNOWLEDGMENT. Preparation of this chapter was supported in part by NIMH/NIDA Centers Grant P50MH43520.

REFERENCES

Bowser, B. P. (1989). Crack and AIDS: An ethnographic impression. *J. Natl. Med. Assoc.* **81**(5): 538–540.

Bowser, B., Fullilove, M. T., and Fullilove, R. (1990). African-American youth and AIDS high-risk behavior, the social context and barriers to prevention. *Youth Soc.* **22**(1):54–66.

Duke, S. I., and Omi, J. (1991). Development of AIDS education and prevention materials for women by health department staff and community focus groups. *AIDS Educ. Prev.* **3**:90–99.

El-Sadr, W., and Capps, L. (1992). The challenge of minority recruitment in clinical trials for AIDS. *J. Am. Med. Assoc.* **267**:954–957.

Fullilove, M. T., and Fullilove, R. (1989). Intersecting epidemics: Black teen crack use and sexually transmitted disease. *J. Am. Med. Women's Assoc.* **44**:146–153.

Fullilove, M. T., Weinstein, M., Fullilove, R. E. I., Crayton, E. J., Goodjoin, R. B., Bowser, B., and Gross, S. (1990). Race/gender issues in the sexual transmission of AIDS. In P. Volberding and M. A. Jacobson (eds.), *AIDS Clinical Review 1990.* New York: Dekker, pp. 25–62.

Fullilove, M. T., Lown, E. A., and Fullilove, R. E. (1992). Crack 'hos and skeezers: Traumatic experiences of women crack users. *J. Sex Res.* **29**:275–287.

Fullilove, M. T., Fullilove, R. E., Smith, M., Winkler, K., Michael, C., Panzer, P. G., and Wallace, R. (1993). Violence, trauma and posttraumatic stress disorder among women drug users. *J. Traumatic Stress* (in press).

Fullilove, R. E., Fullilove, M. T., Bowser, B. P., and Gross, S. A. (1990). Risk of sexually transmitted disease among black adolescent crack users in Oakland and San Francisco, Calif. *J. Am. Med. Assoc.* **263**:851–855.

Labov, W. (1972). *Language in the inner city.* Philadelphia: University of Pennsylvania Press.

Magaña, R. (1991). Sex, drugs and HIV: An ethnographic approach. *Soc. Sci. Med.* **33**:5–9.

Mays, V. M., and Jackson, J. S. (1991). AIDS Survey Methodology with black Americans. *Soc. Sci. Med.* **33**:47–54.

Mead, M. (1969). Research with human beings: A model derived from anthropological field practice. *Daedalus (Boston)* **98**:361–386.

Mieczkowski, T. (1988). Crack distribution in Detroit. Paper presented at the American Society of Criminology Annual Meetings, Chicago.

Raines, H. (December 1, 1991). Grady's gift. *New York Times Sunday Magazine,* pp. 50, 89–90, 98–102.

Thomas, S. B., and Quinn, S. C. The Tuskegee Syphilis Study, 1990 to 1992: Implications for HIV education programs in the black community. *Am. J. Pub. Health.* **81**:1498–1505.

Wallace, R. (1988). A synergism of plagues: "Planned shrinkage," contagious housing destruction, and AIDS in the Bronx. *Environ. Res.* **47**:1–33.

Weissman, G. (1991). Working with pregnant women at high risk for HIV infection: Outreach and intervention. *Bull. N.Y. Acad. Med.* **67**:291–300.

6

Response Bias in Surveys of AIDS-Related Sexual Behavior

JOSEPH A. CATANIA, HEATHER TURNER, ROBERT C. PIERCE, EVE GOLDEN, CAROL STOCKING, DIANE BINSON, and KAREN MAST

1. OVERVIEW

Survey research plays a key role in AIDS behavioral research by describing how AIDS-relevant (sexual or drug) behaviors are distributed, by explicating the conditions that influence high-risk activities, and by providing a basic program evaluation tool. The quality of this work depends on there being reliable and valid methods for assessing self-reported sexual (and drug) behavior. Unfortunately, "sex surveys" suffer from numerous unresolved problems related to participation bias and measurement error (systematic error) (Bentler and Abramson, 1981; Catania *et al.*, 1990a,b; Gagnon, 1988; Green and Weiner, 1977; Miller *et al.*, 1990). Thus, an important priority is to determine which techniques minimize measurement error and maximize participation across the different ethnic groups and subcultures of importance to AIDS investigators (Catania *et al.*, 1990a,b).

JOSEPH A. CATANIA, ROBERT C. PIERCE, EVE GOLDEN, DIANE BINSON, and KAREN MAST • Center for AIDS Prevention Studies, Department of Medicine, University of California, San Francisco, California 94143.   *HEATHER TURNER* • Department of Sociology and Anthropology, College of Liberal Arts, Horton Sciences Center, University of New Hampshire, Endura, New Hampshire 03824-3586.   *CAROL STOCKING* • Center for Clinical Medical Ethics, University of Chicago, Chicago, Illinois 60637.

Methodological Issues in AIDS Behavioral Research, edited by David G. Ostrow and Ronald C. Kessler. Plenum Press, New York, 1993.

The focus of this chapter is on measurement error associated with the specific task of assessing respondents' sexual behavior. Participation bias is obviously a concern to AIDS survey researchers, but the problems in this regard may not be much different from those faced by investigators conducting surveys on other less sensitive topics. [Note this is not the case with respect to laboratory studies of sexual behavior in which strong participation biases have been observed with respect to respondent characteristics, beliefs, and sexual behavior (see for review Catania *et al.*, 1990a).] Indeed, recruitment of respondents is the most difficult task confronting any survey. The point at which most potential respondents refuse to participate often occurs very early in the initial contact, typically before the respondent has heard what the survey is about and most often during the household enumeration (this is particularly problematic in phone surveys where respondents easily assert their lack of interest by simply hanging up the phone). For instance, in a recently completed National AIDS-related survey of nearly 14,000 respondents, we (Catania, 1991) found that over 80% of refusals occurred before respondents heard that the survey was about AIDS-related issues. The largest source of bias in AIDS-related surveys is then not necessarily related to the sensitive nature of the question topics, but reflects the general proclivities of various segments of the population to participate in surveys of any type (also see Groves, 1989, for discussion of how cooperation rates have changed over time). The difficulties in obtaining respondent cooperation are compounded when sampling from culturally diverse groups, different ethnic and age groups. Discussion of these issues goes beyond the scope of this chapter.

1.1. AIDS-Relevant Sexual Behaviors

AIDS-related surveys of sexual behavior in the United States cover the life span from adolescence to old age and include work on all sexual orientation and race/ethnic groups. What sexual behaviors are considered AIDS-relevant? A limited set of behaviors transmit AIDS. Anal and vaginal penetrative intercourse are associated with HIV transmission. People who practice these behaviors with large numbers of partners run an increased risk of infection. The risk of HIV transmission related to oral intercourse and oral–anal sex is uncertain since studies on these behaviors have difficulties acquiring respondents who practice only these activities. Finally, when the objective is expanded to include safe sexual behaviors, all variants of protected (e. g., condom use) penetrative and nonpenetrative sexual activities become relevant.

1.2. Measurement Error and Participation Bias

We review literature on measurement error in studies of human sexual behavior with attention to the problems of gathering sexual information in the context of AIDS. We discuss four general indices of measurement error in assessments of sexual behavior (item refusal, over- and underreporting, and test–retest reliability) and address how these are influenced by respondent, instrument, interviewer, and mode of data collection variables (for general discussion see Bradburn *et al.,* 1978; Groves, 1989; Sudman and Bradburn, 1974, 1983). Measurement error is of critical concern to AIDS research. High levels of measurement error may distort estimates of high-risk sexual practices and, consequently, weaken behavioral epidemiological work in this area. If, for example, large percentages of heterosexuals overreport condom use, then predictions of HIV spread in the heterosexual population will be underestimates. Unreliable (test–retest) assessments pose considerable problems for longitudinal surveys and evaluation research that examine changes in sexual behavior over time, since one cannot be certain if any observed changes in behavior are actual changes or result from the unreliability of the reports. At present, there are insufficient data to determine which techniques minimize measurement error for a given subpopulation of interest.

Before addressing the issues of response bias, some discussion needs to be devoted to the problem of the validity of self-reported sexual behavior. Since there are strong cultural taboos surrounding direct observation of other people's sexual activities, sex researchers rely heavily on self-reports of sexual behavior. Obviously, in addition to minimizing measurement error, we must work toward developing validity indices of self-reported sexual activities that index if a person has performed the behavior (incidence) and how often they have performed it (frequency).

2. VALIDITY OF SELF-REPORTED SEXUAL BEHAVIOR

As we have discussed previously (Catania *et al.,* 1990a), there are a number of reasons to suspect inconsistencies between people's actual sexual behavior and their self-reports in an interview. For instance, privacy needs, embarrassment, and fear of reprisals may motivate people to conceal their true sexual behavior, while others may find it self-enhancing to embellish on their actual sexual experiences. However, even respondents who are highly motivated to provide "truthful" responses may have distorted memories of how often they have actually performed specific sexual behaviors.

Although some laboratory studies have made direct observations of sexual behavior (e. g., Farkas *et al.,* 1978), population surveys of sexual behavior are based solely on self-reports of unknown validity. We have previously reviewed the scant research on the validity of self-reported sexual behavior and on strategies for validating these self-reports (Catania *et al.,* 1990a,b). These strategies rely on biological markers for validation (e. g., Udry and Morris, 1967) and, therefore, cannot be used to assess the accuracy of frequency reports of coitus or nonvaginal intercourse, and are difficult or costly to apply in large population-based surveys. Correlations between partners' reports of how often they have sex over a given time period have also been interpreted as validity coefficients of self-reported sexual behavior (e. g., Clark and Wallin, 1964; Coates *et al.,* 1988; Jacobson and Moore, 1981; Kinsey *et al.,* 1948, 1953; Levinger, 1966). However, this approach has been criticized because the couples' self-reports of their mutual sexual activity still need to be validated against some objective index (Catania *et al.,* 1990a,b). That is, partners' perceptions of their sexual relationship may be of interest in their own right, but they do not provide information on the validity of self-reported sexual events.

Reverse record studies also provide an opportunity for indirectly assessing validity of sexual behavior. For instance, a telephone survey call list might be salted with phone numbers and names of people who have verified sexually transmitted diseases (STD). Examination of the salted respondents in terms of their willingness to report having had an STD over the telephone would provide an indirect measure of people's willingness to report highly sensitive sex-relevant information. This type of reverse record study would require a complex set of procedures to blind the interviewers and study investigators to the identities of the salted respondents. For such a study to work, however, clinic patients would also need to be blind to the true nature of the study. This raises ethical and legal concerns since clinic patients may not be willing to have their phone number and name released by the clinic under any circumstances and their willingness to participate would not be made under conditions that describe the true nature of the study. In some regards this latter problem raises ethical issues that parallel those discussed in Stevenson and colleagues' chapter with respect to double-blind control group experiments.

In general, sex research lacks a gold standard for validating self-reported sexual behavior. Since we do not have a solid validity index of self-reported sexual behavior and large measurement error further undermines the validity of self-reported sexual behavior, the goal of minimizing measurement error becomes all the more important.

3. NEED FOR PRETESTING

Before beginning our discussion of the issues surrounding measurement error associated with assessments of self-reported sexual behavior, it is important to first consider what efforts might be made to head off difficulties associated with these assessments. Pretesting items is considered standard practice for all survey research, yet little systematic research has been conducted to examine the utility of various pretesting techniques. An exception to this observation is recent work by Charles Cannell and colleagues at the University of Michigan (Cannell *et al.,* 1989; Oksenberg *et al.,* 1991). They have developed and experimentally tested a system of pretesting techniques that are easy to use and provide straightforward interpretation of problems posed by individual survey questions for both interviewers and respondents in terms of (1) questions that are difficult to ask, (2) question comprehension, (3) lack of a common understanding of terms and concepts, and (4) difficulty in cognitive processing of information. The three central components of their approach are behavior coding, use of special probes, and special training of pretest interviewers. Pretest interviews are taped and a series of simple behavior codes are used by independent raters to rate each question (e. g., *slight changes:* interviewer read the question with slight changes; *interruption:* respondent interrupted the question reading with an answer; *clarification:* respondent requested clarification, explanation, or repeat of the question). The behavior codes lead to a quantitative assessment of the problems associated with each item. At the end of and occasionally during the interview, selected items are probed. The probes need to be specific to discrete elements of the question (words, phrases), and are used to assess respondents' understandings of question and terms and problems with response categories. In addition, interviewers are given training in how to recognize problems with questions, how to identify the nature of the problems, and how to rate question problems. Cannell *et al.* (1989) have provided a detailed description of these pretesting techniques and report a series of experiments attesting to their utility (also see Oksenberg *et al.,* 1991).

What the Cannell *et al.* (1989) work does not assess are respondents' negative emotional reactions to questions. In AIDS-related surveys the potential may be high for respondents to become upset about questions that ask for intimate details of their sexual experiences. Strong negative reactions to particular items may lead to premature termination of the interview, or in some other way bias responses to subsequent items (e. g., increase "decline to answer" or "don't know" responses). We examined this issue in pretest work for the National AIDS Behavioral Surveys (Catania, 1991). Specifically, we were interested in detecting when during the course of the telephone interview respondents might begin to show signs of emotional distress. Each survey item had as part of the response categories a set of codes that the interviewer could check if the respondent began to show signs of distress (e. g., distress would be indicated if respondent's tone of voice became angry, respondent became belligerent and defensive, respondent broke the phone connection). Since the survey contained a large of number of potentially sensitive questions on AIDS-related behaviors, attitudes, and beliefs, we thought it was important to determine if particular items might be distressing to respondents and, in turn, lead to premature break-offs or in some other way contaminate subsequent questions. What we found was that very few people were upset by questions on sexual behavior, sexual attitudes, and related topics. In part this may have been because respondents knew they could decline to answer questions (although very few did) and, therefore, felt more in control of the interview process. Furthermore, detailed sexual behavior items were asked only of people with some minimal risk factor (e. g., two-plus sexual partners, HIV$^+$, IVDU), which may screen out the most conservative elements of the population who might become distressed about questions that inquire about their specific sexual practices. In surveys that wish to obtain detailed reports of sexual behavior from all respondents or wish to assess more threatening questions (e. g., questions about masturbation are more threatening than questions about intercourse) the issue of emotional upset needs to be revisited. Pretest findings that identify particularly upsetting items might lead to strategies to help prevent emotional distress or positioning of distressing items at the end of the survey to avoid contaminating responses to other survey items.

Focus groups have also been used for pretesting items and have great value as investigators begin to chart the best ways to communicate with underresearched groups on topics that have not been widely investigated. In this regard, focus group methodology provides a useful technique for identifying comprehension problems in survey questions and for eliciting wording that is socially acceptable to respondents (Basch, 1987; Catania, 1991; Folch-Lyon *et al.,* 1981; Folch-Lyon and Trost, 1981; Schearer, 1981; Stycos, 1981). Focus groups have been used successfully in areas related to the type of topics covered by surveys of sexual behavior (e. g., family planning and birth control) with black, white, and Hispanic respondents (Basch, 1987; Catania, 1991; Folch-Lyon *et al.,* 1981; also see Fullilove and Fullilove, this volume). The problems inherent in sampling opinions in group situations aside, the weak link in most focus group research is in obtaining a representative sample that reflects the characteristics of respondents you wish to eventually survey, particularly respondents who may have the most difficulty with item comprehension and terminology. These problems were approached in pretesting the National AIDS Behavioral Surveys in which we conducted a series of six focus groups (Catania, 1991). Focus group participants were randomly selected from a list frame (phone numbers) and screened by phone interview to obtain samples of young and older adults, black and Hispanic respondents, and men and women with at most a high school education. We selected for people with at most a high school education (50% had less than a high school education) under the assumption that these individuals might have the most difficulty with comprehension of the questions and specific terms. Evidence from these focus groups is not without some caveats, however. Obviously the technique for initially sampling focus group respondents, in this case by phone, may be one source of bias in that even under the best conditions some 20–40% of households with phones will fail to participate in any given telephone survey. However, since the planned national survey was to be conducted by telephone we felt that the bias introduced by sampling focus group members by telephone would be somewhat parallel to what we would expect in the actual survey. Thus, it may be important to recruit focus group participants using procedures similar to those intended for recruiting respondents in the actual survey. However, additional attrition-related bias may be introduced since, by necessity, focus groups will involve some degree of travel by respondents to go from home or work to the data collection site. Requiring respondents to travel to a research site has been found to generate biased samples with respect to sexual attitudes and behavior (Kaats and Davis, 1971). Nevertheless, the results from the focus groups can be extremely useful. One way to test the results of the focus groups is to conduct a second pretest (based on the focus group findings) under the exact conditions in which you plan to collect the actual survey. Again the rule of obtaining representativeness with respect to the actual survey respondents, particularly of respondents who may have potential problems, is important. Utilizing pretest procedures such as those described previously (e. g., Cannell *et al.,* 1989) within this second pretest will provide further documentation of problem items and the need to reword or drop items.

4. INDICES OF MEASUREMENT ERROR

4.1. Overview

Measurement error may hamper AIDS prevention efforts by biasing estimates of the prevalence of high-risk sexual behaviors, lead to misidentification of at-risk populations, and by biasing estimates of the statistical relationships between variables. Measurement error associated with self-reported sexual behavior may occur in a number of different ways: (1) Respondents may refuse to answer a question, (2) respondents may underreport their actual activity levels by indicating that they have never performed a behavior they have in fact performed, (3) respondents may admit performance of the behavior, but then substantially underreport the actual frequency of that activity, and (4) respondents may report behaviors (type or frequency) never performed (overreport). Given the lack of a gold standard validity index for self-reported sexual behavior, it is difficult to detect when respondents are over- or underreporting their sexual behavior in any absolute sense. Relative assessments of over- and underreporting of sexual behavior can be obtained, however, when comparing different data collection modes (e. g., Blair *et al.,* 1977; Bradburn *et al.,* 1978).

Item refusal may be easier to assess in terms of an absolute quantity. Comparison of refusal rates across modes may, however, prove somewhat complicated by the fact that some respondents find it more socially acceptable and less confrontational to report nonperformance rather than refuse to answer a question. Current evidence suggests that self-presentation bias differs between data collection modes in surveys of sexual behavior (see Catania *et al.,* 1990a). Thus, comparisons of refusal rates between modes should also include data on the rate of answering "never" or "zero" to behavior questions. Past studies of sexual behavior have typically not provided both refusals and never/zero rates for sexual behavior items.

Refusal rates (i. e., refusing to answer a question) are the most frequently reported index of measurement error in sexuality surveys. Refusal rates for sexual items in self-administered questionnaires (SAQs) (adult samples) range from 6% to 13% for items assessing the frequency of vaginal intercourse, 7% to 19% for masturbation items (Bradburn *et al.,* 1978; Catania *et al.,* 1986; Johnson and DeLamater, 1976), and have averaged about 6% for assessments of numbers of sexual partners in the past year (Michael *et al.,* 1988). Comparable data for face-to-face and telephone interviews have not been published.

Nonresponders (i. e., those who refuse to answer some or all sex questions) in sex surveys are reported to be older, less educated, and have lower reading ability than responders (Johnson and DeLamater, 1976; for young adults). In addition, nonresponders have less sexual experience (direct or vicarious) and, therefore, may be sexually more inhibited than responders (Catania *et al.,* 1986; see Self-Presentation Section). Not all findings fit these general observations. Michael *et al.* (1988), for example, found that refusal rates for questions on numbers of sexual partners were highest for never-married men in their 30s (11.4%).

4.2. Nonresponse to Sex Questions in Telephone Surveys

We employed data from the National AIDS Behavioral Survey (NABS; Catania, 1991) to examine the extent of nonresponse to various sexual questions and to determine if responders and nonresponders differ in some important way. Responders and nonresponders were compared on various demographic characteristics and on a number of psychosocial measures including: a brief measure of sexual self-disclosure ("Do you think that talking about sex in an AIDS survey is very easy to do, kind of easy, kind of hard, or very hard to do?"), perceived survey confidentiality ("How much do you agree or disagree that surveys conducted by universities or colleges will keep your answers confidential or private?"), church attendance ("Over the last year, how often have you gone to church or other types of religious meetings or services?": 1+/week, 1–3/month, <1/month, don't go), acculturation (Hispanics only), and recent survey experience ["How many surveys have you participated in over the last 6 months, including telephone, mail, and face-to-face interviews (excluding current interview?")].

Findings show remarkably little missing data on any of the sexual behavior questions asked in the survey, ranging from zero to 1.2%. For example, only 0.1% of central city respondents refused to indicate whether they were sexually active, 0.5% refused to give their sexual orientation, and 0.6% and 0.1% respectively refused to say how often they had had vaginal or anal intercourse in the past 6 months. Less than 1% of younger respondents (18–49 years of age) and 1.2% of older (50+ years of age) central city respondents refused to indicate the number of sexual partners they had in the past 5 years. The national sample showed similar percentages of missing data. Demographic differences between responders and nonresponders were also minimal. Only minor age variations were evident, with 1.5% of the lowest age group (18–29) and 2.9% of the highest age group (60–75) refusing to answer one or more sex items. Social-psychological comparisons showed respondents with low sexual disclosure (found it "hard" or "very hard" to talk about sex) to be more likely to refuse to answer sex items than respondents who indicated greater ease of sexual disclosure. Specifically, 3.4% of "low" disclosure respondents declined to answer one or more sex items, while only 1.1% of the "high" disclosure group refused to answer any items with sexual content. Perceived confidentiality of surveys also showed some significant but minor differences, with 1.3% of respondents with high perceived confidentiality and 3.5% of respondents with low perceived confidentiality refusing to answer at least one sex item. There were no differences in the tendency to decline to answer sex questions between respondents showing different levels of prior survey experience, acculturation (Hispanics only), and church attendance.

In general, results from the NABS suggest that in terms of questions about being currently sexually active (yes, no), sexual orientation, numbers of sexual partners (past 5 years, past year, past 6 months), vaginal and anal intercourse, and condom use (past 6 months), very few respondents declined to answer or said they didn't know the answer to those questions. The general sexual activity and sexual orientation items and numbers of partners questions were asked of all respondents and results for these questions are therefore the most generalizable. In brief, it appears that once respondents agreed to participate in the survey, they were generally willing to answer these types of sexual behavior questions. However, questions on vaginal or anal intercourse and condom use were asked only of people with some minimal HIV risk factor (two-plus sexual partners/year, received a blood transfusion between 1978 and 1985, were HIV+, used i.v. drugs in the past 5 years, or had a primary sexual partner with one of these characteristics). Consequently, it cannot be concluded that people who lack a risk factor and who may be more sexually conservative (i. e., in the NABS those lacking a risk factor were typically mutually monogamous or sexually inactive) would also have low rates of item refusals on questions about specific sexual activities.

4.3. Test–Retest Reliability

Test–retest correlations provide an index of measurement error in terms of the stability of people's estimates of their sexual activities for some standard interval of time (i. e., both reports should refer to the same time period). [The correlations between partners' reports of how often they have sex over a given time period have been interpreted as reliability coefficients of self-reported sexual behavior (e. g., Clark and Wallin, 1964; Coates *et al.*, 1988; Kinsey *et al.*, 1948, 1953), but these correlations are less than ideal as a measure of interobserver reliability (see Catania *et al.*, 1990a).] The few studies that have examined test–retest correlations for sexual behavior questions have investigated a wide range of behaviors for gay men and heterosexual adults and adolescents.

For gay men, test–retest coefficients have ranged from 0.40 to 0.91 across different types of sexual behaviors including reports of numbers of sexual partners, oral sex behaviors, anal intercourse (insertive, receptive, with/without condoms), and miscellaneous anal activities (e. g., fisting, fingering) (Coates *et al.*, 1986; Saltzman *et al.*, 1987; for review see Catania *et al.*, 1990a). The wide range in values underscores the importance of not assuming that high reliability for one sexual activity measure necessarily confers high reliability on measures of other sexual behaviors. For heterosexual adults, test–retest correlations have also ranged widely (0.30–0.90) with higher reliabilities found for incidence items (i. e., have you ever performed?) than frequency items and lower values for items that require recall for long (a year) versus short (a month) time periods (Catania *et al.*, 1990a; Kauth *et al.*, 1991). Test–retest coefficients for heterosexual adolescent reports of coital frequency, masturbation frequency, and condom use are relatively high (2-month retrospective reports; in the 0.80 to 0.98 range) with black adolescent males evidencing the lowest reliability scores (Catania *et al.*, 1990a; Rodgers, 1982). Since adolescents probably have less sexual experience and fewer sexual encounters than adults for a given period of time, the higher test–retest coefficients for adolescents relative to adults may reflect their having less information to recall and fewer contaminating events (e. g., inclusion of events outside the recall period).

Although the existing test–retest data are uniform in endorsing the quality of retrospective reports of different sexual behaviors, test–retest offers one route by which memory problems and techniques to enhance recall of sexual behaviors can be studied (see Croyle and Loftus, this volume). Studies are needed that examine reliability for different retrospective reporting periods across specific sexual behaviors using common reporting periods for each assessment, for different age groups, ethnic/racial populations, and with an emphasis on differential recall problems of people with different levels of sexual experience. In general, incidence reports of sexual behavior have high levels of test–retest reliability, but test–retest coefficients of frequency reports evidence considerable variability across different types of sexual activities and deteriorate the longer the retrospective reporting period.

5. RESPONDENT INFLUENCES ON MEASUREMENT ERROR

Respondent variables concern properties of the person that influence the primary task of giving information. Respondent variables include elements of recall, self-presentation bias, motivational issues, and question comprehension. In the following sections we focus on four memory-related issues: the vividness and complexity of the material to be recalled, inferential recall strategies, and emotional influences on recall. Issues of self-presentation bias and respondent motivation will also be discussed. The topic of respondent comprehension is deferred to a later section on instrument influences on measurement error (see Section 6.2).

5.1. Recall: Vividness, Complexity, Inferential Strategies

One of the least understood areas of sex research is the effect that memory has on the task of recalling past sexual experiences (see Croyle and Loftus, this volume). Difficulties with recalling past sexual events, fluctuations over time in the ability to recall sexual events (e. g., in longitudinal studies), and the unintentional inclusion of sexual events from time periods outside those being inquired about would increase measurement error associated with assessments of sexual activities. The recall of sexual events is probably dependent on the length of the recall period, vividness of the events to be recalled, the difficulty of the task involved in recalling past events, and the respondents' motivation to perform the task of recalling past experiences.

Although many respondents report being able to clearly remember certain sexual milestones, many details of our past sexual experiences may become fuzzy with time. Memories of sexual events that have a high personal salience may be more easily remembered. However, the salience of any particular sexual encounter may decrease considerably when the complexity of those encounters increases. That is, a person may have greater difficulty in recalling occurrences of specific sexual acts if they have a large number of sexual partners, and large and highly variable sexual behavioral repertoires (see Catania *et al.,* 1990a; Coates *et al.,* 1986). Moreover, some sexual events may be very salient yet so emotionally painful (e. g., date rape) that they remain repressed at least in terms of what respondents are willing to relate to an interviewer (see Section 5.2). Lastly, particularly salient sexual fantasies may, for some respondents, become confused with actual events and inadvertently be included in self-reports of, for example, numbers of sexual partners.

Given the fallibility of people's memory for sexual events, one important methodological question is: how should we ask sexual questions or structure their order to maximally enhance recall? Although a number of strategies have been put into practice, they have not been examined empirically (Croyle and Loftus, this volume, provide insights into how this might be done). For instance, it has not been established whether we may begin a sexual history with questions about respondents' most recent sexual experiences or their earliest experiences, nor have the relative merits of global retrospective reports versus partner-by-partner assessments been examined.

How do respondents compute estimates of their sexual behavior? In general, respondents rely on inferential methods to compute behavioral estimates particularly when the length of the reference period or the frequency of occurrence of a behavior increases (Bradburn *et al.,* 1987). Two broad strategies, decomposing and the availability heuristic, have been observed in research contexts not dealing with sexuality (Bradburn *et al.,* 1987). In general, sex researchers have not examined how respondents calculate their number of sexual partners and compute behavioral frequencies across partners for particular periods of time. It is essential that we have an understanding of these processes, particularly in terms of the biases different "guesstimating" methods have on reports of specific sexual activities.

5.2. Recall: Emotional Issues

As discussed, the degree of personal salience of a sexual encounter may influence ease of recall. Strong emotions at the time of a particular encounter may enhance the salience of that event. Pleasurable and negative emotions associated with one's sexual encounters may, however, differentially influence recall. For instance, within the same marital dyad, sexually satisfied partners report higher levels of activity than unsatisfied partners (Clark and Wallin, 1964; Levinger, 1966). Presumably events associated with highly positive emotions are more likely to be recalled than events coupled with negative feelings. In this regard, we might understand the typical finding that women tend to report fewer sexual partners than men, in part because women are the recipients of more negative sexual experiences. For instance, women are more likely to experience rape (Hall and Hirschman, 1991; Malamuth *et al.*, 1991) with estimates of nearly one in three women having been date-raped (Hall *et al.*, 1991). These speculations need to be examined empirically. In general, negative or positive sexual feelings may bias reports by coloring the person's recall of specific sexual episodes. How emotional states at the time of interview influence the degree and direction of measurement error are issues for further investigation.

5.3. Self-Presentation Bias

Self-presentation bias in sex research reflects the underlying values that a culture or specific subculture place on revealing sexual experiences to others (Catania *et al.*, 1986, 1990a). Given that people wish to present themselves in a positive light, self-presentation bias may lead to either over- or underreporting of a particular sexual behavior depending on whether that behavior has a positive or negative social value. For instance, young adults in today's Western culture may find it difficult to admit to being virgins. Pre-AIDS, gay men may have readily admitted to having unprotected anal intercourse, but may be more reticent to report such now. These various scenarios suggest that sexual behaviors vary in their degree of social desirability depending on what it means for the respondent to reveal performance of that activity. We have previously reviewed findings and conceptual issues relating social desirability to self-reports of sexual behavior (Catania *et al.*, 1990a). A number of studies indicate that sexual questions are threatening for some people, which, in turn, influences their willingness to report their sexual experiences (Bolling, 1976; Bolling and Voeller, 1987; Bradburn *et al.*, 1978; Catania *et al.*, 1986). Hypotheses concerning ethnic, sexual orientation, and gender differences in self-presentation bias with respect to reporting sexual behavior have been derived, but not systematically tested (see Catania *et al.*, 1990a,b). For instance, Hispanic individuals relative to Anglos may be more sexually conservative and, therefore, may be less willing to reveal sexual activity to an interviewer. Conversely, Hispanic culture may hold machismo values that lead to overreporting of sexual behavior, particularly by males. There is a significant need for research on social structural differences in self-presentation bias associated with specific sexual activities.

Under what conditions are people likely to bias their answers about sexual behavior in a socially desirable direction? Several studies suggest that respondents are more likely to admit to sexual behavior, particularly proscribed sexual activities, under private conditions that avoid face-to-face contact with an interviewer [telephones, self-administered questionnaires (SAQs), computer-administered surveys; Czaja, 1987–88; Millstein and Irwin, 1983]. However, it is more difficult to use SAQs or obtain telephone interviews with

IVDUs and it is not apparent to what extent prior work in the sexual survey area is generalizable to minority populations, the elderly, adolescents, and gay/bisexual men and women (Catania *et al.,* 1990a). Similarly, it is unclear how different types of question structures and formats influence self-presentation bias, although evidence is accumulating to suggest that non-judgmental presentation of sexual questions coupled with familiar wording and open-ended response formats may reduce presentation bias (Blair *et al.,* 1977; Bradburn and Sudman, 1979; Johnson, 1970).

Minimizing presentation bias through procedural adjustments is one approach to the problem. However, a complementary tack is to measure self-presentation bias. Measures of the tendency to make socially desirable responses have a long research history that is replete with measurement and conceptual problems (Bradburn and Sudman, 1979; Catania *et al.,* 1990a; Larsen *et al.,* 1976; Martin and Greenstein, 1983; Millham, 1974; Shulman and Silverman, 1974). Another approach that has been empirically tested and shows some promise is to directly assess people's willingness to disclose their sexual behaviors, since self-disclosure is the central issue (Catania *et al.,* 1986; Herold and Way, 1988; see for review Catania *et al.,* 1990b). Measures of sexual self-disclosure tendencies have not been employed in AIDS research, but would be of obvious value in assessment of underreporting of sexual activity. Obviously, these measures do not provide an index of who is likely to overreport sexual behavior. In brief, self-presentation bias is a critical concern in AIDS-related behavioral research, yet it is poorly understood with respect to self-reports of specific sexual activities across sex, age, sexual orientation, and cultural subgroups at risk for AIDS. These are not trivial issues, since they directly impact the ability to achieve a clear understanding of the conditions that facilitate changes in sexual behavior and, consequently, the ability to evaluate behavioral interventions.

5.4. Motivation

How motivated people are to perform the role of respondent may be another source of measurement error. Highly motivated respondents may make greater effort in thinking about the content of each question and their responses to those questions. Less motivated participants may offer more "don't know" and "decline to answer" responses or give less thoughtful answers. Differences in motivation would seem to be of importance in situations where respondents need to make greater effort to recall past sexual behaviors (e. g., given large numbers of partners). From the standpoint of altruistic and self-preservation motives, groups at highest risk for HIV infection may represent those most motivated to work with the investigator to arrive at useful answers. However, respondents motivated by high levels of self-interest may not always be the best respondents in terms of providing accurate responses. If, for example, respondents believe that research participation will increase their chances of obtaining access to new experimental treatments for HIV, then some highly motivated respondents may bias their responses in unknown directions so as to facilitate continued contact with the investigator.

The development of procedural techniques that will motivate respondents to be open and truthful about their sexual behavior is an area that has received some research attention. Singer (1978a,b; Singer and Frankel, 1982) has conducted a number of studies that examine how respondents' motivation to respond to sensitive questions on sexual behavior and other topics is influenced by informed consent procedures. In general, she has found that greater assurances of confidentiality may have a slightly positive effect on response rates to questions about sexual behavior. Singer also found that disclosing the purpose of the study may decrease nonresponse to sexual items, but this is not universally true, particularly when the purpose of the study is far removed from the concerns of respondents (e. g., a methodological study; Singer and Frankel, 1982). However, the gains achieved by long detailed explanations of the study appear to be quite minimal and there is some question as to how much respondents actually cognitively process what they are being told during the informed consent procedures.

At present, issues of respondent motivation are the most poorly understood aspects of methodological research. How do we measure respondents' motivations to provide full and complete information? Moreover, can we modify the relevant motives so as to mobilize the most advantageous conditions for collecting sexual information? These are important concerns that strike at the center of the participant–investigator relationship, yet are unexplored in an area of research that likely elicits extremes of respondent motivation.

6. INSTRUMENT VARIABLES

Instrument variables include issues of terminology, question wording, properties of question structure, and order effects. Instrument variables may often overlap with properties of the respondent and interviewer. The instrument may elicit reactions from the interviewer that, in turn, influence how respondents answer questions about their sexual behavior. For instance, interviewers who are uncomfortable with various sexual behaviors may, when asking questions about those activities, provide respondents with cues that suggest that the interviewer holds negative opinions about those sexual behaviors; this belief may reduce respondents' motivation to answer questions and enhance self-presentation bias. Lastly, instruments of varying lengths and complexity place differential demands on the respondents' memory and motivation to perform the task.

Language is the operational system by which questions and answers are transmitted between interviewer and respondent. Consequently, the respondent's comprehension of sexual terms used in the interview is of substantial importance to measurement error. Because of the interplay between question terminology and respondent comprehension, we discuss comprehension issues here instead of under respondent influences on measurement error.

6.1. Order Effects

A common assumption is that question sensitivity should increase progressively across items; subjects are then gradually desensitized to more intimate items. Sensitive items presented too early may lead to greater measurement error (Bradburn and Sudman, 1983). Alternatively, respondents may lose motivation over the course of an interview and evidence increased measurement error on items at the end of an interview. Finding the right balance between interview length and order requires pretesting, where the focus is on respondents' perceptions of the task and their actual responses to the questions (see Orne, 1969).

Prior studies have failed to find that order effects influence measurement error for sexual questions in either SAQs (Catania *et al.*, 1986) or face-to-face interviews (DeLamater, 1974; DeLamater and MacCorquodale, 1975). These studies are based on college students and young adult samples and may not be generalizable to adolescents and the rest of the adult population (see Catania *et al.*, 1986, 1990a). Lastly, surveys that do not focus on sexual topics have found that SAQs may be less susceptible to order effects than other data collection modes (Bishop *et al.*, 1988). Identifying when order effects are likely to occur may, in part, require an appreciation of how the sequencing of questions influences the social meanings of the behavior and, thereby, affects self-presentation bias. Johnson (1970) found that married couples reported higher levels of extramarital coitus when the behavioral items were preceded by a nonjudgmental "attitudes toward extramarital coitus" battery than with the reverse order. Thus, appropriate sequencing may reassure the respondent that it is acceptable, under interview conditions, to admit to socially undesirable activities. One untested hypothesis in this area is that the respondent's trust in the interviewer's ability to be accepting of them may be enhanced by beginning questionnaires with items that reflect a nonjudgmental view of the target behaviors or wording behavioral questions so that all possible variants are nonjudgmentally presented (Bradburn and Sudman, 1983; Catania *et al.*, 1990b). The insertion of explanatory material for questions whose purpose is not immediately apparent to respondents has also been suggested as technique for providing respondents with adequate justification for asking questions that, by themselves, may seem overly intrusive (Catania *et al.*, 1990a).

6.2. Terminology and Question Structure

One of the least understood problems of sex research is that of selecting workable terminology for different sexual behaviors. Investigators have previously mapped, to some degree, the sexual terminologies of various populations (homosexuals: Rodgers, 1972; black teenagers: Folb, 1980; Mexicans: DeUsandizaga Y Mendoza, 1973; black adults: Andrews and Owens, 1973), but the generalizability of this work is unknown and may be dated. An extensive mapping of sexual terminologies across subpopulations and, as with Spanish-speaking peoples, across dialects may be needed (see Catania *et al.*, 1990a,b). It is uncertain, however, to what extent such a mapping is needed. It may be that the standard terms used in surveys of sexual behavior such as penis, vagina, anal intercourse, when accompanied by some brief explanation, are understandable to the vast majority of the population in the United States. Focus group and telephone pretest work conducted for the NABS, described earlier, suggested that respondents did understand standard sexual terms. Ford and Norris (1991) also found that standard terms such as penis, vagina, and anus were understood by low-income black and Hispanic adolescents, although Hispanic women had some comprehension difficulties. As the authors note, their study is based on a small convenience sample ($n = 64$) and may not be generalizable beyond the age groups studied. More extensive pretesting work such as that described by Cannell *et al.* (1989) is probably needed to fully elucidate the meanings given to common sexual terms and to identify preferred terms that respondents will feel most comfortable with in an interview situation. Nevertheless, even if only a small minority of respondents fail to understand standard sexual terms it still may be important to consider techniques that make sexual questions understandable to these respondents. A number of approaches have been suggested including having the interviewer provide translations from standard to more familiar slang terms, by verbally describing the sexual activity in question, or by showing respondents drawings or pictures of the behavior in question. These approaches may be limited, however, in that some respondents may be too embarrassed to ask about a sexual term they do not understand or become upset by being shown graphic depictions of sexual acts. With SAQs, standard and slang terms can be built into definition sheets that are administered with the questionnaire. The usefulness of definition sheets is obviously reduced when respondents have problems with reading comprehension.

Past research has indicated that familiar wording (e. g., using the phrase love making instead of vaginal intercourse) may decrease measurement error when respondents are asked to generate alternative terms or phrases for standard sexual terms (Blair *et al.*, 1977; Bradburn and Sudman, 1979; Sudman and Bradburn, 1983). Nevertheless, the effects on self-reported sexual behavior relating to differences in word familiarity are not as pronounced as the effects for question structure (Blair *et al.*, 1977; Bradburn and Sudman, 1979; Sudman and Bradburn, 1983). Further, the decision to use familiar sexual terms is not clear-cut. Some respondents report more comfort with standard than slang terms for sexual behavior, and asking respondents what kinds of sexual terminology they would like the interviewer to use may place additional demands on the interviewer and would not work for SAQs. Research is needed to examine the issue of terminology more closely. Prevalence studies are needed that assess comprehension across diverse populations of currently used standard terms for sexual behavior. In any case, investigators should conduct pilot studies that focus on respondents' understandings and perceptions of sexual terms to be employed in the study.

Bradburn *et al.* (1978; Blair *et al.*, 1977) have examined how different question lengths and response formats influence self-reported sexual behavior in a national survey of adults. They found that longer questions with open response formats lead to higher reports of vaginal intercourse than short questions with closed response formats. Since this work is based predominantly on adult heterosexual white respondents, the generalizability of the results to minority populations, IVDUs, homosexuals, and adolescents needs to be examined. In addition, it would be important to investigate other techniques for asking sexual questions. For example, loading questions by asserting that the behavior being asked about is not uncommon has been suggested as a means of reducing self-presentation bias associated with reporting behaviors perceived to be deviant (Groves, 1989, p. 471; Sudman and Bradburn, 1983, p. 75). In addition, Kinsey *et al.* (1948) recommended that questions about sexual behavior should assume the behavior, an approach that Sudman and Bradburn (1983) also recommend for behaviors that may typically be underreported, but not for activities that may be overreported. These various approaches need to be subjected to experimental verification for the specific case of asking sexual questions.

7. MODE EFFECTS

7.1. Overview

Much of what is known about AIDS-related sexual activity and the correlates of these behaviors is based on data collection techniques whose limitations or superiority for gathering sexual information are poorly understood.

The AIDS-related sex surveys to date have utilized a wide range of techniques including face-to-face interviews in household or clinic settings (e. g., Detels *et al.*, 1989; Martin, 1987; Schechter *et al.*, 1988; Winkelstein *et al.*, 1987; see for review Catania *et al.*, 1989b), telephone interviews (Catania, 1991; Catania *et al.*, 1991; Levy and Albrecht, 1989; Strunin and Hingson, 1987), and SAQs (Baldwin and Baldwin, 1988; Catania *et al.*, 1989a; McKusick *et al.*, 1985). Diary approaches have not been used in any large-scale AIDS-related behavior surveys that we are aware of.

The study of mode effects revolves around two basic questions (Groves, 1989): how do variations in the properties of a given mode influence measurement error, and how do different modes of data collection compare in their effects on measurement error? Although these two fundamental issues have been examined in numerous other health and behavioral contexts, very little of this work has focused on the assessment of sexual behavior (Groves, 1989).

Perhaps of central importance to sex surveys are mode differences in (1) the degree of privacy extended to respondents as they answer questions about sexual behavior, (2) the degree of anonymity afforded the respondent in terms of being unidentifiable, and (3) the degree of credibility the study's representatives achieve with respect to the respondents' belief that the questions concerning sexual behavior have a legitimate purpose and are not simply voyeuristic (or have criminal intent).

High credibility, and greater privacy and anonymity presumably decrease measurement error associated with responses to sensitive questions (Bradburn and Sudman, 1979). Credibility perceptions may vary from believing the interview is legitimate science, that it is a prank, or represents criminal intent. Anonymity and privacy may vary according to the extent that respondents believe the investigator can identify them, can connect answers with personal identifiers, and can see or hear them during the interview. The various modes provide different mixes of anonymity, privacy, and credibility dependent on the extent to which a given mode uses visual and auditory communication channels and limits procedural variations (e. g., interview length, authentication materials).

In asking sexual questions, it is unclear whether any mode has a distinct advantage over any other mode of data collection. For example, relative to telephone surveys, FTFIs may produce higher interviewer credibility by providing visual cues such as supporting letters and identification badges, and since FTFIs can typically have greater length than telephone interviews, FTFIs may provide more time to facilitate the respondent's trust in the interviewer. However, by reducing visual contact between the investigator and respondent, telephone surveys and SAQs may enhance anonymity and privacy more than FTFIs (Bradburn and Sudman, 1979; Czaja, 1987–88). Further, some individuals may attribute higher credibility to telephone interviews than FTFIs because the idea of admitting a stranger (interviewer) into their home elicits fears of being victimized in some fashion (Levy and Albrecht, 1989). Nevertheless, telephone surveys of sexual behavior must contend with the "obscene caller" phenomenon, which might be offset by providing call-back numbers or use of advance letters that increase the interviewer's credibility. Relative to verbal interview approaches, SAQs may vary along a wider range of privacy–credibility–anonymity combinations depending on the conditions under which the respondent receives and completes the SAQ (e. g., in a face-to-face situation with an interviewer-facilitator present versus mailed to respondents). Although the need to examine mode differences in credibility and privacy has an intuitive appeal, direct measures of respondents' perceptions of credibility and privacy associated with sex surveys have not been contrasted across modes. Mode preference studies have been conducted, but the results are typically biased toward the mode of assessment used to collect the preference measures (Groves, 1989), and have not addressed the specific issues of privacy, anonymity, and credibility in the context of asking sex questions.

7.2. Self-Administered Questionnaires

SAQs have a number of inherent advantages over other modes in that, under appropriate conditions, they provide considerable privacy for the respondent, one person can administer SAQs to large groups of people simultaneously, and they are inexpensive to use in group situations (e. g., school classes, health clinics). These advantages are offset by a number of problems including being limited by respondents' reading ability, the investigator's ability to employ language understandable to a wide range of respondents, and provide little opportunity to probe ambiguous responses. Several studies indicate that respondents are more willing to disclose sexual information on SAQs than in FTFIs (Catania *et al.,* 1986; Millstein and Irwin, 1983), but this is not a universal finding (DeLamater and MacCorquodale, 1975). In brief, SAQs provide a useful but limited tool for conducting AIDS-related sex research.

7.3. Telephone Interviews

Telephone surveys provide a useful tool for assessing AIDS-related behaviors, although they may be of limited utility in surveys of difficult-to-reach groups such as intravenous drug users and street youth who are unlikely to have residential telephones. For general population surveys, however, telephone surveys can provide good coverage. Some 97% of households in the United States have telephones (Groves, 1989) and a recent NABS (Catania *et al.,* 1991) obtained a 70% cooperation rate at the national level and a 65% cooperation rate when sampling central city areas in major metropolitan cities. Both samples oversampled minorities and the elderly, two groups that often show low cooperation rates across modes.

Past work has provided a basis for believing that telephone surveys may work well in collecting sensitive information (Czaja, 1987–88). Recent mode comparison surveys in Great Britain and France (Bajos *et al.,* 1991; McQueen *et al.,* 1989) indicate that telephone interviews produce response levels to questions on sexual behavior (e. g., numbers of partners, same gender sex, condom use) at or above levels reported in face-to-face interviews. Research on other sensitive topics including drunk driving arrests and bankruptcy filings also indicates that telephone surveys provide completed interviews at levels comparable or better than those achieved by standard FTFIs, face-to-face with a randomized response format, and SAQs (Bradburn and Sudman, 1979). Several studies suggest that telephone surveys yield response rates comparable to other methods and produce good-quality data on other sensitive topics (e. g., birth control questions) (Coombs and Freedman, 1964; Groves, 1989; Hochstim, 1967; Kegeles *et al.,* 1969; Levy and Albrecht, 1989; Rogers, 1976). Lastly, in the NABS (Catania *et al.,* 1991), we found that 1% or less of respondents declined to answer sensitive questions on sexual behavior and HIV testing even though they were told that declining to answer a question was an option.

Despite the encouraging findings discussed above, de Leeuw and van der Zouwen's (1988) review of the literature on response styles in telephone and FTFIs (none assessed sexual behavior) indicated considerable ambiguity in the findings, with some studies showing telephone and others FTFIs to be the superior method (also see Bradburn and Sudman, 1979; Hochstim, 1967; Kegeles *et al.,* 1969). However, these reviews do not take into account the conceptual difficulties in comparing studies that, although they all involve mode comparisons, are assessing very different topics (e. g., health behavior, drunk driving, bankruptcy, psychological states, income, political attitudes, voting behavior) that most likely differ in terms of perceived sensitivity/threat. It may be that particularly bland topics are assessed equally well by whatever mode is used, extremely sensitive topics will produce large mode differences in response bias, and moderately sensitive topics will show response differences across modes, but the differences will not be clear-cut and from study to study may evidence a great deal of variability. This set of hypotheses may help explain some of the inconsistencies past reviews have observed across mode comparison studies.

7.4. Face-to-Face Household Interviews

Since Kinsey, FTFIs have often been used in surveys of adult sexual behavior. The evidence reviewed previously suggests that FTFIs are comparable to other modes in collecting data on sexual behavior, although, at times, they may produce data of inferior quality. It is unclear, however, why FTFIs sometimes fail where other modes succeed, but, in part, it may be that since FTFIs involve both visual and auditory social contexts, they may heighten self-presentation bias. Nevertheless, FTFIs may achieve greater credibility and trust in the eyes of the respondent, and may produce advantages with regard to training respondents in the use of different response scales and correcting misperceptions. Efforts to maintain these desirable features of the FTFI, but decrease self-presentation bias, are under way through the use of tape recorder-administered surveys and other mechanical devices that reduce interviewer–respondent contact. These technical innovations may prove to have merit over other approaches for reducing embarrassment, such as the random response techniques, that have not improved reporting in sexuality surveys over that obtainable from standard FTFIs (Zelnik *et al.*, 1981). Considerable work needs to be conducted to assess the advantages of FTFIs in surveys of sexual behavior across different social groups. This is an important issue since some groups of respondents may be best accessed through FTFIs (e. g., IVDUs).

7.5. Diaries

Since diaries can be used to gather retrospective reports over very brief time intervals (e. g., within hours of a sexual encounter a person could record details in a diary), the common problems of retrospective data (forgetting and telescoping) are reduced. Diaries have been found to produce improvements in responses to items in general health surveys (Verbugge and Depner, 1980), have relatively high completion rates, and are useful even with respondents with little formal education (low-education respondents, however, tend to drop out sooner; Sudman and Lannom, 1980). Sudman and Lannom (1980) compared diaries with FTF and telephone interviews in the collection of general health information and found that diaries produced better detailed responses to health questions, greater accuracy on some types of questions, and diaries that are regularly retrieved from respondents by an interviewer are easier to code and have the most complete data and detailed information (i. e., in their study this was the result of interviewer editing conducted at the time of the monthly visit). Though diaries may provide more precision than other methods, to date, diaries have not been reported to have been used in AIDS behavioral studies.

8. INTERVIEWER VARIABLES

Characteristics of the interviewer (gender, age, ethnicity), interviewer role demands and behavior during the course of the interview (Sudman and Brad-

burn, 1974) may influence measurement error. Past work suggests that interviewer effects are particularly salient when the task reflects the social relationships involved in the interview (Hatchett and Schuman, 1975; Schuman
and Converse, 1971; Sudman and Bradburn, 1974). Sexuality interviews may
be particularly sensitive to interviewer effects, but prior studies have found
few effects for interviewer variables on responses to sexual questions (Darrow
et al., 1986; DeLamater, 1974; DeLamater and MacCorquodale, 1975; Johnson and DeLamater, 1976; Singer *et al.,* 1983). One exception is that young
adult female respondents have been found to report less current sexual behavior to male than female interviewers (DeLamater, 1974). These findings
are somewhat at variance with Abramson and Hanschumacher's (1978) results,
which indicated that male respondents gave significantly more sexual verbalizations in the presence of a male than a female interviewer, and female
respondents provided low levels of sexual verbalizations across interviewer
conditions. Catania *et al.* (1990b) recently reported data on IVDUs collected
by Dale Chitwood (University of Miami HIV Center) who found that differences in reporting specific types of sexual behavior between gender-matched
and -unmatched groups generally occurred for categories of behavior divergent
from traditional penis-in-vagina intercourse, and most notably for anal sexual
activities. In general, a higher proportion of respondents, regardless of gender,
reported sexual behaviors to female interviewers than to male interviewers.
However, more women than men were influenced by gender of the interviewer.
While significantly more sexual behaviors were reported to females by both
female and male respondents, the reasons for this are not clear. The female
interviewers may have been perceived as more sympathetic and less threatening
than the male interviewers. In addition, there were differences between male
and female interviewers in that female interviewers had been with the project
longer and one female interviewer had a more relevant job history (i. e., an
interviewer in an STD clinic). It may be that because of their background
and longevity with the project, the female interviewers were more comfortable
asking sensitive sexual behavior questions and, thus, respondents were less
inhibited in their responses.

   Overall, the literature on interviewer factors in sexuality research provides
little guidance for the survey researcher. Singer *et al.* (1983) suggest that interviewer factors may be less salient in telephone interviews as opposed to
face-to-face interviews, but this conclusion is not definitive. It is still unclear
as to when it is necessary to match ethnic, sexual orientation, gender, and
age characteristics of interviewer and respondent (see Catania *et al.,* 1990a).
The effects of interviewer role demands and performance in sexuality surveys
are still inadequately understood. At present there are no recognized standards
by which to judge the quality of interviewers' techniques in conducting sexual
interviews, and it is unclear what techniques, if any, investigators presently

employ for improving the quality of sex interviewing abilities. In part, the absence of clear gender-of-interviewer effects on measurement error in past studies may reflect the fact that, despite claims to the contrary, the interviews may have been consistently of marginal quality. Techniques such as those developed for pretesting by Cannell *et al.* (1989) may be useful for objectively assessing interview training and performance in conducting sex interviews.

9. CONCLUSIONS

The work discussed here touches on various methodological issues of import to surveys of sexual behavior. A number of investigators have previously reviewed literature in this area and the interested reader is directed to these for further discussion (Catania *et al.,* 1990a,b; Gagnon, 1988; Green and Weiner, 1977). Below we summarize conclusions from prior reviews and the current chapter, which, in total, emphasize the need for methodological research on numerous fronts with regard to assessing AIDS-relevant sexual behavior.

- Although some excellent methodological studies have been conducted, much of this work is in need of replication across various ethnic, age, and AIDS-risk groups.
- More systematic methods of pretesting questions that assess sexual behavior (and related constructs) need to be incorporated in future AIDS-related surveys. This work may add some costs to the overall project, but this extra cost is minimal compared with the price that is paid by having items that are incomprehensible to the respondent or that yield responses that are incomprehensible to the investigator.
- One priority is to map the sexual terminology that different groups of people comprehend and feel comfortable using when asking and answering questions about their sexual activities. Without a comprehensive understanding of the appropriate terminology to be employed in asking sex questions, it is more difficult to untangle other potential influences on measurement error. Despite the fact that work needs to progress in this area, recent investigations suggest that terminology problems may not be a major concern; this is an assertion that should be backed up in any given study by rigorous pretesting work.
- It is also important to determine how to best present AIDS-related sex research to prospective respondents so as to reduce the threat associated with answering questions about sex, and, correspondingly, enhance participation.

- As in surveys of other types of behavior, human sexuality surveys must also confront problems of recall accuracy. Work is needed that examines how recall accuracy is influenced by length of the recall period, personal salience of past sexual events, emotions associated with one's sexual partner(s) and behavior, task complexity (e. g., with respect to recalling behaviors performed with multiple sexual partners), the relative frequency of the specific behavior being assessed, the respondents' motivation to perform the task, and the types of inferential methods respondents use to provide their behavioral estimates.
- Self-presentation bias may also be a significant barrier to obtaining accurate estimates of sexual behavior. Past studies suggest that privacy concerns, question structure, and question wording may impact on self-presentation bias in sex research. These findings require replication across different AIDS-relevant populations, and further work is needed to develop procedures to reduce self-presentation bias as well as to construct relevant measures of self-presentation bias.
- Research concerning mode influences on measurement error is needed. The advantages of different modes with respect to measurement error in sexuality surveys are unclear. This work is warranted in particular because the high costs of conducting surveys limit efforts to regularly monitor levels of risk behavior over time with repeated cross-sectional and longitudinal surveys. In particular, face-to-face household probability surveys are very expensive and it is unlikely that current funding sources would be able to fund the needed survey work if all studies were to be based on FTFI methods. However, telephone and mail SAQ surveys offer low-cost alternatives. As the National Academy of Science's report indicates (Miller *et al.*, 1990), the limitations and advantages of these low-cost alternatives to face-to-face surveys have not been adequately examined.
- Research should also go forward on examining the biasing effects of properties within modes. For example, within-mode studies are needed to examine for interviewer effects on measurement error. Very few studies have examined interviewer effects in AIDS-related sex research.
- The development of more exacting validity measures of self-reported sexual behavior remains a major challenge. Current validity indices are unable to achieve one-to-one correspondence with self-reports of sexual behavior (e. g., STD rates, condom sales, urine analysis for sperm).

In summary, the amount of work that needs to be conducted in this area is daunting. However, much of this work can be conducted in parallel fashion. For instance, work on semantic and memory issues is easily integrated into experiments examining mode effects either as preliminary steps or as separate conditions within a larger experimental design. What is critical is that this work be replicated across and within age groups, gender, sexual orientation, racial groups, and other relevant risk groups (e. g., IVDUs).

ACKNOWLEDGMENT. This research was supported in part by NIMH grants MH39553, MH46240, MH43892 and NIMH/NIDA Center grant MH42459.

REFERENCES

Abramson, P., and Handschumacher, I. (1978). Experimenter effects on responses to double-entendre word. *J. Pers. Assess.* **1978**:592–596.

Andrews, M., and Owens, P. (1973). *Black language.* West Los Angeles: Seymour–Smith.

Bajos, N., Spira, A., Ducot, B., Leridon, H., and Riandey, B. (1991). Sexual behavior in France: Feasibility study. In *VII International Conference on AIDS,* Abstract Book Vol. 1, Abstract MD4063 (p. 405). Florence, June 1–7.

Baldwin, J. D., and Baldwin, J. A. (1988). Factors affecting AIDS-related sexual risk-taking behavior among college students. *J. Sex Res.* **25**(2):181–196.

Basch, C. (1987). Focus group interview: An underutilized research technique for improving theory and practice in health education. *Health Educ. Q.* **14**(4):411–448.

Bentler, P., and Abramson, P. (1981). The science of sex research: Some methodological considerations. *Arch. Sex. Behav.* **10**:225–251.

Bishop, G., Hippler, H. J., Schwartz, N., and Strack, F. (1988). A comparison of response effects in self-administered and telephone surveys. In R. Groves, P. Biemer, L. Lyberg, J. Massey, W. Nicholls, II, and J. Waksberg (eds.), *Telephone survey methodology.* New York: Wiley, pp. 321–340.

Blair, E., Sudman, S., Bradburn, N., and Stocking, C. (1977). How to ask questions about drinking and sex: Response effects in measuring consumer behavior. *J. Market. Res.* **14**:316–321.

Bolling, D. (1976). Heterosexual anal intercourse, an illustrative case. *J. Fam. Pract.* **3**:557–558.

Bolling, D., and Voeller, B. (1987). AIDS and heterosexual anal intercourse. *J. Am. Med. Assoc.* **258**:474.

Bradburn, N., and Sudman, S. (1979). *Improving interview method and questionnaire design.* San Francisco: Jossey Bass.

Bradburn, N., and Sudman, S. (1983). *Asking questions: A practical guide to questionnaire design.* San Francisco: Jossey Bass.

Bradburn, N., Sudman, S., Blair, E., and Stocking, C. (1978). Question threat and response bias. *Public Opinion Q.* **42**:221–234.

Bradburn, N., Rips, L., and Shevell, S. (1987). Answering autobiographical questions: The impact of memory and inference on surveys. *Science* **236**:157–161.

Cannell, C., Oksenberg, L., Kalton, G., Bischoping, K., and Fowler, F. (1989). *New techniques for pretesting survey questions* (NCHSR #HS 05616). Survey Research Center, University of Michigan.

Catania, J. (1991). The National AIDS Behavioral Surveys: Methodological overview. In *American Psychological Association Meetings,* San Francisco, June.

Catania, J., McDermott, L., and Pollack, L. (1986). Questionnaire response bias and face-to-face interview sample bias in sexuality research. *J. Sex Res.* **22**:52–72.

Catania, J., Coates, T., Greenblatt, R., Dolcini, M., Kegeles, S., Puckett, S., Corman, M., and Miller, J. (1989a). Predictors of condom use and multiple-partnered sex among sexually active adolescent women: Implications for AIDS-related health interventions. *J. Sex Res.* 26:489–501.

Catania, J., Coates, T., Kegeles, S., Ekstrand, M., Guydish, J., and Bye, L. (1989b). Implications of the AIDS risk-reduction model for the gay community: The importance of perceived sexual enjoyment and help-seeking behaviors. In V. M. Mays, G. W. Albee, and S. F. Schneider (eds.), *Primary prevention of AIDS: Psychological approaches.* Beverly Hills: Sage, pp. 242–261.

Catania, J., Gibson, D., Chitwood, D., and Coates, T. (1990a). Methodological problems in AIDS behavioral research: Influences on measurement error and participation bias in studies of sexual behavior. *Psychol. Bull.* 108(3):339–362.

Catania, J., Gibson, D., Marin, B., Coates, T., and Greenblatt, R. (1990b). Response bias in assessing sexual behaviors relevant to HIV transmission. *Eval. Progr. Plan.* 13:19–29.

Catania, J., Coates, T., Stall, R., Bye, L., Kegeles, S., Capell, F., Henne, J., McKusick, L., Morin, S., Turner, H., and Pollack, L. (1991). Changes in condom use among homosexual men in San Francisco. *Health Psychol.* 10(3):190–199.

Clark, A., and Wallin, P. (1964). The accuracy of husbands' and wives' reports of the frequency of marital coitus. *Popul. Stud.* 18:165–173.

Coates, R., Soskolne, C., Calzavara, L., Read, S., Fanning, N., Shephard, F., Klein, M., and Johnson, J. (1986). The reliability of sexual histories in AIDS related research: Evaluation of an interview administered questionnaire. *Can. J. Public Health* 77:343–348.

Coates, R., Soskolne, C., Calzavara, L., Read, S., Fanning, M., Shephard, F., Klein, M., and Johnson, J. (1988). Validity of sexual contacts of men with AIDS or an AIDS-related condition. *Am. J. Epidemiol.* 128:719–728.

Coombs, L., and Freedman, R. (1964). Use of telephone interviews in a longitudinal fertility study. *Public Opinion Q.* 28:112–118.

Czaja, R. (1987–88). Asking sensitive behavioral questions in telephone interviews. *Int. Q. Community Health Educ.* 8:23–32.

Darrow, W., Jaffe, H., Thomas, P., Haverkos, H., Rogers, M., Guinan, M., Auerbach, D., Spira, T., and Curran, J. (1986). Sex of interviewer, place of interview, and responses of homosexual men to sensitive questions. *Arch. Sex. Behav.* 15:79–88.

DeLamater, J. (1974). Methodological issues in the study of premarital sexuality. *Sociol. Methods Res.* 3(1):30–61.

DeLamater, J., and MacCorquodale, P. (1975). The effects of interview schedule variations on reported sexual behavior. *Sociol. Methods Res.* 4:215–236.

de Leeuw, E., and van der Zouwen, J. (1988). Data quality in telephone and face to face surveys: A comparative meta-analysis. In R. Groves, P. Biemer, L. Lyberg, J. Massey, W. Nicholls, II, and J. Waksberg (eds.), *Telephone survey methodology.* New York: Wiley, pp. 283–298.

Detels, R., English, P., Visscher, B., Jacobson, L., Kingsley, L., Chmiel, J., Dudley, J., Eldred, L., and Ginzburg, H. (1989). Seroconversion, sexual activity, and condom use among 2915 HIV seronegative men followed for up to 2 years. *J. AIDS* 2:77–83.

DeUsandizaga Y Mendoza, P. (1973). In B. Costa-Amic (ed.), *el Chingolés: Primer Diccionario Del Lenguaje Popular Mexicano* [*The first dictionary of popular Mexican sexual slang*]. Mexico: Miembro de la Cámara Nacional de la Industria Editorial.

Farkas, G., Sine, L., and Evans, I. (1978). Personality, sexuality, and demographic differences between volunteers and nonvolunteers for a laboratory study of male sexual behavior. *Arch. Sex. Behav.* 7(6):513.

Folb, E. (1980). *Runnin' down some lines: The language and culture of black teenagers.* Cambridge, Mass.: Harvard University.

Folch-Lyon, E., and Trost, J. (1981). Conducting focus group sessions. *Stud. Fam. Plan.* **12**:443–449.

Folch-Lyon, E., de la Macorra, L., and Schearer, S. (1981). Focus groups and survey research on family planning in Mexico. *Stud. Fam. Plan.* **12**:409–432.

Ford, K., and Norris, A. (1991). Methodological considerations for survey research on sexual behavior: Urban African American and Hispanic youth. *J. Sex Res.* **28**:539–555.

Gagnon, J. (1988). Sex research and sexual conduct in the era of AIDS. *J. AIDS* **1**(6):593–601.

Green, R., and Weiner, J. (1977). Methodology in sex research. In *NIMH.* Chevy Chase, Md.: DHHS.

Groves, R. (1989). *Survey errors and survey costs.* New York: Wiley.

Hall, G., and Hirschman, R. (1991). Toward a theory of sexual aggression: A quadripartite model. *J. Consult. Clin. Psychol.* **59**:662–669.

Hall, G., Hirschman, R., and Beutler, L. (1991). Introduction to special section on theories of sexual aggression. *J. Consult. Clin. Psychol.* **59**:619–620.

Hatchett, S., and Schuman, H. (1975). White respondents and race-of-interviewer effects. *Public Opinion Q.* **39**:523–528.

Herold, E., and Way, L. (1988). Sexual self-disclosure among university women. *J. Sex Res.* **24**: 1–14.

Hochstim, J. (1967). A critical comparison of three strategies of collecting data from households. *J. Am. Stat. Assoc.* **62**:976–989.

Jacobson, N., and Moore, D. (1981). Spouses as observers of the events in their relationships. *J. Consult. Clin. Psychol.* **49**(2):269–277.

Johnson, R. (1970). Extramarital sexual intercourse: A methodological note. *J. Marriage Fam.* **32**:279–282.

Johnson, W., and DeLamater, J. (1976). Response effects in sex surveys. *Public Opinion Q.* **40**: 165–181.

Kaats, G., and Davis, K. (1971). Effects of volunteer biases in studies of sexual behavior and attitudes. *J. Sex Res.* **7**(1):26–34.

Kauth, M., St. Lawrence, J., and Kelly, J. (1991). Reliability of retrospective assessments of sexual HIV risk behavior: A comparison of biweekly, three-month, and twelve-month self-reports. *AIDS Educ. Prev.* **3**(3):207–214.

Kegeles, S., Fink, C., and Kirscht, J. (1969). Interviewing a national sample by long distance telephone. *Public Opinion Q.* **33**:412–419.

Kinsey, A., Pomeroy, W., and Martin, C. (1948). *Sexual behavior in the human male.* Philadelphia: Saunders.

Kinsey, A., Pomeroy, W., and Martin, C. (1953). *Sexual behavior in the human female.* Philadelphia: Saunders.

Larsen, K., Martin, H., Ettinger, R., and Nelson, J. (1976). Approval seeking, social cost and aggression: A scale and some dynamics. *J. Psychol.* **94**:3–11.

Levinger, G. (1966). Systematic distortion in spouses' reports of preferred and actual sexual behavior. *Sociometry* **29**:291–299.

Levy, J., and Albrecht, G. (1989). Methodological considerations in research on sexual behavior and AIDS among older people. In M. Riley, M. Ory, and D. Zablotsky (eds.), *AIDS in an aging society: What we need to know.* Berlin: Springer.

McKusick, L., Wiley, J. A., Coates, T. J., Stall, R., Saika, G., Morin, S., Charles, K., Horstman, W., and Conant, M. (1985). Reported changes in the sexual behavior of men at risk for AIDS, San Francisco, 1982–1984: The AIDS behavioral research project. *Public Health Rep.* **100**(6):622–628.

McQueen, D., Gorst, T., Nisbet, L., Robertson, B., Smith, R., and Uitenbroek, D. (1989). *A study of lifestyle and health* (Interim Report No. 1). Research Unit in Health and Behavioral Change, University of Edinburgh, 17 Teviot Place, Edinburgh, EH1 2QZ, United Kingdom.

Malamuth, N., Sockloskie, R., Koss, M., and Tanaka, J. (1991). Characteristics of aggressors against women: Testing a model using a national sample of college students. *J. Consult. Clin. Psychol.* **59**:670–681.

Martin, H., and Greenstein, T. (1983). Individual differences in status generalization: Effects of need for social approval, anticipated interpersonal contact and instrumental task abilities. *J. Pers. Soc. Psychol.* **45**:641–662.

Martin, J. (1987). The impact of AIDS on gay male sexual behavior patterns in New York City. *Am. J. Public Health* **77**:578–581.

Michael, R., Laumann, E., Gagnon, J., and Smith, T. (1988). Number of sex partners and potential risk of sexual exposure to HIV. *Morbidity and Mortality Weekly Report* **37**:565–568.

Miller, H., Turner, C., and Moses, L. (1990). *AIDS: The second decade.* Washington, D.C.: National Academy Press.

Millham, J. (1974). Two components of need for approval score and their relationship to cheating following success and failure. *J. Res. Pers.* **8**:378–392.

Millstein, S., and Irwin, C. (1983). Acceptability of computer-acquired sexual histories in adolescent girls. *J. Pediatr.* **103**(5):815–819.

Oksenberg, L., Cannell, C., and Kalton, G. (1991). New strategies for pretesting survey questions. *J. Off. Stat.* **7**(3):349–365.

Orne, M. (1969). Demand characteristics and the concept of quasi-controls. In R. Rosenthal and R. Rosnow (eds.), *Artifact in behavioral research.* New York: Academic Press, pp. 143–149.

Rodgers, B. (1972). *The queen's vernacular: A gay lexicon.* San Francisco: Straight Arrow Books.

Rodgers, J. (1982). The rescission of behaviors: Inconsistent responses in adolescent sexuality data. *Soc. Sci. Res.* **11**:280–296.

Rogers, T. (1976). Interviews by telephone and in person: Quality of responses and field performance. *Public Opinion Q.* **40**:51–65.

Saltzman, S., Stoddard, A., McCusker, J., Moon, M., and Mayer, K. (1987). Reliability of self-reported sexual behavior risk factors for HIV infection in homosexual men. *Public Health Rep.* **102**:692–697.

Shearer, B. (1981). The value of focus group research for social action programs. *Stud. Fam. Plan.* **12**:407–408.

Schechter, M., Craib, K., Willoughby, B., Douglas, B., McLeod, A., Maynard, M., Constance, P., and O'Shaughnessy, P. (1988). Patterns of sexual behavior and condom use in a cohort of homosexual men. *Am. J. Public Health* **78**:1535–1538.

Schuman, H., and Converse, J. (1971). The effects of black and white interviewers on black responses in 1968. *Public Opinion Q.* **35**:44–68.

Shulman, A., and Silverman, I. (1974). Social desirability and need for approval: Some paradoxical data and a conceptual re-evaluation. *Br. J. Soc. Clin. Psychol.* **13**:27–32.

Singer, E. (1978a). The effect of informed consent procedures on respondents' reactions to surveys. *J. Consum. Res.* **5**:49–57.

Singer, E. (1978b). Informed consent: Consequences for response rate and response quality in social surveys. *Am. Sociol. Rev.* **43**:144–162.

Singer, E., and Frankel, M. (1982). Informed consent procedures in telephone interviews. *Am. Sociol. Rev.* **47**:416–427.

Singer, E., Frankel, M., and Glassman, M. (1983). The effect of interviewer characteristics and expectations on response. *Public Opinion Q.* **47**:68–83.

Strunin, L., and Hingson, R. (1987). AIDS and adolescents: Knowledge, beliefs, attitudes and behavior. *Pediatrics* **79**:825–828.

Stycos, J. (1981). A critique of focus groups and survey research: The machismo case. *Studies Fam. Plan.* **12**:450–456.

Sudman, S., and Bradburn, N. (1974). *Response effects in surveys.* Chicago: Aldine.

Sudman, S., and Bradburn, N. (1983). *Asking questions: A practical guide to questionnaire design.* San Francisco: Jossey Bass.

Sudman, S., and Lannom, L. (1980). *Health care surveys using diaries* (DHHS Publication PHS 80-3279, pp. 16–20). National Center for Health Survey Research.

Udry, J., and Morris, N. (1967). A method for validation of reported sexual data. *J. Marriage Fam.* **29**:442–446.

Verbugge, L., and Depner, C. (1980). *Methodological analyses of Detroit health diaries* (DHHS Publication PHS 80-3279, pp. 144–158). National Center for Health Survey Research.

Winkelstein, W., Samuel M., Padian, N., Wiley, J., Lang, W., Anderson, R., and Levy, J. (1987). The San Francisco men's health study: III. Reduction in HIV transmission among homosexual/bisexual men, 1982–86. *Am. J. Public Health* **76**:685–689.

Zelnik, M., Kantner, J., and Ford, K. (1981). *Sex and pregnancy in adolescence.* Beverly Hills: Sage.

Recollection in the Kingdom of AIDS

ROBERT T. CROYLE and
ELIZABETH F. LOFTUS

1. INTRODUCTION

Several years ago, the award-winning author and filmmaker Peter Davis took a look into the "trenches of the imaginary AIDS kingdom" (Davis, 1987). He went straight to the New York bars where young people go to make new acquaintances, and interviewed patrons. He talked to—among others—three 24-year-old men (Tom, Dick, and Harry), all of whom were worried about contracting AIDS. Each had been out of college for a couple of years and had gone on to become a building supply salesman, a veterinarian, and a medical student. Of the three, only Tom reported wearing a condom the last time he had sex, which was with a prostitute who made him use one. Harry, the med student, reported that he carried condoms with him all the time, but didn't always use them. Davis also talked to "Alice, Betty, and Carol," three 23-year-old women in advertising. Betty reported that she hadn't used a rubber in 8 years, not since her first sexual experience when she was 15. "Believe me, I don't want to go through that again," she added. Alice claimed to have used one once, but didn't like it. Carol added, "We all believe in precautions, but we don't necessarily take them." She drew an analogy to cigarette smoking. "Like I know cigarettes are harmful and have killed a lot more people than AIDS, but I haven't stopped smoking them."

The gloomy picture of condom use being painted by Peter Davis's interviews is somewhat different from the optimistic picture a reader gets from

ROBERT T. CROYLE • Department of Psychology, University of Utah, Salt Lake City, Utah 84112. *ELIZABETH F. LOFTUS* • Department of Psychology, University of Washington, Seattle, Washington 98195.

Methodological Issues in AIDS Behavioral Research, edited by David G. Ostrow and Ronald C. Kessler. Plenum Press, New York, 1993.

a recent introductory psychology text (Roediger *et al.*, 1991). The text reports on data published in the 1980s, which say that about half of adolescents have had intercourse by the age of 16. We also learn that sexual practices are changing: "Because herpes and AIDS . . . are currently incurable, adolescents have increased their use of condoms and altered their sexual activity."

Which is it? Is the use of condoms really up? If so, by how much? Are people really altering their sexual activities? Regardless of whether people are providing information on these topics to an inquiring journalist during an informal interview, or to a researcher who is gathering data for publication, people necessarily use their memories to respond. The journalist and researcher care, or at least should care, about the reliability of those memories. How reliable is memory of condom use, acts of intimacy, exchanges of blood, or any information that is important in the kingdom of AIDS? There seems to be little doubt that the role of memory in the task of recalling AIDS-related information is one of the least understood areas of sex research (Catania *et al.*, 1990).

Our goal in this chapter is to describe briefly general information about how memory works that could be relevant to the AIDS problem. Within the general field of memory, there is a more specific literature on health-related memories. Respondents in health memory research have occasionally answered questions about AIDS-related information, but more often they have been probed for their recollections of other symptoms, illness episodes, and physician communications. These findings could provide clues to the reliability of the memories that are central to AIDS.

In a few cases, attempts have been made to improve memory for health-related information. Sometimes these methods work. Would they also work when the topic is past sexual behaviors or frequency of condom use? This is one issue we tackle in our section on research needs in AIDS-related reporting and memory.

2. THE FIELD OF MEMORY

There is no question that people must rely on memory to answer the kinds of questions that AIDS researchers care about. For example, they rely on memory when asked about the nature and frequency of their sexual contacts (Jewell and Shiboski, this volume). They rely on memory when asked questions like, "Do you know anyone who suffers from AIDS?" or "How many people have you known personally, either living or dead, who came down with the disease called AIDS?"

2.1. Two Forms of Long-Term Memory

Before discussing specific kinds of memories, it is helpful to say something in general about how memory researchers conceptualize memory. Information in long-term memory takes a variety of forms. It includes general knowledge about the world, such as the fact that AIDS is a deadly disease, or that anal intercourse is a high-risk sexual activity. But it also includes personal experiences (e. g., "I didn't use a condom the last time I had sex"). Tulving (1972) coined a useful distinction between these two classes of memories; he labeled the former kind "semantic memories" and the latter "episodic memories." In his words:

> Episodic memory receives and stores information about temporally dated episodes or events, and temporal-spatial relations among these events. . . . Semantic memory is the memory necessary for the use of language. It is a mental thesaurus, organized knowledge a person possesses about words and other verbal symbols, their meanings and referents, about relations among them, and about rules, formulas, and algorithms for the manipulation of these symbols, concepts, and relations. [pp. 385–386]

In other words, episodic memory contains information about life experiences. It is a memory of one's personal history—information that is associated with a particular time or place. The information about a personal homosexual experience at Christmastime in 1985 is episodic. Semantic memory has to do with one's general factual knowledge. Words, concepts, facts that a person knows without necessarily knowing how or when they were first encountered or acquired fall into this category. When a respondent understands a question asked by a researcher, such as "With how many different partners have you had anal penetrative intercourse?" he or she may be using both semantic memory (to understand the terminology) and episodic memory (to retrieve the specific episodes).

Tulving conceived of episodic and semantic memory as two information-processing systems that (1) selectively receive information from perceptual and cognitive systems, (2) retain various aspects of that information, and (3) transmit that information when it is needed. The two systems are thought to differ in the type of information that is stored, the conditions and consequences of retrieval, and possibly vulnerability to interference.

In his subsequent formulation, Tulving (1983) presented an expanded set of features that distinguish episodic and semantic memory. One important distinguishing feature is the vulnerability of information to change. Information stored in the episodic system is more vulnerable—it is changed, modified, and lost more readily—than information in the semantic system. You might retain quite accurately the semantic memory fact that anal intercourse is a high-risk sexual behavior, but not retain specific episodes of high-risk sexual behaviors from your past. Why? One reason is that the information in the semantic system is overlearned (ingrained through frequent practice and use) while information in the episodic system is typically based on single episodes. Moreover, Tulving would claim, the relatively looser organization of the information in the episodic (e. g., unrelated personal experiences) relative to the semantic system (e. g., the names of close relatives) may contribute to its greater vulnerability. A final source of the ease with which information in the episodic system is modified is the richness of combinations of cognitive elements characterizing any particular episode. In contrast, the information in semantic memory is more streamlined.

Tulving was careful to note that the hypothesis of differential vulnerability to interference of the two systems holds only on the average. Generally speaking the episodic system displays greater vulnerability. However, it is entirely possible that many episodes will be remembered better than many parts of semantic knowledge. Thus, your first sexual experience might be a particularly well-remembered episode, while certain semantic facts (e. g., capitals of South American countries) might not be.

2.2. Memory Errors

When people try to recall specific episodes from the past (say, the number of different sexual partners during the previous 12 months) a number of memory errors can occur. First, an episode can be forgotten. Even something as important as a hospitalization can elude attempts at recovery in as short a time as a year. This was shown clearly in a project that asked people to remember their own hospitalizations (Public Health Service, 1965 as cited in Loftus, 1982). The respondents were approximately 1500 persons who had been discharged from a hospital in the preceding year. Surprisingly many people failed to report their hospitalization. Although fewer than 5% of hospitalizations were not reported if the interview occurred within several weeks of hospital discharge, closer to 20% of hospitalizations were not reported if the interview occurred roughly a year after discharge.

There are other kinds of memory errors, besides simple forgetting, that could lead to erroneous answers to a question about recent sexual partners. One of these is "telescoping." Survey respondents are frequently asked to report events that occurred during a specific period of time (e. g., "During the last six months, how often did you . . ."), referred to as a "reference period." Forward telescoping occurs when a person remembers an event as having occurred more recently than it actually did; backward telescoping occurs when a person remembers an event as having occurred longer ago than it actually did. The evidence suggests that forward telescoping for crimes, accidents, hospitalizations, and other significant events is a more common problem than backward telescoping. In fact, two types of forward telescoping have been observed. In one study, investigators attempted to verify the dates provided by survey respondents for previously reported crimes. The data revealed that about 20% of those that were verified in police records occurred prior to the beginning of the reference period provided to respondents (Garofalo and Hindelang, 1977). When a respondent pulls into the reference period an incident that actually occurred earlier, this is known as external telescoping.

Another common telescoping error is that of internal telescoping. This occurs when the incident belongs in the reference period, but when respondents are asked for the month of occurrence, they recall it as occurring more recently than it did. Internal forward telescoping was observed in a study that began with a victimization survey, and matched reported victimizations to police records. Over 200 crime incidents reported to survey interviewers in Portland, Oregon, in 1974 were matched with official crime reports of the same incidents (Schneider et al., 1978). Of 203 incidents for which respondents could recall a given month of occurrence, 49% were placed in a month other than the one in which the incident occurred. While some internal backward telescoping occurred, the net tendency was for 18% of the events to be telescoped forward. For all crimes, the net average telescoping was 2.24 months forward.

A major question is why people remember a robbery that happened last January as if it happened last March. One plausible hypothesis is that it has to do with rehearsal. People's most vivid experiences (e. g., significant health events, death of loved ones) tend to be rehearsed (Rubin and Kozin, 1984). Perhaps the relative apparent recency arises from those subsequent rehearsals. To fully understand external and internal telescoping errors, however, we must know much more about them. Some memory researchers believe that the reasons for these seemingly similar errors may not be the same. Internal telescoping errors may arise from a different cognitive mechanism than external telescoping errors.

Aside from "plain old" forgetting and telescoping, there are some other common errors of memory that are worth attention. When people have an experience, and are later exposed to new relevant information, the new information can affect their earlier memories. Research conducted both by the first author and by others has shown that this new information can become incorporated into older memories. If the person reads someone else's version of the event, or is asked a series of leading questions about the event, these have the potential for contaminating the person's original memory. When exposed to misleading postevent information, subjects in memory experiments have misrecalled the color of a car that was green as being blue, a yield sign as a stop sign, broken glass or tape recorders that never existed, and even something as conspicuous as a barn when no barn was ever seen (Loftus, 1979). This research on the malleability of memory suggests that some information residing in a respondent's memory may be altered or contaminated

by postevent input. This work constitutes evidence for the particular vulnerability of episodic memories about which Tulving hypothesized. This means
that even the best laid plans of researchers for gathering accurate data may
be stymied by the reconstructive and malleable nature of memory. Recognizing
that a leading question can affect its answer cannot undo earlier contamination
of memory, but at least it can avoid further contamination.

3. HEALTH-RELATED MEMORIES

Traditional studies of episodic memory outside the health domain undoubtedly have implications for AIDS researchers, but those within the health
domain may link more clearly. In the health domain, one known memory
error is that people underreport chronic health conditions and the use of
health care resources associated with them (Jabine, 1987).

For example, in one study, the recollections of members of a health-
maintenance organization (HMO) gathered during a telephone interview were
compared with information obtained from their medical records (Loftus *et
al.*, 1992). A major finding was that when people tried to recall their visits
(or the visits of their spouses) over the previous year, they underreported the
number of visits. In one study, people failed to remember roughly 60% of
their actual visits. Which visits did they forget? One might presume that most
of them would be the less recent visits, but this was not necessarily the case.
Of the forgotten visits, 27% were from the most recent 4-month period, 33%
of them were visits from 5 to 8 months earlier, and 40% of them were visits
from 9 to 12 months earlier.

Means and Loftus (1991) hypothesized that this underreporting stems
from differences in the way that recurring and isolated personal events are
represented in memory. Over time there is a tendency for memories to lose
details and for similar events to meld together or get lost. Neisser (1986) made
a similar point when he suggested that the properties that are invariant across
repetitions of an event (or across similar events) may become more accessible
than individual event occurrences. Based on this conceptualization, Means
and Loftus reasoned that in the health domain, repeated visits of a particular
type (e. g., to the dentist or allergist) might lead to the development of a molar
memory or generic script that might be relatively easy to describe. It would
be harder, however, to access memories of specific dentist or allergist visits
and to retrieve information unique to such a visit. Support was found for
these intuitions. When patients' memories were checked against medical record
information, it was clear that individual health events within a group of recurring, similar events were much less likely than nonrecurring events to be
recalled (see also Means *et al.*, 1988).

This study also found that people used different strategies in responding to questions about their doctor visits depending on both the type and frequency of an event. For repetitive events, it is common for people to estimate rather than recall unique episodes. Moreover, when there are more than three visits of a particular kind, use of strategies other than event recall becomes common. We will return to this issues when we discuss AIDS-related memories.

Underreporting is common when people recall doctor visits. However, with other health-related information, overreporting can be the more significant problem. In one study of the ability of 660 people to accurately report on their own recent health procedures (e. g., eye exam within the last 6 months), massive overreporting occurred. Overreporting ranged from a low of about 7% for a mammogram to a high of nearly 20% for a flu vaccination. It was common for reports of a given procedure to be twice as great as the actual number of procedures within the 6-month period (Loftus *et al.,* 1990).

Research conducted by public health investigators has provided a number of lessons concerning memory for health behaviors. Many of these studies use a test–retest strategy rather than verification. Individuals might be asked, for example, to keep a daily diary of food consumption over several days. Several weeks or months later, they are asked to recall their average level of consumption for the same period. One finding from this type of research is that current behavior is often a better predictor of retrospective reports than the original, concurrent assessment. This has frequently been observed in epidemiological studies of diet (e. g., Wu *et al.,* 1988). Ross (1989) has argued that individuals have implicit theories of stability and change concerning themselves that serve as guides when inferring past behavior. When individuals believe that they have consistently behaved in a certain manner, memory errors will tend to exaggerate the similarity between the present and the past. This is the type of effect frequently observed in the dietary behavior studies.

4. IMPROVING MEMORY

Several recent studies involve attempts to improve memory for health-related experiences. Sometimes the attempts work, sometimes they don't. The good news first.

Asking more than one question often leads to more accurate reports. Consider the problem of overreporting of procedures that has been found in several studies. When people were asked whether they had a physical exam, for example, during a particular reference period, say 2 months, overreporting occurred. A simple technique reduced overreporting. The technique entailed asking people about the procedure twice, first in connection with a different reference period (e. g., physical exam within the last 6 months) and then in connection with the reference period of interest (e. g., physical exam within the last 2 months) (Loftus et al., 1990). Why do two questions lead to better reporting? A "precision" hypothesis was supported: The two-time-frame questioning procedure helps because it conveys to the respondent that the interviewer wants greater precision in dating than the single-time-frame question implies.

For the problem of recurring events, there is, happily, a partial cure, revealed in a study of actual patients who were trying to remember their doctor visits. The technique was designed to (1) help people decompose their molar memories of groups of similar events into individual events and (2) place all remembered health events into a personal timeline. The intervention more than doubled the proportion of recurring events on the medical record that was recalled. In addition, the technique increased the proportion of events that could be dated and the accuracy of dates recalled (Means and Loftus, 1991; see also Means et al., 1988).

Now some bad news. For several years, researchers were interested in the order in which subjects probed their memory for a series of events. For example, do they recall doctor visits over a reference period in a forward (chronological) order, a backward (reverse chronological) order, or some other order (e. g., significant events first)? Would they be more accurate and complete if they were urged to use one order versus another? There were theoretical reasons to predict an advantage for forward over backward, and different theoretical reasons to predict just the opposite. To date, several studies have examined this issue, with conflicting results. Loftus et al. (1992) found a trend for backward order to be better than forward or free recall for the recall of medical-provider visits. On the other hand, Jobe et al. (1990) found recall to be best if people were allowed to recall medical-provider visits in whatever order they chose, rather than when instructed to use a forward or backward order. Whether the apparent inconsistency in findings relates to the differences in subject sample (HMO members versus general population), differences in extent of visits (few versus many), or some other aspects, recommendations about recall order remain premature until these issues are sorted out.

More bad news came from a series of studies designed to explore a technique for improving memory for voting behavior (Abelson et al., 1992). It is well known in the world of voting behavior that people who are asked whether they voted in the last election often claim they did when they did not. The percentage of false alarms (saying you voted when you didn't) is often astoundingly high, in the neighborhood of 25 to 30%. By contrast, the rate of misses (saying you didn't vote when you did) is low, typically less than 5%. Since the accuracy of memory for health-related behaviors was improved by asking two questions instead of one, it was reasonable to hypothesize that two questions might also improve memory for voting behavior. To test this hypothesis, Abelson *et al.* (1992) asked all subjects whether they voted in a previous election. Half the subjects were asked an introductory question prior to the critical question. More specifically, the target question for all respondents was, "Did you vote in the 1986 elections for United States Congress last November?" Half the respondents were first asked, "Thinking back over the last four national elections, that is, the presidential elections of 1980 and 1984, and the congressional elections of 1982 and 1986, did you vote in any of these elections?" The results were disappointing; no impact of the double questioning technique was found, either in this study or in two others that tried modifications of the procedure.

The voting research did produce an interesting result, however, that could potentially have bearing on the recollections of AIDS-related behaviors. In short, the result is that overreporting got worse with longer delays. For example, in one study, the false alarm rate was 16% when respondents were asked about an election that occurred 2 weeks earlier. However, when asked about that same election 6 1/2 months earlier, the false alarm rate rose to 40%. Moreover, Abelson *et al.* (1992) found that habitual voters were more apt to falsely claim they voted. One explanation for this finding is that people will fill the gaps in their memory with socially desirable "memories." As more time passes, and memory grows weaker, it becomes easier for an individual to recruit memories from other sources (e. g., prior voting experiences) to fill those gaps.

5. AIDS-RELATED ISSUES

5.1. Special Problems with AIDS-Related Memories

It is well known that the AIDS virus is spreading in this country among i.v. drug addicts and sexually promiscuous people (Gallo, 1990). Thus, the people from whom we especially want accurate information are people who have experienced recurring, similar events. The sexual patterns of gay men may also tend to be more complex than those of adolescents or heterosexual adults (Catania *et al.*, 1990). As we saw, memory for recurrent experiences is especially poor, because groups of similar events tend to meld together in the mind. The recent focus on AIDS has also led investigators to develop measures of a wider variety of sex and drug-use behaviors than had been previously studied (e. g., Darke *et al.*, 1991). This only increases the backlog of questions that need to be validated.

But there is a further problem related to memory that is special to AIDS. Given that the AIDS virus can cause dementia (Navia *et al.*, 1986), what hope do we have of gathering accurate information from people whose memory systems may already be impaired? Traditionally, neurological problems were assumed to be limited to HIV-positive individuals who had already developed AIDS. Recent research, however, has documented verbal long-term memory deficits in HIV-positive individuals who have yet to manifest any other symptoms of AIDS (Lunn *et al.*, 1991).

Although a discussion of the neuropsychological aspects of AIDS-related memory is well beyond the scope of this chapter, we will discuss briefly three other domains of psychological research that are especially relevant to surveys concerning the mental health aspects of AIDS. Our intent is not to provide a comprehensive review but to highlight lines of research that have encountered many of the same problems now faced by AIDS mental health researchers.

5.2. Recall of Stressful Life Events

One important area of study in AIDS mental health research is stressful life events. Over the past two decades, many studies have examined the relationship between stressful life events and disruptions of physical or mental health (Lazarus and Folkman, 1984; Thoits, 1983). Because chronic stress and social disruption have been associated with suppression of immune function (O'Leary, 1990), several investigators have begun to examine the possible role of life events in the development and progression of AIDS.

Unfortunately, the evidence concerning the reliability and validity of life stress reports is not encouraging. Although many of these problems can be attributed to the inherent inaccuracy of category checklists (Raphael *et al.*, 1991), recall errors also play an important role. In one study that used college students, Klein and Rubovits (1987) had subjects complete a stressful event checklist (Sarason *et al.*, 1978) every 5 weeks for 5 months. Subjects were then asked to complete the same checklist for the entire 5-month period. Agreement between the concurrent (5-week) and retrospective reports occurred for only 52% of the event categories. One of the most surprising findings from this study concerned the reporting of deaths among family members. Ten deaths were reported, but only four were reported at both a 5-week and the 5-month assessment.

The Klein and Rubovits study did provide some data that were encouraging for those interested in conducting methodological research on reporting accuracy. One concern about test–retest studies is the possibility that reliability and validity are overestimated because participants have recorded ongoing events so that investigators can later verify retrospective reports. Keeping a diary may encourage rehearsal and elaborate encoding, and therefore increase subsequent memory performance. Memory performance at the final retrospective assessment might be misleading for another reason. Subjects may simply recall their previous reporting of an event rather than the event itself.

Fortunately, Klein and Rubovits included a control group that completed only the final, retrospective assessment. They found that the number and type of events reported by the control group did not differ significantly from those of the other study participants.

One of the most significant problems in this type of research is "falloff," which refers to the decrease in the number of events reported as more distal time periods are used. Falloff has frequently been documented in studies that use test–retest methods for assessing retrospective reporting reliability (e. g., Casey *et al.*, 1967). One study that utilized a national probability sample found that falloff was rapid for the previous 12 months, but began to level off afterward (Funch and Marshall, 1984). Although the falloff phenomenon is consistent with the well-documented relationship between passage of time and memory performance, telescoping may also contribute to falloff. Despite the gloomy picture, partial remedies are available. Research has shown that falloff can be decreased through an interviewer's use of extensive probes (Brown and Harris, 1982).

5.3. Recall of Sexual Behaviors

Catania *et al.* (1990) reviewed what little research there is concerning the validity of self-reported sexual behavior. The main barrier against validity research in this domain is verification. Some investigators have interviewed sex partners as a means of assessing the validity of self-reports (e. g., Coates *et al.*, 1988). When Coates *et al.* (1988) compared reports of AIDS cases with reports of healthy partners, the cases reported more risky activities than did their partners. The investigators suggested that partners may have been motivated to forget risky activities to preserve the assumption that they were uninfected. But without true verification, this interpretation is simply speculation.

Test–retest studies can suggest some of the variables that are likely to affect reporting accuracy. Test–retest coefficients may vary substantially across different sex behaviors and across different ethnic groups. Saltzman *et al.* (1987) examined test–retest reliability among 116 gay males who utilized a community health center. The median test–retest interval was slightly less than 5 weeks. Analyses revealed moderate levels of reliability on most of the measures. For example, participants were asked to report the frequency of insertive anal intercourse without a condom during the previous 6 months. Responses were coded into five categories from "never" to "four or more times per week." The percentage agreement for the two answers was 66% (kappa = 0.53). Items that asked about perceived change were less reliable than measures of frequency.

Unfortunately, no useful biological indices for relevant sexual behavior are available. Given that an assessment of recall errors depends on the availability of an effective verification procedure, very little can be said about the actual extent of memory failures in studies of sexual behavior. The paucity of research on validity in this domain should decrease within the next few years as more test–retest findings are reported from cohort studies now under way.

5.4. Recall of Everyday Events

Research on memory for everyday events is unfamiliar to most public health investigators, despite the fact that it is highly relevant to the study of health behavior. In contrast to research on stressful life events and sexual behavior, studies of everyday event memory have provided several important insights that may prove extremely useful for the study of AIDS risk behavior. Some of the most interesting work has been conducted by investigators who used themselves in longitudinal single-subject designs.

One example of single-subject research was reported by Linton (1982), who studied her own memory for 6 years. She wrote down two events every day. Every month she tested her memory of two events that were randomly selected from the entire diary. The test required Linton to estimate the chronological order of the two events and the dates of the two events. One of the interesting findings from this study was that Linton had no recollection whatsoever of many of the events she later read about in her diary. She also found that memories for more recent events seemed to be organized chronologically, but that memories for more distant events were organized categorically, especially when they occurred frequently (e. g., chores, meetings, meals). These frequent events blended together and could not be distinguished from one another. This suggests that older memories for everyday events are more likely to be integrated into semantic memory; therefore, specific information about dates is not remembered but inferred (e. g., "In those days, I usually had meetings on Mondays").

Wagenaar (1986) conducted a similar study of everyday memory. He recorded *who, what, where,* and *when* for each of 2400 events, and rated each events, commonality, emotionality, and pleasantness. To test himself, he provided one cue (e. g., *what* information) and then tried to fill in the other information about the event. He found that recall could be improved by providing himself with additional cues. Pleasant events were remembered better than unpleasant ones (see also Matlin and Stang, 1978). Uncommon and emotionally involving events were also more likely to be remembered. Of all the memory cues, *when* (providing a date) was the least effective and *what* was the most effective. In other words, when he was reminded first of a specific event or behavior, it was easier to fill in information about where and with whom it happened. On the other hand, only a few landmark events were precisely dated in memory (see Cohen, 1989, for further discussion of auto-biographical memory research).

More recent studies of everyday events have been more comprehensive in their approach. One of the most informative was conducted by Skowronski et al. (1991). Sixty-seven subjects recorded one event daily for 10 weeks. As they recorded the event, subjects rated it for pleasantness and typicality for that person. The study also incorporated an unusual feature. Subjects kept a second event diary in which they recorded events for a second person who they saw frequently. This allowed the investigators to test whether the variables studied affected self memories differently than memories concerning others.

The findings replicated and extended the earlier research. Pleasant events were more likely to be recalled than were unpleasant events, but this effect was limited to self events. Both pleasant and unpleasant events were recalled significantly better than neutral events. Events that were atypical for the person were recalled better than typical ones. Women were somewhat better than men in remembering the date of an event, and self events were dated more accurately than other events. Although subjects were generally poor at dating events, the more an individual could remember about an event, the more able he or she was to reconstruct the date accurately.

What can we say about AIDS survey methods based on the literature on everyday events? First, it appears that pleasant events may be disproportion-ately represented in memory-based self-reports. Because emotionally signifi-cant events are recalled better than neutral ones, it may make sense to assess this factor at the time of recall. This may be especially important for sexual encounters. We should point out, however, that some data suggest that emo-tionality is a more important factor among young adults than among older adults. For older adults, the best-remembered events seem to be those that they have thought about or discussed the most (Cohen and Faulkner, 1988).

Second, it is clear that questions that require a respondent to date events that are not highly unusual or significant measure a respondent's guessing strategy rather than his or her experience. This guessing strategy may simply reflect an individual's self-concept, which can include both accurate and in-accurate beliefs about how their behavior has changed over time. Memory research also suggests that retrieval cues other than dates should be used more often in surveys. Often, investigators have access to objective data that can be used as landmarks or retrieval cues. For example, important events that have verifiable dates could be used to ask a respondent about events that occurred before or after the event (rather than the date of the event). The Wagenaar (1986) study described above suggests other aspects of events that might be used as memory cues.

6. ETHICAL ISSUES IN STUDYING AIDS-RELATED MEMORY

In addition to the general ethical issues discussed elsewhere in this volume (Stevenson *et al.*), the study of AIDS-related memories raises some unique ethical concerns. Research on memory has shown that emotion plays a complex role in the organization and retrieval of personal memories (Bower, 1981). Ever since Freud developed his theory of repression, many have assumed that distressing memories are often held below awareness in order to prevent the anxiety associated with them. If this is true, then testing and applying techniques to enhance memory may have some negative consequences for study participants.

Consider a survey respondent whose closest lover died of AIDS. The respondent now seems to have largely recovered from this trauma, and he is getting on with his life. For this particular individual, coping well means not remembering or thinking about this important relationship that ended tragically. Along comes the zealous survey researcher who is determined to apply the latest techniques for enhancing the accuracy of this respondent's memory for AIDS-related behaviors and exposure. After the interviewer applies these techniques and obtains the desired responses, the relationship between the interviewer and interviewee ends. Now the respondent is left with rekindled emotions, vivid recollections, and a renewed sense of loss and despair.

Is this a realistic scenario? Anecdotal reports from survey administrators indicate that questions upset respondents less often than many critics assume. Unfortunately, we don't have a lot of good data to address this question. Most of the accounts of traumatic memory and its rejuvenation come from clinical case reports. Although some evidence suggests that a mechanism like repression may operate in the human memory system (Erdelyi, 1985), we know very little about the effects of uncovering "repressed" memories. We raise the issue here not to alarm investigators but to suggest that the immediate and delayed impact of intrusive questioning about sensitive matters are poorly understood and are worthy of further study.

7. RESEARCH NEEDS

Clearly, memory failures play a critical role in the validity of AIDS research. This is troubling both for mental health investigators and for those concerned with the etiology of the disease itself. As Catania *et al.* (1990) have noted, ". . . important behavioral routes of HIV transmission might be overlooked because of recall problems that increase measurement error and, therefore, reduce the statistical significance of such routes in models predicting HIV transmission" (p. 345).

What kinds of methodological research on AIDS-related reports would be most useful at this juncture? The biggest gaps appear in the domain of sexual behaviors. One of the lessons learned from methodological research in nutritional epidemiology is that you can't assume that people have encoded all the relevant information in the first place. What study participant ever expected to be asked about the amount of broccoli they consumed or their use of butter and cooking oil? As we mentioned earlier, respondents often develop strategies for inferring past behaviors based, in part, on their knowledge of current behaviors and their memory of preferences and patterns (Bradburn et al., 1987; Croyle et al., 1992). This isn't all bad, for many case–control studies have found that even inferred "memories" can result in a reasonably accurate report. We should keep in mind, however, that many respondents who attempt to recall the frequency of a complex pattern of sexual behaviors may be engaging similar inference strategies that we need to be familiar with. Once the most effective strategies are determined, they can be provided to a respondent by the interviewer.

Given that verification of sexual behavior reports is usually impossible, how can we design studies to examine the role of bias and error? Research in other domains of health memory has shown that a great deal can be learned by examining the relative impact of psychological variables on memory-based reports. Catania et al. (1990) suggest several: the relative frequency of the behavior, emotions associated with one's sexual partner, and the number of different partners, among others. We believe that the test–retest methodology that has been used so frequently in other domains holds promise in the AIDS domain. Unfortunately, most of the reliability studies concerning sexual behavior published so far have not asked respondents to report on the same reference period. Low correlations between test and retest could indicate a poor instrument, a change in sexual behavior, poor memory, or any combination of the three.

Earlier we discussed research concerning the effects of leading questions on memory. Memory itself can be changed when a respondent is asked questions that imply facts about an event that are untrue. This means that survey questions must be carefully checked for underlying assumptions. One way to examine the long-term impact of questions on AIDS-related memory would be to vary the presence of questions within a diary study. When later retrospective assessments are obtained, the investigator could test whether frequently repeated questions produce retrospective reports that are different than less frequently used questions.

Given the promising findings from other research on health-related memory, we suggest a two-pronged approach to addressing problems in risk behavior assessment. Research on the role of memory in AIDS-related surveys should focus not only on documenting its failures but also on improving its performance. Therefore, test–retest studies should include imbedded experiments that test both old and new methods for helping people retrieve and report accurate AIDS-related information. The best experiments will be those that are derived from widely accepted theories of memory and information processing. Theoretically based tests of different question strategies are more cost-effective and efficient than the atheoretical trial-and-error experiments so often reported in previous research.

Research on health-related memory has focused on three content areas: doctor–patient communication, dietary behavior, and health events. All three bodies of research have documented substantial problems in memory performance. Nevertheless, some progress has been made in all three domains toward understanding and improving memory performance. Patients' memories of physician communications can be improved by increasing the message's organization and simplicity (Ley, 1982). Dietary recall can be improved through the use of probes, decomposition, and context reinstatement (Fisher and Quigley, 1992). Memory for health events can be improved through the use of multiple time frames, decomposition, and landmarks (Loftus *et al.,* 1990). All of these domains were at one time characterized by frustrated investigators faced with seemingly intractable problems of measurement. Although the process has been a slow and painful one, each domain has manifested significant progress toward conquering the enemies of good memory.

Now we are faced with a new problem to which we can apply the theories and methods of cognitive psychology. This challenge is surely to be our greatest challenge yet. Given the extensive behavioral AIDS research already under way, understanding and improving memory for AIDS-related behaviors and symptoms is a goal that can't be achieved too soon. Survey methodologists and cognitive psychologists have shown what they can do when they join efforts. By combining our efforts with those of the public health research community, we can do our part in the fight against AIDS.

ACKNOWLEDGMENTS. The authors acknowledge the support of grants HS 05521 from the National Center for Health Services Research and Health Care Technology Assessment, HS 06660 from the Agency for Health Care Policy and Research, and MH43097 from the National Institute of Mental Health.

REFERENCES

Abelson, R. P., Loftus, E. F., and Greenwald, A. G. (1992). Attempts to improve the accuracy of self-reports of voting. In J. Tanur (ed.), *Questions about survey questions: Meaning, memory, expression, and social interactions in surveys.* New York: Russell Sage.

Bower, G. (1981). Mood and memory. *Am. Psychol.* **6**:129–148.

Bradburn, N. M., Rips, L. J., and Shevell, S. K. (1987). Answering autobiographical questions: The impact of memory and inference on surveys. *Science* **236**:157–161.

Brown, G. W., and Harris, T. (1982). Fall-off in the reporting of life events. *Soc. Psychiatry* **17**: 23–28.

Casey, R. L., Masuda, M., and Holmes, T. H. (1967). Quantitative study of recall of life events. *J. Psychosom. Res.* **11**:239–247.

Catania, J. A., Gibson, D. R., Chitwood, D. D., and Coates, T. J. (1990). Methodological problems in AIDS behavioral research: Influences on measurement error and participation bias in studies of sexual behavior. *Psychol. Bull.* **108**:339–362.

Coates, R. A., Calzavara, L. M., Soskolne, C. L., Read, S. E., Fanning, M. M., Shepherd, F. A., Klein, M. H., and Johnson, J. K. (1988). Validity of sexual histories in a prospective study of male sexual contacts of men with AIDS or AIDS-related condition. *Am. J. Epidemiol.* **128**:719–728.

Cohen, G. (1989). *Memory in the real world.* Hillsdale, NJ: Erlbaum.

Cohen, G., and Faulkner, D. (1988). The effects of ageing on perceived and generated memories. In L. W. Poon, D. C. Rubin, and B. Wilson (eds.), *Cognition in adulthood and later life.* London: Cambridge University Press.

Croyle, R. T., Loftus, E. F., Klinger, M. R., and Smith, K. D. (1992). Reducing errors in health-related memory: Progress and prospects. *Information and Behavior* Brunwick, NJ: Transachon Books, Vol. 4, pp. 255–268.

Darke, S., Hall, W., Heather, N., Ward, J., and Wodak, A. (1991). The reliability and validity of a scale to measure HIV risk-taking behaviour among intravenous drug users. *AIDS* **5**:181–185.

Davis, P. (1987). Exploring the kingdom of AIDS. *New York Times Magazine,* May 31.

Erdelyi, M. H. (1985). *Psychoanalysis: Freud's cognitive psychology.* San Francisco: Freeman.

Fisher, R. P., and Quigley, K. L. (1992). Applying cognitive theory in public health investigations: Enhancing food recall with the cognitive interview. In J. Tanur (ed.), *Questions about survey questions: Meaning, memory expression, and social interaction in surveys.* New York: Russell Sage.

Funch, D. P., and Marshall, J. R. (1984). Measuring life stress: Factors affecting fall-off in the reporting of life events. *J. Health Soc. Behav.* **25**:453–464.

Gallo, R. C. (1990). My life stalking AIDS. *Discover* (Special Issue).

Garofalo, J., and Hindelang, M. J. (1977). *An introduction to the National Crime Survey.* Washington, D.C.: U.S. Department of Justice.

Jabine, T. B. (1987). Reporting chronic conditions in the National Health Interview Survey, a review of tendencies from evaluation studies and methodological studies. *Vital and health statistics,* Series 2, No. 105 (DHHS Publ. PHS 87-1379). Washington, D.C.: U.S. Government Printing Office.

Jobe, J. B., White, A. A., Kelley, C. L., Mingay, D. J., Sanchez, M. J., and Loftus, E. F. (1990). Recall strategies and memory for health care visits. *Milbank Q.* **68**:171–189.

Klein, D. N., and Rubovits, D. R. (1987). The reliability of subjects' reports of life events inventories: A longitudinal study. *J. Behav. Med.* **10**:501–512.

Lazarus, R. S., and Folkman, S. (1984). *Stress, appraisal, and coping.* Berlin: Springer.

Ley, P. (1982). Giving information to patients. In J. R. Eiser (ed.), *Social psychology and behavioral medicine.* New York: Wiley, pp. 339–373.

Linton, M. (1982). Transformations of memory in everyday life. In U. Neisser (ed.), *Memory observed: Remembering in natural contexts.* San Francisco: Freeman, pp. 77–91.

Loftus, E. F. (1979). The malleability of human memory. *Am. Sci.* **67**:312–320.

Loftus, E. F. (1982). Memory and its distortions. In A. G. Krant (ed.), *G. Stanley Hall Lectures.* Washington, DC: APA Press, pp. 119–154.

Loftus, E. F., Klinger, M. R., Smith, K. D., and Fiedler, J. (1990). A tale of two questions: Benefits of asking more than one question. *Public Opinion Q.* **54**:330–345.

Loftus, E. F., Smith, K., Klinger, M., and Fiedler, J. (1992). Memory and mismemory for health events. In J. M. Tanur (ed.), *Questions about survey questions: Meaning, memory, expression, and social interactions in surveys.* New York: Russell Sage.

Lunn, S., Skydsbjerg, M., Schulsinger, H., Parnas, J., Pederson, C., and Mathiesen, L. (1991). A preliminary report on the neuropsychologic sequelae of human immunodeficiency virus. *Arch. Gen. Psychiatry* **48**:139–142.

Matlin, M. W., and Stang, D. J. (1978). *The Pollyanna principle.* Cambridge, Mass.: Schenkman.

Means, B., and Loftus, E. F. (1991). When personal history repeats itself: Decomposing memories for recurrent events. *Appl. Cogn. Psychol.* **5**:297–318.

Means, B., Mingay, D. J., Nigam, A., and Zarrow, M. (1988). A cognitive approach to enhancing health survey reports of medical visits. In M. M. Gruneberg, P. E. Morris, and R. N. Sykes (eds.), *Practical aspects of memory: Current research and issues.* New York: Wiley, Vol. 1, pp. 537–542.

Navia, B. A., Jordan, B. D., and Price, R. W. (1986). The AIDS dementia complex, I: Clinical features. *Ann. Neurol.* **19**:517–524.

Neisser, U. (1986). Nested structure in autobiographical memory. In D. C. Rubin (ed.), *Autobiographical memory.* London: Cambridge University Press, pp. 71–81.

O'Leary, A. (1990). Stress, emotion, and human immune function. *Psychol. Bull.* **108**:363–382.

Public Health Service (1965). *Reporting of hospitalization in the health interview survey.* Washington, D.C.: U.S. Government Printing Office (DHEW-HSM Publication No. 73-1261).

Raphael, K. G., Cloitre, M., and Dohrenwend, B. P. (1991). Problems of recall and misclassification with checklist methods of measuring stressful life events. *Health Psychol.* **10**:62–74.

Roediger, H. L., Capaldi, E. D., Paris, S. G., and Polivy, J. (1991). *Psychology,* 3rd ed. New York: Harper Collins.

Ross, M. (1989). Relation of implicit theories to the construction of personal histories. *Psychol. Rev.* **96**:341–357.

Rubin, D. C., and Kozin, M. (1984). Vivid memories. *Cognition* **16**:81–95.

Saltzman, S. P., Stoddard, A. M., McCusker, J., Moon, M. W., and Mayer, K. H. (1987). Reliability of self-reported sexual behavior risk factors for HIV infection in homosexual men. *Public Health Rep.* **102**:692–697.

Sarason, I. G., Johnson, J. H., and Siegel, J. M. (1978). Assessing the impact of life changes: Development of the Life Experiences Survey. *J. Clin. Consult. Psychol.* **46**:932–946.

Schneider, A. L., Griffith, W. R., Sumi, D. H., and Burcart, J. M. (1978). *Portland forward record check of crime victims.* Washington, D.C.: U.S. Department of Justice.

Skowronski, J. J., Betz, A. L., Thompson, C. P., and Shannon, L. (1991). Social memory in everyday life: Recall of self-events and other-events. *J. Pers. Soc. Psychol.* **60**:831–843.

Thoits, P. A. (1983). Dimensions of life events that influence psychological distress: An evaluation and synthesis of the literature. In H. Kaplan (ed.), *Psychosocial stress: Trends in theory and research.* New York: Academic Press, pp. 33–103.

Tulving, E. (1972). Episodic and semantic memory. In E. Tulving and W. Donaldson (eds.), *Organization of memory.* New York: Academic Press, pp. 381–403.

Tulving, E. (1983). *Elements of episodic memory.* London: Oxford University Press.

Wagenaar, W. (1986). My memory: A study of autobiographical memory over six years. *Cogn. Psychol.* **18**:225–252.

Wu, M. L., Whittemore, A. S., and Jung, D. L. (1988). Errors in reported dietary intakes. *Am. J. Epidemiol.* **128**:1137–1145.

Comments on Croyle and Loftus's Recollections in the Kingdom of AIDS

ROBYN M. DAWES

What they say is, of course, correct. The problem is to use their insights and results to answer the question that the late Clyde Coombs characterized as the basic philosophical question: "What do we do next?" Memories are inaccurate. Moreover, this inaccuracy relates not just to random processes, but also to systematic ones that can be specified, described, and studied—and that have predictable results. Therefore, AIDS researchers who gather retrospective reports of behavior should do what?

In his recent American Psychological Society address, Ebbe Ebbesen (1991) suggested that the generic answer to this question should be "nothing." After pointing out that the success of physics stems in large part from good measurement—of independent and dependent variables—that permits generalization from what happens in laboratory situations to those outside, he argued that in the absence of such measurement, it is inappropriate to generalize to "real world" problems (e. g., in courtroom settings) from our theory-driven experimental results (where "theory" often predicts merely the direction

ROBYN M. DAWES • Department of Social and Decision Sciences, Carnegie Mellon University, Pittsburgh, Pennsylvania 15213.

Methodological Issues in AIDS Behavioral Research, edited by David G. Ostrow and Ronald C. Kessler. Plenum Press, New York, 1993.

of our results). Reading Croyle and Loftus, we find no measurement of the independent variables, while the measurement of the dependent variables involves crude indices of recall accuracy, often changing from study to study. Moreover, even in those studies devoted to the control of effects (e. g., of forward telescoping by asking a previous question about a longer time interval), the effects are purely directional. If we were to agree with Ebbesen, we might just give up worrying about recall inaccuracy in the kingdom of AIDS, at least for the next couple hundred years, by which time the problem may have resolved itself—one way or another.

Another approach is to measure the effects of variables somewhat arbitrarily assessed in terms of their statistical effects; then, no matter where the numbers come from, we can state that *certeris paribus* certain variables "account for" certain amounts of change in others. (The standard analysis of a regression equation, for example, does not involve the meaning of the independent and dependent variables, but how much of a change in the dependent is brought about by unit changes in each of the independent ones.) Unfortunately, however, the generalization of statistical results involves strong assumptions—most particularly that the *same* population is randomly sampled on multiple occasions. But we're interested in different parts of the river, and in the same part at different times. When taken literally, the assumption that we are sampling from a well-specified population—let alone the assumption that we can generalize to the population parameters, or to new samples on the assumption that both samples are truly random—is ludicrous in most of the contexts we study. I mean the term "ludicrous" literally. Yet we trudge ahead with our t tests, our p values, and our eta squares to demonstrate the existence and magnitudes of our effects. If we're statistically sophisticated, we can point out that the standard statistical assumptions are sufficient to guarantee the validity of our inferences but are not necessary. So we do what? Take the results on faith?* And then there is still the lingering problem of a population from which we're sampling, which is reasonable only in such contexts as the random sampling of voting intentions of potential voters. Ebbesen is at least one-up on this approach. In accepting the Newtonian definition of mass as the ratio of force to the acceleration of a body in a frictionless atmosphere unperturbed by other gravitational forces, we at least don't have to worry about specifying the population of such atmospheres

---

* Most researchers evaluate the statistical assumptions with the data itself by performing various "tests" of the "goodness" of these assumptions about the population sampled. They then worry only if the data itself leads to the rejection of one or more of these assumptions. Because the standard rejection criterion is the demonstration of a "significant" violation of an assumption, such a procedure misuses the logic of the significance test. In effect, it involves accepting a *specific* null hypothesis on the basis of a failure to reject it.

(denotatively, i. e., other than by definition), and we certainly don't have to worry about how to sample randomly from them (and we *do* have good definitions and measurements of "force" and "acceleration.")

I would like to suggest that neither the measurement nor the statistical models are correct for *our* field, and for this reason the work summarized by Croyle and Loftus Croyle is quite valuable in it. What we have is consistency across *qualitatively diverse contexts.* Moreover, this consistency yields generalizations about memory—even though these generalizations are often expressed with mere words. Now of course a lot of verbal description in social science is pure junk ("words, words, words"—Hamlet), because when the phenomenon is examined without the words, it either disintegrates or turns into a platitude believed by our great-great-grandmothers (many of which may also—like them—disintegrate if viewed in too harsh a light). But here, we have some pretty good distinctions about what will affect memory and how, at least in terms of predicting the existence, direction, and occasionally the relative magnitude of inaccuracy.

As I have argued elsewhere (Dawes, 1992), this consistency across qualitatively diverse contexts may be the best goal in our "science." My prime example was the consistency in comparing statistical prediction versus clinical prediction. If statistical prediction were superior to clinical *only* in predicting academic success, or future violence, or parole violation, or business bankruptcy, or final psychiatric diagnosis, or marital happiness, etc., then we would not be so impressed. (At least, I would not be.) But when we find a uniformity in the comparison of prediction modes across a variety of human outcomes (Dawes *et al.,* 1989), we are impressed. We are especially impressed when we find that there are no exceptions except in areas in which the clinical prediction is based on more (often much more) information than is the statistical one, and that these exceptions occur only in the areas of medicine and business. (In psychology, apparently, more is less.) Moreover, we find this consistency despite different measures used in the various studies to assess even variables claimed to be "the same" (through a verbal definition), and across time when in fact "the population" changes—if ever it were originally well-specified, except trivially as the sample in the context studied.

I have suggested that we regard each study (not each subject in each) as a sample of $n = 1$, but even then we are faced immediately again with the question of specifying the population from which we're sampling (and certainly not randomly). What is "the population of judgment tasks predicting human outcomes?" [Critics of the results often want to include chess, or hypothetical studies in clinical psychology not yet conducted involving sufficient "ecological validity" to allow "really" expert clinicians to demonstrate what they "really" can do, while ignoring the studies that have actually been conducted in which they really can't; for an example of the latter suggestion, see Matarazzo's

(1990) defense of the "psychological portraits" he presents in courtrooms, which must be valid because simple predictions and categorizations previously presented in courtrooms aren't.] I have no answer to this nagging question. We're left with the same problem that we face when we agree with people that every judgment must be made "in context," but neither we nor the people giving the advice know exactly which of the multiple possible contexts in which each judgment is embedded should be considered. Nevertheless, this search for consistency across diversity does exist and forms the basis of our generalizations—many of which turn out to be correct when examined! I think we should accept that approach, just as (to come back to Ebbesen) physicists accepted their field long before Bridgman decided it was based on operational definitions or Campbell specified how measurement had a firm basis in concatenation.

So accepting the generalizations as valid, we can ask what they imply about memory in the AIDS kingdom. Application neither through precise measurement nor through direct statistical generalization is possible. Thus, what I propose is a *direct* study to determine the effects of the systematic inaccuracies discussed by Croyle and Loftus on subjects' retrospective recall of behaviors relevant to the spread of HIV. Here, I endorse the view that "inaccuracy" is defined relative to some purpose; that is, simply knowing, for example, that a particular type of event may be telescoped by—on the average—X months is important only to the extent that it affects the *conclusions* of a researcher asking subjects to recall this event. As, for example, Croyle and Loftus write at one point about inference effects in memory: "This isn't all bad, for many case–control studies have found that even inferred 'memories' can discriminate between large study groups." The question is, of course, whether a particular purpose of the research is to discriminate between such groups. Diet is an excellent example. Peoples' recall of dietary input over the previous 2 weeks is influenced by their habitual eating habits (Smith *et al.,* 1991). If, however, the purpose of the researcher in collecting recall for the previous 2 weeks is to discriminate between groups with different dietary habits, such an influence does not result in a "bad" inaccuracy. In fact, it may even be desirable!

What I propose is first to have the most active AIDS researchers who base conclusions on retrospective memory (e. g., through surveys) meet and reach some agreement (not necessarily a clear or unanimous one) on what they desire to learn from collecting reports based on such memory. Then, a large study of the relevant populations should be conducted in which the subjects are asked to report behaviors on a continuing basis—e. g., through repeated surveys of a brief former time period or through diary. The behaviors reported would be those of most importance to the researchers' potential conclusions. Then these same subjects would be surveyed on a retrospective basis for the same time periods, perhaps by people who are not easily identified with those collecting the original concurrent reports. Thus, the systematic discrepancies—*and their importance for potential conclusions*—can be assessed directly.

The actual design of this prospective/retrospective study cannot, however, be quite that simple. As Croyle and Loftus point out: (1) making systematic reports may affect behavior and (2) recall may be to some extent of the reports made rather than of the behavior itself. To determine the possible effects of report making on behavior, it is necessary to have a comparison group (C_1) that makes retrospective reports alone. The possible effect of recalling the reports rather than the behavior must be assessed by *two* additional comparison groups. The first (C_2) engages in retrospective recall *first* and provides concurrent behavioral reports *later*. That would appear to be a strange activity were it not for the third comparison group (C_3) that provides concurrent reports at both points in time, i. e., both at the time the major group provides them and at the time comparison group C_2 does. This C_3 group does not provide retrospective reports at all, but does provide the researchers with an estimate of how intra- and interindividually *consistent* the behavior is across the two time periods. What can then be assessed is the accuracy and bias of the people in group C_2 by comparing its members' reports of the previous

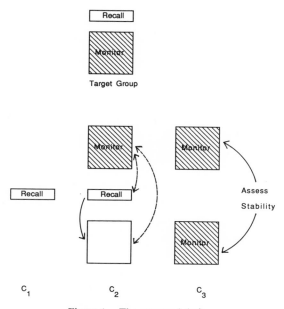

Figure 1. The proposed design.

time period with their subsequent concurrent reports in light of the knowledge of this consistency. (The comparison is analogous to partial correlation, and may in fact use partial correlation techniques.) The reports of those in C_2 are, however, "uncontaminated" by having made the previous concurrent reports. This design is presented in Fig. 1.

That's it. The "methodologists' joy" is to suggest what others should— or might profitably—do, without doing it themselves. In this instance, what others could do would cost millions. I suggest that because survey researchers and many others in the kingdom of AIDS research are compelled to use retrospective recall in much of their work, these would be millions well spent. My suggestion is unbiased by any concerns that I might wish to receive any money to do such a study myself.

REFERENCES

Dawes, R. M. (1992). Comment: Quandary: Correlation coefficients and contexts. In L. Montada, S. H. Filipp, and M. J. Lerner (eds.), *Life crises and experiences of loss in adulthood.* Hillsdale, N.J.: Erlbaum, pp. 521–529.

Dawes, R. M., Faust, D., and Meehl, P. E. (1989). Clinical versus actuarial judgment. *Science* **243**:1668–1674.

Ebbesen, E. (June 16, 1991). Talk presented at the Annual Meeting of the American Psychological Society, Washington, D.C.

Matarazzo, J. (September, 1990). Presidential address: Psychological assessment versus psychological testing. *Am. Psychol.* **45**(9):999–1017.

Smith, A. F., Jobe, J. B., and Mingay, D. J. (1991). Retrieval from memory of dietary information. *Appl. Cogn. Psychol.,* Vol. 5, 269–296.

III

Analysis and Modeling Issues

Using Surveillance Data for Assessing and Projecting the AIDS Epidemic

VICTOR DE GRUTTOLA and MARCELLO PAGANO

1. INTRODUCTION

Systems for surveillance of AIDS exist in the United States and other countries. Since 1982, the Centers for Disease Control (CDC) has collected information on AIDS cases concerning dates of AIDS diagnosis and report, diseases present, demographics, risk factors for transmission, HIV antibody test, and date of death. The CDC provides public use data sources that enable investigators to explore their own hypotheses concerning epidemic trends; although the geographic information only describes the region in which the AIDS case occurred, no specific information about states or cities is available. Nonetheless, the public-access data permit analyses of trends in incidence of AIDS over time and by region or risk category as well as analyses of survival after AIDS diagnosis. Using surveillance data bases requires sophisticated analyses; even seemingly straightforward comparisons, such as rates of growth of the epidemic by sex or risk category, require complex methods. The reason for this is that changes over time in the definition of AIDS, in reporting lag, or in treatment have a profound effect on estimates of trends. In this report, we consider these problems in detail as well as ways to adjust for them in analyses of surveillance data.

VICTOR DE GRUTTOLA and MARCELLO PAGANO • Department of Biostatistics, Harvard School of Public Health, Boston, Massachusetts 02115.

Methodological Issues in AIDS Behavioral Research, edited by David G. Ostrow and Ronald C. Kessler. Plenum Press, New York, 1993.

Surveillance data bases are unique in that they attempt to cover entire populations; the AIDS surveillance data base collected by the CDC contains information on over 180,000 cases. Because of a recent change that includes having a CD4 count below $200/mm^3$ in the AIDS case definition, Dr. James Curran of the CDC has projected that this number could soon double (quoted by Mireya Navarro, 1991). The problem with such data, however, is that they arise from many different systems for collection involving many different agencies. Therefore, the quality of such data is likely to be highly variable. Analytical methods must be robust to the uncertainty in data quality and must take into account the heterogeneity in completeness and reporting lag over regions, time, or patient characteristics. Although problems arise because of such variability, people who are likely to be excluded from coverage in a surveillance data base are also likely (perhaps even more likely) to be excluded from other sources of information such as clinical trials.

2. AIDS DEFINITION

Surveillance of AIDS is complicated by the fact that the progression of HIV disease is extremely heterogeneous; there are many pathologies related to HIV that vary greatly in severity and prognosis. The AIDS case definition was chosen for its specificity; public health officials attempted to limit the definition to conditions that could not have any other cause besides HIV. As a result, the AIDS definition is not based on the degree of severity of disease. Kaposi's sarcoma, which has always been an AIDS-defining condition, may be fairly benign and treatable, whereas life-threatening pulmonary tuberculosis was not AIDS defining until 1993. In addition, the definition has changed on two occasions prior to 1993 (1985 and September, 1987) to include new conditions as well as presumptive diagnosis of conditions that had previously required laboratory confirmation (CDC, 1987). The 1985 change in definition had relatively little impact on AIDS incidence, but the 1987 change had a substantial effect since 8–12% of AIDS cases diagnosed among men who have sex with men in 1988–89 met only the new conditions (Karon and Berkelman, 1991). In addition, the new conditions such as wasting and dementia had a greater effect on people infected with HIV through i.v. drug use than through homosexual contact. The consequence is that the diagnosis of AIDS is not based on a single type of biological event, but on the first of many possible events. Thus, the time until AIDS diagnosis must be seen as a problem of competing risks, each of which varies over time since infection and chronologic time. The risks are affected by secular trends, such as the decline in incidence of Kaposi's sarcoma, as well as by prophylactic treatments. In addition, the change in definition produces discontinuities in reporting. At the time of the change, prevalent as well as incident cases that meet the new definition may be reported. Therefore, before we can consider how to take into account the effect of changes in definition on analyses, we must first consider the effect of reporting delay under a constant definition.

3. REPORTING DELAY AND TIME TREND ANALYSIS

In order to estimate the time trend of any aspect of an epidemic, one must take into account the fact that cases of AIDS are not reported immediately, and that some cases are never reported at all. Delays in reporting can be a function of chronologic time of diagnosis (age of the epidemic), medical condition, geographic region, and risk group. We can accommodate the reporting delay by using only data that appear to be nearly complete, perhaps by considering only cases diagnosed 2 or more years prior to time of analysis. If we want to make inference about more recent trends, we must estimate the reporting delay distribution, and then augment the number of reported cases by the number that we expect to have been diagnosed but not yet reported. Of course, some cases will never be reported, but if this proportion is fixed, it will not affect the time trends (see discussion below).

One problem with estimating reporting delay is that the observed data on reporting arise from a right-truncated distribution, i. e., we are only aware of reporting delays that are shorter than the time from diagnosis to the time of analysis; we obviously don't know about cases that will be reported in the future. As a consequence, all attempts to compensate for the effect of reporting delay depend on some assumptions about the future, which are essentially extrapolations from the past. Under the assumption that the distribution is stationary over chronologic time, the estimation is straightforward (Lagakos *et al.,* 1988; Karon *et al.,* 1989). Because of changes over time in reporting systems, however, such as the change from passive to active surveillance or the use of death certificates in certain geographic regions, the reporting delay may depend on other factors; and this dependence must be modeled. Suggestions for how to model this dependence have been made by Brookmeyer and Liao (1990), Harris (1990), Pagano *et al.* (in press), and Kalbfleisch and Lawless (1991). The change in the reporting delay distribution over chronologic time may be one of the most important.

The methodologies mentioned above are all similar in that they require a model for the dependence of reporting on a factor such as chronologic time or region. One approach is a loglinear model to describe the dependence. We introduce the following notation: Let $p(t = j | z)$ be the probability of reporting at time j for covariate z (which may be chronologic time, region, risk group, etc.). We model the dependence of $p(t | z)$ as

$$p(t = j \,|\, z) = \exp(\eta_j(z))/\Sigma \, \exp(\eta_j(z))$$

where

$$\eta_j(z) = 0 \qquad \text{if } j = 0$$

$$\eta_j(z) = \alpha_j + z^T \beta_j \qquad \text{if } 1 \le j \le T$$

and α_j and β_j are the parameter vectors.

Lagakos *et al.* (1988), Kalbfleisch and Lawless (1991), and Brookmeyer and Liao (1990) consider transformation of the data so that right-truncated observations become left-truncated observations. The advantage of the approach by Pagano *et al.* (in press) is that data can be both truncated and censored. It also yields a more realistic estimate of the uncertainty and graphical diagnostics useful for model checking. It is related to the approach of Harris (1990) but differs in that the latter requires some constraints on the reporting distribution.

We display the results of the analyses of reporting trend for data reported through the end of 1990 to the CDC. Figure 1 shows the tendency for reporting delay to increase in the Northeast and West, but not in rural areas and in the South. Figures 2 and 3 show the similar regional trends for the major risk groups: men who have sex with men (MSM) and intravenous drug users (IVDU). Note that the reporting delay is greater in most regions for the IVDU

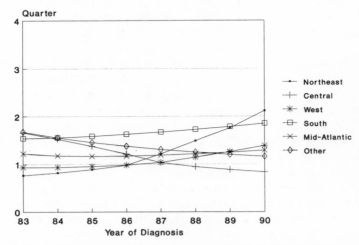

Figure 1. The medians of the reporting distributions for the total AIDS population: Northeast, Central, West, South, mid-Atlantic, and other (areas with population less than 1 million).

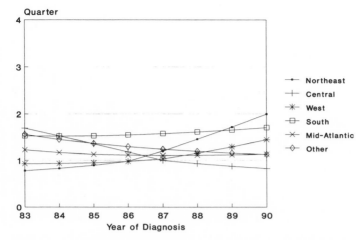

Figure 2.   The medians of the reporting distributions for the MSM risk group.

than for the MSM. Figure 4 shows the U.S. incidence of AIDS as adjusted by the time-invariant and the time-varying reporting delay estimates. Note that the correction for reporting delay that assumes that the delay distribution is stationary can give misleading results concerning current epidemic trends. Figures 5 and 6 show the incidence for MSM and IVDU adjusted in the two

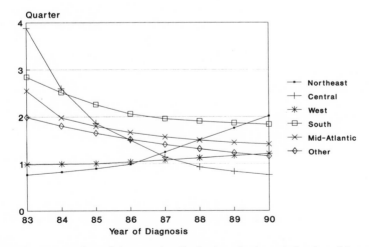

Figure 3.   The medians of the reporting distributions for the male i.v. drug risk group.

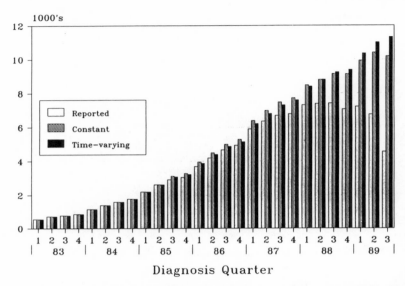

Figure 4. USA AIDS incidence by quarter of diagnosis. Clear bars show reported AIDS incidence; striped bars, AIDS incidence adjusting for a constant reporting delay; solid bars, AIDS incidence adjusting for a logistic (time-varying) reporting delay.

different ways. Figure 7 shows the reported incidence and the two kinds of adjusted incidence for New York City.

Regardless of which modeling approach is chosen, one must use whatever information one has about the nature of the reporting systems when compensating for reporting delay. Any anomalous period that can be recognized such as when a system was being changed should be noted; the delay data from these times might be handled differently, so that they would not contribute to long-term trends.

The approach to estimation of distributions that have arbitrary censoring and truncation is useful for estimating other distributions of interest such as survival after AIDS diagnosis (see below) or latency between infection and onset of disease for cases in which the infection time is known.

Change in Definition

Even if the definition had not changed, monitoring trends would present a challenge, but the combination of changes in definition, secular trends in reporting, and discontinuities in reporting resulting from the definitional change makes this problem very thorny. Compensating for the changes in

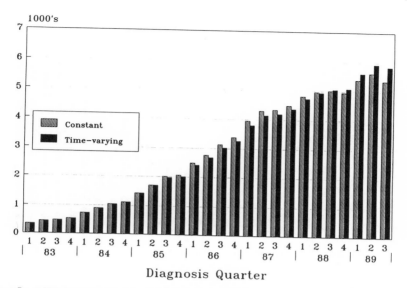

Figure 5. AIDS incidence by quarter of diagnosis for MSM. Striped bars show AIDS incidence adjusting for a constant reporting delay; solid bars, AIDS incidence adjusting for a logistic (time-varying) reporting delay.

definition requires modeling of the different competing risks, and we need more information to make development of such models possible. Projections are especially affected by such developments because they are sensitive to recent trends.

To describe the information that is needed to compensate for changes in definition, we introduce notation. The time of reporting of AIDS might be considered a convolution of three random variables:

$$a_{bc} = i + l + t$$

where i is the time of HIV infection, l is the time from infection to old-definition AIDS (ODA), and t is the reporting delay. After the change in definition, the time of reporting of AIDS is modeled as

$$a_{ac} = i + z + t$$

where $z = \min(l, m)$ and m is the time to conditions that meet the new but not the old definition of AIDS (NDA). In addition to AIDS reporting, surveillance also provides dates of death reporting,

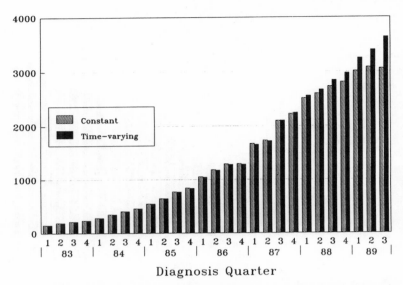

Figure 6. AIDS incidence by quarter of diagnosis for IVDU. Striped bars show AIDS incidence adjusting for a constant reporting delay; clear bars, AIDS incidence adjusting for a logistic (time-varying) reporting delay; solid bars, reported AIDS incidence.

$$d = a + s + t_d$$

where d is the time of death reporting, a is the time of AIDS diagnosis, s is the survival after AIDS diagnosis (by either new or old definition), and t_d is the death reporting delay.

There are two different ways that we can try to compensate for the change in definition. The first is to try to estimate what the incidence would have been, had the new definition of AIDS (NDA) been used from the start. This is equivalent to estimating the distribution of a_{ac} for the entire observation period, taking into account those individuals who died with NDA without ever developing ODA. The second is to estimate what the incidence after the change would have been had the old definition of AIDS remained in effect. This is equivalent to estimating the distribution of a_{bc} for the period after the change in definition. In either case, one needs estimates of the joint distribution $F(l, m, s \mid i, z)$. This distribution cannot be estimated from surveillance data alone, which only provide information on l (before the change) and z (afterward). In fact, accurate estimation would require a cohort followed since the start of the epidemic for ODA, NDA, and death, for whom at least some of the seroconversion times were known. Even then, we might not be sure that

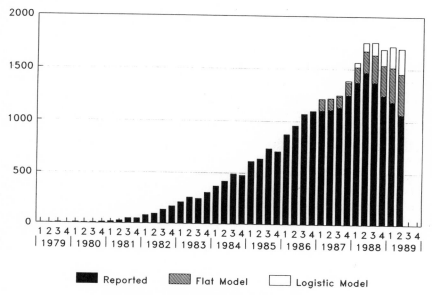

Figure 7. AIDS incidence for New York City.

the experience of such a cohort would generalize to populations as a whole. Surveillance data could be made more useful if dates of all three events (onset of NDA, onset of ODA, death) and reporting delays for these events were collected. In this case, one could try to estimate these probabilities from surveillance. The likelihood for such data would present a complex blend of censoring and truncation, but by making various assumptions about dependence on chronologic time, we might be able to estimate the relevant probabilities.

One simpler approach is to assume that the transition probabilities for the transitions shown graphically below have been stable over time. While this is unlikely to be completely true, it at least enables us to use some available, although incomplete, information.

$$HIV^+ \rightarrow NDA \rightarrow Death$$

In addition, one needs to know the effect of being diagnosed with NDA or ODA on reporting delay. A discontinuity in reporting probably occurred at the time of the change in definition, since there were undoubtedly prevalent as well as incident cases of NDA that were reported. This may have produced the unexpected high incidence in the last quarter of 1987 in New York, for example (Pagano *et al.*, 1992).

In the absence of such analysis, adjustment for reporting delay must be ad hoc; all we can really expect are analyses of sensitivity to different assumptions about the effect of the definitional change. Available data are sparse, but there is some useful information. One study of death certificates in New York City found that about 6% of the apparently HIV-related deaths in 1986 were from NDA with no mention of ODA (New York City Department of Health, personal communication). As stated above, it appears that among MSM, about 8–12% of cases of AIDS diagnosed in 1988–89 met only NDA conditions. From a cohort followed in San Francisco, it appears that about half of such people die before development of an ODA condition; the median time for development of such a disease was estimated to be 27 months (Karon and Berkelman, 1991). A rough adjustment accounting for the cases of NDA that never developed ODA before 1987 might be to augment the observed incidence of ODA before 1987 by a fixed percentage. To adjust for the fact that some of the cases of ODA developed NDA first, one might move a percentage of the ODA cases back in time.

The challenges in assessing epidemic trends are increased by the recent changes in the AIDS case definition to allow a CD4 count below $200/mm^3$. Since this definition requires monitoring of events with no clinical manifestations, it reflects individual medical choices more strongly than did the previous definition. Adjustment for the change in definition is complicated by the fact that the changes impact very differently on different demographic and risk groups.

One way to avoid the dependence on the AIDS definition for monitoring trends is to monitor death certificates. This requires consideration of the degree to which HIV caused death or contributed as an underlying cause of death. Only about 70 to 90% of people with life-threatening HIV infection were reported as AIDS cases in 1987 in New York, and this may be lower for IVDU (Stoneburner *et al.*, 1988).

4. SHORT-TERM PROJECTIONS

There are three different approaches to short-term projections. The first involves numerical extrapolation of AIDS incidence. This has the advantage of requiring no modeling assumptions about the epidemic, but has the disadvantage that it does not make use of other available information. In addition, it makes an implicit assumption that the mathematical form of the epidemic trend (e. g., polynomial, sigmoidal) is correct and will continue to be so in the future. A second approach arises from attempts to model the dynamics of the epidemic. This approach has the advantage of being able to incorporate all available information about the epidemic, but has the disadvantage that no comprehensive model of the epidemic exists, and if one did it would require estimation of an enormous number of parameters to be useful. In addition, there would not be a way to validate such a model.

For these reasons, the most useful way to make short-term projections may be to use a deconvolution or "back-calculation approach" first proposed by Brookmeyer and Gail in 1988. This approach relies on the fact that the observed AIDS incidence arises from a convolution of two other distributions, the distribution of time of HIV infection and the latency distribution between HIV infection and onset of AIDS. Estimates of the latency distribution are available for several cohorts, and AIDS incidence rates are available from surveillance. From these, one can deconvolve to get the HIV infection incidence over time, although this estimate is not stable for the years immediately preceding the end of the observation period for AIDS incidence. The distribution of HIV infection can then be convolved with the latency to produce projections into the future that will arise from infections that occurred before a given point in time. The problem with this approach is that numerical deconvolution is notoriously unstable; many different combinations of latency and infection-time distributions may explain the AIDS incidence data equally well. In addition, if one wishes to project all AIDS cases, one must make assumptions about the rates of recent HIV infection. Nonetheless, even fairly different distributions will provide fairly similar short-term projections.

An additional problem arises from the fact that the latency distribution is not stationary over chronologic time. The effect of treatments and other exposures will undoubtedly change this distribution. Furthermore, there is considerable uncertainty in the estimation of this distribution, which should be reflected in the uncertainty of the projections—something that is not well handled by published solutions.

To describe the deconvolution methods, we first present some notation. Let a_i be the observed AIDS incidence in quarter i, n_i the number of people infected in quarter i, and p_{ij} the probability that a person infected in quarter i has a latency period of j. $E(a_j)$ refers to the expected number of cases of AIDS in the jth interval:

$$E(a_1) = n_1 p_{11}$$

$$E(a_2) = n_1 p_{12} + n_2 p_{21}$$

$$E(a_3) = n_1 p_{13} + n_2 p_{22} + n_3 p_{31}$$

$$\vdots$$

$$E(a_n) = n_1 p_{1n} + n_2 p_{2n-1} + \cdots + n_n p_{n1}$$

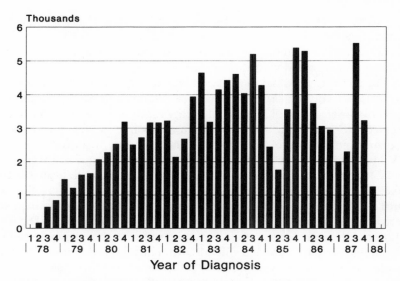

Figure 8. HIV incidence estimate. Result of ridge regression with weight 0.5.

Two approaches to deconvolution have been described, backcalculation by Brookmeyer and Gail (1988) and a regression decomposition method (Pagano *et al.,* 1992). The approach to short-term projection developed by Brookmeyer and Gail differs from the regression approach in its underlying assumptions as well as in its number of parameters. It assumes that the number of AIDS cases per year is independently distributed and follows a multinomial distribution. The infection times are assumed to be distributed as a step function, which requires a specification of "knots" for the incidence curve of infection; these knots are the times of changes in the step function. The regression decomposition approach, by contrast, models the covariance of the AIDS incidence explicitly. This approach estimates the number of infections in each calendar year, without assuming that this number follows any given functional form.

In the regression decomposition approach, the covariance of (a_j, a_{j+m}) is modeled as $-\sum n_k p_{jk} p_{j+m,k}$. Although a least-squares estimate for n is available, it is very sensitive to the choice of p. Therefore, one might consider an alternative ridge regression estimator.

The regression decomposition is more flexible because of the larger number of parameters and the lack of a need to impose a structure on the infection time distribution. It should produce more realistic estimates of variance for the n, because of the lack of imposed structure and the explicit modeling of the covariance of a_j, which are not assumed to be independent. An example of an estimate of the HIV infection incidence is shown in Fig. 8. Figure 9 shows the reported and adjusted incidence until mid-1989 and the projected incidence after 1989 according to three different assumptions about rate of infection after 1986; no new cases, 5000 per year, and 10000 per year. The projected incidence is obtained by extending the convolution described above into the future; of course, this approach requires assumptions about the future number of infections, but the short-term results are not too sensitive to these assumptions.

5. SURVIVAL AFTER AIDS DIAGNOSIS

Surveillance data bases provide much information about survival that is not available from any other source, since patients who enroll in clinical trials or observation studies may not be typical of all patients, but virtually all deaths are reported in the United States. Although dates of death are generally accurately reported, the delay in reporting may be considerable, and information on death reporting delay is not always available. Therefore, we cannot be certain whether or not patients not yet reported as dead are still alive. In this case the random variable, survival time plus reporting time, is right-truncated. Methods similar to those for reporting delay can be used to estimate the survival time; once again the dependence of survival on chronologic time and other variables must be modeled.

Use of surveillance data for analyses of survival requires a particularly high level of data quality for other reasons as well. Since HIV patients are at risk of many conditions, it is important to establish which AIDS-defining condition occurred first in chronologic time and to establish the date of onset accurately. Since patients may be concerned about confidentiality, the date of the first AIDS-defining condition may never be known; and AIDS reported much later. In addition, time of onset of AIDS depends not only on the actual onset of disease, but also on the availability of medical resources for establishing diagnoses.

Nonetheless, it is possible to estimate some general trends in survival from surveillance data. From analyses of survival data from the national CDC surveillance data base, it appears that significant increase in survival over chronologic time of AIDS diagnosis between 1984 and 1989 is mostly confined to MSM who were diagnosed with pneumocystis carinii pneumonia (PCP) (Tu et al., 1991). On the average there was a 14% reduction in mortality each year for the PCP patients and about 5% for conditions other than Kaposi's sarcoma (KS) and PCP. A separate analysis of the improvement in survival before and after 1987 showed a reduction of 28 and 35% in mortality for IVDU and non-IVDU after 1987. Note that the trend toward improvement

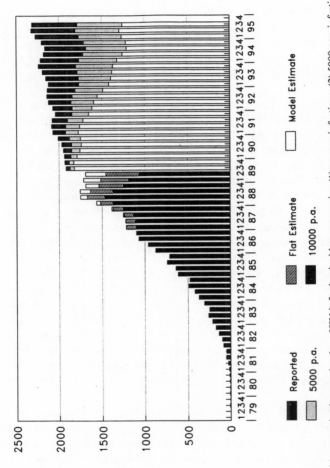

Figure 9. AIDS incidence projections under three HIV infection incidence scenarios: (1) no new infections, (2) 5000 new infections *per annum* (p.a.), and (3) 10000 new infections p.a. These accompany the observed and estimated, according to the logistic model for reporting, incidence numbers to date.

in survival began before the introduction of AZT and PCP prophylaxis in 1987 and 1988.

6. COMBINING DATA FROM DIFFERENT SOURCES

Surveillance data can often be combined with other sources to increase the power and scope of analyses. The example described above uses external estimates of latency for short-term projections. In many states, screening of newborn blood produces estimates of the number of infected women giving birth. This can be combined with surveillance data to provide estimates of the risk of AIDS over time to children born to HIV-infected mothers and to provide short-term projections of AIDS incidence (De Gruttola *et al.*, 1991).

In addition, combining surveillance data bases with information from death registration can provide important checks on quality of data as well as permit estimation of survival. Completeness of reporting can be ascertained by determining the proportion of cases in which AIDS is mentioned in the death certificate that have been reported. Accuracy of information can be evaluated by comparing demographic information in the two systems. In addition, one can try to make some inference about the number of patients for whom HIV is a contributing cause of death, and determine whether this proportion varies by the type of case.

7. CONCLUSION

Surveillance data bases are necessary for assessing epidemic trends as well as the public health impact of medical policy and of treatment advances. Use of such information is not straightforward, however, because of the enormous number of factors that affect reporting systems. Therefore, sophisticated statistical techniques are required for understanding and using these important sources of information.

ACKNOWLEDGMENTS. We thank Dr. John Karon of the Centers for Disease Control for information and many helpful comments. This research was supported in part by grant 1-R29-AI28905 and AI28076.

REFERENCES

Brookmeyer, R., and Gail, M. H. (1988). A method for obtaining short-term projections and lower bounds on the size of the AIDS epidemic. *J. Am. Stat. Assoc.* **83**:301–308.

Brookmeyer, R., and Liao, J. (1990). The analysis of delays in disease reporting: Methods and results for the acquired immunodeficiency syndrome. *Am. J. Epidemiol.* **132**:355–365.

Centers for Disease Control. (1987). *Morbidity and Mortality Weekly Report* **36**, No. 1S.

De Gruttola, V., Tu, X., and Pagano, M. (1991). Pediatric AIDS in New York City: Estimating the distributions of infection, latency and reporting delay and projecting future incidence. Presented at the Meetings of the East North American Region of the Biometrics Society, March, 1991.

Harris, J. E. (1990). Reporting delays and the incidence of AIDS. *J. Am. Stat. Assoc.* **85**:915–924.

Kalbfleisch, J., and Lawless, J. (1991). Regression models for right truncated data with application to AIDS incubation times and reporting lags. *Stat. Sin.* **1**:19–32.

Karon, J., and Berkelman, R. (1991). The geographic and ethnic diversity of AIDS incidence trends in homosexual/bisexual men in the United States. *J. AIDS.* **4**:1179–1181.

Karon, J., Devine, O., and Morgan, W. (1989). Predicting AIDS incidence by extrapolating from recent trends. In C. Castillo-Chavez (ed.), *Mathematical and Statistical Approaches to AIDS Epidemiology.* Berlin: Springer-Verlag.

Lagakos, S., Barraj, L., and De Gruttola, V. (1988). Nonparametric analysis of truncated survival data, with application to AIDS. *Biometrika* **75**:515–523.

Navarro, M. (1991). US widens rules of who has AIDS. *The New York Times,* August 8, 1991, D21.

Pagano, M., De Gruttola, V., MaWhinney, S., and Tu, X. M. (1992), The HIV epidemic in New York City: Projecting AIDS incidence and prevalence. In N. Jewell, K. Dietz, & F. V. Birkhäuser, *AIDS Epidemiology: Methodologic Issues.*

Pagano, M., Tu, X. M., De Gruttola, V., and MaWhinney, S. Analysis of censored and truncated data: Estimating current AIDS incidence from surveillance data. *Biometrics,* (in press).

Stoneburner, R., Des Jarlais, D., Benezra, D., Gorelkin, L., Sotheran, J. L., Friedman, R., Schultz, S., Marmor, M., Mildvan, D., and Maslansky, R. (1988). A larger spectrum of HIV-1-related disease in intravenous drug users in New York City. *Science* **242**:916–919.

Tu, X., Meng, X., and Pagano, M. (1991). The AIDS epidemic: Estimating the survival distribution from surveillance data. Technical Report, Department of Biostatistics, Harvard School of Public Health, 677 Huntington Ave., Boston, Mass. 02115.

Comment on De Gruttola and Pagano's Using Surveillance Data for Assessing and Projecting the AIDS Epidemic

John M. Karon

Surveillance data are useful in answering public health questions about the human immunodeficiency virus (HIV) epidemic. The data tell us which groups (geographic, racial/ethnic, sex, age, transmission risk) are most affected by the epidemic. Analyses based on the surveillance data provide projections of future AIDS cases, as well as estimates of AIDS and HIV prevalence (CDC, 1990; CDC, 1992b). These data also show changes in mortality patterns over time (Harris, 1990).

De Gruttola and Pagano discuss basic issues involved in using AIDS surveillance data based on their experience in analyzing data from New York City. In this comment, I add insight gained from analyzing national data. Unless otherwise specified, "AIDS" refers to conditions meeting the 1987 surveillance definition for AIDS (CDC, 1987).

1. AIDS SURVEILLANCE DATA

In the United States, each person meeting the AIDS surveillance definition must be reported to the local, state, or territorial health department. Health departments submit information (without names or other personal identifiers) to the Centers for Disease Control (CDC), including demographic data (age, sex, race/ethnicity, and geographic area of residence at diagnosis), transmission ex-

JOHN M. KARON • Division of HIV/AIDS, National Center for Infectious Diseases, Centers for Disease Control, Atlanta, Georgia 30333.

Methodological Issues in AIDS Behavioral Research, edited by David G. Ostrow and Ronald C. Kessler. Plenum Press, New York, 1993.

posure factors, AIDS-defining diseases present, date of diagnosis of the first of these diseases, HIV test results, and (if the patient has died) date of death. Health departments update their reports when additional information is collected. Subsequent death is reported, but usually subsequently diagnosed diseases are not.

Analyses using transmission exposure category should consider AIDS patients with no identified risk (NIR). Of patients diagnosed during 1990 and reported through December 1992, approximately 4.4% (4.0% of men, 7.4% of women) had NIR; for patients diagnosed during 1991, 5.6% (5.2% of men, 8.8% of women) had NIR. The proportions of NIR cases with various exposure risks can be estimated from interviews conducted with some of these persons (Green, Karon, and Nwanyanwu, 1992). HIV transmission resulting from heterosexual contact is much more common and that in injecting drug users (IDUs) is less common among patients without a risk reported initially than among patients with a reported risk.

Information on each reported AIDS case is available on diskettes for MS-DOS microcomputers. The data include the information described above, plus dates of report for AIDS and for death (if the patient has died). Two demographic variables are grouped to preserve confidentiality. Age at diagnosis has nine categories (5-year intervals for ages 20–49). Residence at diagnosis has six categories: metropolitan statistical areas (MSAs) with 1990 population > 1,000,000 are grouped into five census regions; the remaining group is the rest of the United States combined. A weighting variable is also included to allow the user to adjust for estimated AIDS reporting delays. Selected tables are available for each state and Puerto Rico, as well as each MSA with 1990 population > 500,000.

This information can be obtained from the Division of HIV/AIDS (E–48), Centers for Disease Control and Prevention, Atlanta, Georgia 30333. Information is currently updated twice each year (in January and July). Other data for states, cities, or counties should be requested from the corresponding health department.

2. THE 1987 AIDS SURVEILLANCE DEFINITION

As De Gruttola and Pagano point out, recent trends in AIDS incidence cannot be interpreted without taking into account the change in the AIDS surveillance definition in September of 1987. The definition was modified in two ways. For some diseases [including *Pneumocystis carinii* pneumonia (PCP)], a presumptive instead of a definitive (pathologically confirmed) diagnosis is accepted if the patient has a positive HIV antibody test. In addition, diseases were added to the surveillance definition; the most important of these are wasting syndrome, HIV encephalopathy (dementia), and disseminated *Mycobacterium tuberculosis*. Future analyses of AIDS incidence trends will need to take into account the expansion of the AIDS surveillance definition in January 1993 (CDC, 1992a). The potential effect of this expansion is discussed in a later section.

The 1987 definition change increased reported AIDS incidence. For cases diagnosed after 1987, the proportion satisfying only the expanded definition is greatest in IDUs, cases attributed to heterosexual contact, and children; in blacks and Hispanics; and in women. In each of these groups, this proportion increased each year during 1988–1991.

In considering the effect of the case definition change, it is probably better to focus on the diseases diagnosed by using a "consistent" case definition, comprising all cases with a disease included in the pre-1987 definition. For example, any case with a diagnosis of PCP (whether definitive or presumptive) satisfies the consistent definition. This definition excludes cases reported only on the basis of some combination of coccidioidomycosis, *Cytomegalovirus retinitis,* HIV encephalopathy, *Mycobacterium tuberculosis,* disseminated or extrapulmonary *Mycobacterium* of other species, Salmonella septicemia, wasting syndrome, or (for pediatric patients) bacterial infections.

The proportions of cases not satisfying the consistent definition vary among transmission exposure groups and have been increasing over time. Of all cases diagnosed during 1986, 4.7% did not satisfy the consistent definition. This increased to 11% of cases diagnosed during the second half of 1987, 14% of cases diagnosed during the second half of 1989, and 17% of cases diagnosed during the second half of 1991 (cases reported through December 1992). Cases diagnosed in homosexual or bisexual men who are not IDUs are somewhat less likely, and cases diagnosed in IDUs and in children more likely, to satisfy the consistent definition.

As De Gruttola and Pagano note, data are available from San Francisco on the effect of the 1987 definition change on AIDS incidence satisfying the consistent definition (Karon *et al.,* 1993). These data are not necessarily representative of other areas in the United States, as most of the persons studied in San Francisco are white men reporting sexual contact with other men.

De Gruttola and Pagano suggest taking the definition change into account by modifying AIDS incidence before late 1987. The proportion of cases not consistent with the pre-1987 definition increases over time, so it may be better to modify only the numbers of nonconsistent cases (e. g., using the estimates from San Francisco). Resulting estimates would need to be scaled up to reflect trends in the total numbers of reported cases.

3. REPORTING DELAYS AND COMPLETENESS OF REPORTING

De Gruttola and Pagano show that recent AIDS incidence trends cannot be interpreted without adjusting for reporting delays. Long-term trends must also consider changes in completeness of reporting.

AIDS surveillance data underestimate the extent of severe symptomatic HIV disease in two ways. Some diagnosed AIDS cases are never reported to CDC; based on special studies, CDC currently estimates that 85–90% of all diagnosed cases are reported (Rosenblum *et al.,* 1992). In addition, some HIV-infected persons die without meeting the AIDS surveillance definition. This may be more likely in IDUs than in other transmission groups (Stoneburner, 1989). Using cause-specific mortality information from death certificates, Buehler *et al.* (1990) estimated that 70–90% of the deaths attributable to HIV infection during 1987 in male U.S. residents 25–44 years of age were reported to the AIDS surveillance system. Based on this analysis, reported AIDS cases probably represented about 75% of severe health problems associated with HIV infection during 1987 (CDC, 1990). The analyses of Buehler *et al.* suggest that AIDS case reporting probably became more complete during the mid to late 1980s.

De Gruttola and Pagano's Fig. 4 shows clearly the need to adjust for reporting delays in any analysis that includes recent AIDS incidence. Reporting delays vary among geographic regions (Brookmeyer and Liao, 1990) and also among groups defined by transmission risk and race/ethnicity. Typically, approximately half of all cases ultimately reported are reported within 3 months after the month of diagnosis. Approximately 70, 80, and 95% are reported within 6 months, 12 months, and 3 years, respectively. Rosenberg (1990) describes a simple computational method for estimating reporting delays in a single group if these delays are not changing over time.

Although De Gruttola and Pagano suggest that there are time trends in reporting delays, such trends may be difficult to model and impossible to separate from changes in completeness of reporting. Knowledge of the surveillance system suggests that important factors affecting reporting delays may be temporary, such as changes in personnel levels in specific locations or deadlines for reporting enough cases to meet legislative requirements for funding. Estimates of reporting delays incorporating time trends, therefore, might not be accurate. For example, De Gruttola and Pagano's analyses suggest that a time trend in reporting delays affects estimated AIDS incidence for the first three quarters of 1989. We now know the numbers of AIDS cases ultimately to be reported for these quarters of 1989 quite accurately. In estimating reporting delays, CDC presently assumes that delays are homogeneous over time (Karon *et al.,* 1989) but may vary among groups defined by geographic region, race/ethnicity, sex, and mode of transmission. Based on cases reported through December 1992, CDC estimates that the number of AIDS cases diagnosed in the United States during the first three quarters of 1989 that ultimately will be reported are (rounded to the nearest 100) 9,700, 10,300, and 10,200, respectively; these estimates are much closer to De Gruttola and Pagano's "constant" than the "time-varying" estimates (their Fig. 4).

I recommend, therefore, that analyses of AIDS incidence not use incidence during the latest two or three calendar quarters, especially for restricted geographic areas. This procedure may be better than modeling trends in reporting delays and certainly is easier computationally. In addition, anyone analyzing AIDS or HIV surveillance data from a small geographic region should be familiar with local data collection procedures.

4. THE 1993 AIDS SURVEILLANCE DEFINITION

CDC expanded the AIDS surveillance definition on January 1, 1993, by adding two types of criteria for persons with laboratory-confirmed HIV infection (CDC, 1992a):

1. a CD4+ T-lymphocyte count of <200 cells/μL or a CD4+ percentage <14 in a person who has not been diagnosed with a condition in the 1987 AIDS surveillance definition (hereafter termed "severe immunosuppression"); and
2. pulmonary tuberculosis, recurrent pneumonia, and invasive cervical cancer.

As a result, many HIV-infected persons will be reported to CDC AIDS surveillance substantially earlier than they would have if the definition had not been changed. Estimates of the median time from the onset of severe immunosuppression to a diagnosis of 1987 AIDS range from <12 to >24 months in different studies; this time is longer in persons using antiretroviral therapy or prophylactic therapy to prevent the development of *Pneumocystis carinii* pneumonia (CDC, 1992b; Table 4). In one large study, the median time from the *diagnosis* of severe immunosuppression to the diagnosis of 1987 AIDS was 15 months during 1990–1991 (CDC, 1992b; Appendix).

The effect of changing the AIDS surveillance definition has been predicted from a stochastic model incorporating these data and back-calculation results (CDC, 1992b). Adding severe immunosuppression to the definition is expected to have a much larger effect than adding the other three conditions. The most immediate effect will result from the approximately 50,000 persons with prevalent diagnosed severe immunosuppression in January 1993 (HIV-infected persons without AIDS [according to the 1987 definition] who were diagnosed as severely immunosuppressed before January 1993 and had not yet developed AIDS as of then). The effect of adding the other three conditions is expected to be relatively small (CDC, unpublished data).

Although the data required to evaluate the effect of the change were not yet available when this comment was completed (March 1993), the effects are unlikely to be uniform. State and local AIDS surveillance practices vary, and the requirement for reporting of CD4+ T-lymphocyte counts in HIV-infected persons by laboratories also vary among states. As a result, there are likely to be geographic differences in the effect of the new AIDS surveillance definition on trends in AIDS incidence. Differences in access to medical care for HIV-infected persons (Moore *et al.*, 1991) may also result in differences in the effect of the new definition among groups defined by mode of transmission, by race, and by sex. It is also likely that the new AIDS surveillance definition will have a greater effect in later years, as was the case for the 1987 definition change.

5. METHODS FOR ESTIMATING HIV PREVALENCE AND PREDICTING AIDS CASES

Extrapolation and transmission models are unlikely to yield accurate short-term projections for AIDS cases. The substantive basis for extrapolation was the long and variable period from HIV infection to AIDS (the incubation period; median duration, approximately 10 years). As a result, trends in AIDS incidence would persist: a sudden change in HIV incidence would not affect AIDS incidence for several years, and the effect of the change in HIV incidence would appear over a period of many years. The current use of prophylactic therapy that can delay the onset of AIDS, however, means that AIDS incidence trends can change quite rapidly, making extrapolation unreliable. Transmission models require a detailed understanding of the HIV epidemic and values for many parameters, many of which are very hard to estimate.

Back-calculation is now the modeling method of choice for estimating HIV seroprevalence and predicting future AIDS incidence. Implementing this method, however, poses statistical, epidemiologic, and computational problems (Brookmeyer, 1991; Rosenberg and Gail, 1991). Many issues must be considered in carrying out back-calculation (CDC, 1990). In particular, it is essential to allow for the effect of prophylactic therapy on the incubation period distribution (Gail *et al.*, 1990). Estimates of HIV incidence obtained from back-calculation must be evaluated carefully. Because relatively few persons develop AIDS within 3 years after HIV infection, HIV incidence estimates for the most recent 3 years obtained from back-calculation are imprecise. Annual or quarterly HIV incidence estimates may be implausibly variable, as in De Gruttola and Pagano's Fig. 8, unless a smoothness criterion is incorporated in the estimation procedure (Bacchetti, 1991). Roughness does not necessarily make the resulting AIDS case projections less accurate, however. Adjustments for mortality and incomplete reporting must be made if

HIV incidence estimates from back-calculation are used to estimate HIV seroprevalence (CDC, 1990).

6. ESTIMATING SURVIVAL AFTER A DIAGNOSIS OF AIDS

AIDS surveillance data can be used to detect patterns of survival after a diagnosis of AIDS. Several factors must be considered in analyzing the survival data, however.

Some deaths in reported AIDS patients are never reported to CDC. Hardy and the Long-term Survivor Collaborative Study Group (1991) found that, of 780 apparent long-term (3 year) survivors in whom AIDS was diagnosed before 1984, 61% were known dead and only 15% could be determined to be alive in January of 1987. Since at least 90% of reported persons with AIDS diagnosed during each half-year during January 1981 through June 1986 are reported dead (CDC, 1993), death reporting is probably at least 90% complete for reported AIDS cases. Unreported deaths may tend to be among patients with longer survival after an AIDS diagnosis, as longer survival gives patients more time to move away from the location where AIDS was diagnosed.

Two aspects of the data for reported deaths must also be considered. Approximately 12% of reported AIDS cases have the same dates (month) for AIDS diagnosis and death. These cases represent an unknown mix of patients with very short survival, with a delayed diagnosis (AIDS undiagnosed until death), and with an earlier but unreported diagnosis.

The other caveat regards analyses by disease. Surveillance data do not necessarily include all diseases diagnosed (see the description of the surveillance data). Two published analyses by disease used supplementary data: Harris (1990) used data not available on the current surveillance data set, and Lemp et al. (1990) used extensive data collected in San Francisco.

Finally, just as for AIDS cases, reporting delays and completeness of reporting must be considered in analyzing deaths. Reporting dates for deaths are available only for deaths reported starting in October of 1987. Preliminary analyses suggest that reporting delays for deaths and AIDS cases are similar. Some public health departments are improving their methods for collecting and using death certificates, however, so completeness of reporting for both AIDS cases and deaths may be improving.

REFERENCES

Bacchetti, P. (1990). Estimating the incubation period of AIDS by comparing population infection and diagnosis patterns. *J. Am. Stat. Assoc.* **85**:1002–1008.

Brookmeyer, R. (1991). Reconstruction and future trends of the AIDS epidemic in the United States. *Science* 253:37–42.

Brookmeyer, R., and Liao, J. (1990). Statistical modelling of the AIDS epidemic for forecasting health care needs. *Biometrics* 46:1151–1163.

Buehler, J. W., Devine, O. J., Berkelman, R. L., and Chevarley, F. (1990). Impact of the human immunodeficiency virus epidemic on mortality trends in young men, United States. *Am. J. Public Health* 80:1080–1086.

Centers for Disease Control. (1987). Revision of the CDC surveillance case definition for acquired immunodeficiency syndrome. *MMWR* 36(Suppl. 1S):1S–15S.

Centers for Disease Control. (1990). HIV prevalence estimates and AIDS case projections for the United States: Report based upon a workshop. *MMWR* 39(RR-16):1–31.

Centers for Disease Control and Prevention (1992a). 1993 revised classification system for HIV infection and expanded surveillance case definition for AIDS among adolescents and adults. *MMWR,* 41(RR-17):1–19.

Centers for Disease Control and Prevention (1992b). Projections of the number of persons diagnosed with AIDS and the number of immunosuppressed HIV-infected persons—United States, 1992–1994. *MMWR* 41(RR-18):1–29.

Centers for Disease Control and Prevention (1993). HIV/AIDS surveillance: U.S. AIDS cases reported through December 1992. Division of HIV/AIDS, National Center for Infectious Diseases. February, 1993:1–23.

Gail, M. H., Rosenberg, P. S., and Goedert, J. J. (1990). Therapy may explain recent deficits in AIDS incidence. *J. AIDS* 3:296–306.

Green, T. A., Karon, J. M., and Nwanyanwu, O. C. (1992). Changes in AIDS incidence trends in the United States. *J. AIDS* 5:547–555.

Hardy, A. M., and the Long-term Survivor Collaborative Study Group. (1991). Characterization of long-term survivors of acquired immunodeficiency syndrome. *J. AIDS* 4:386–391.

Harris, J. E. (1990). Improved short-term survival of AIDS patients initially diagnosed with Pneumocystis carinii pneumonia, 1984 through 1987. *J. Am. Med. Assoc.* 263:397–401.

Karon, J. M., Buehler, J. W., Byers, R. H., Farizo, K. M., Green, T. A., Hanson, D. L., Rosenblum, L. S., Gail, M. H., Rosenberg, P. S., and Brookmeyer, R. (1993). *Projections of the numbers of persons diagnosed with AIDS and of immunosuppressed HIV-infected persons, United States, 1992–1994: Statistical methods and parameter estimates.* (U.S. Department of Health and Human Services publication HIV/NCID/10-92/028). Atlanta, Georgia, 1993.

Karon, J. M., Devine, O. J., and Morgan, W. M. (1989). Predicting AIDS incidence by extrapolating from recent trends. In C. Castillo-Chavez (ed.), *Mathematical and Statistical Approaches to AIDS Epidemiology.* Berlin: Springer-Verlag, pp. 58–88.

Lemp, G. F., Payne, S. F., Neal, D., Temelso, T., and Rutherford, G. W. (1990). Survival trends for patients with AIDS. *J. Am. Med. Assoc.* 263:402–406.

Moore, R. D., Hidalgo, J., Sugland, B., and Chaisson, R. E. (1991). Zidovudine and the natural history of the Acquired Immunodeficiency Syndrome. *NEJM* 324:1412–1416.

Rosenberg, P. S. (1990). A simple correction of AIDS surveillance data for reporting delays. *J. AIDS* 3:49–54.

Rosenberg, P. S., and Gail, M. H. (1991). Backcalculation of flexible linear models of the human immunodeficiency virus infection curve. *Appl. Stat.* 40:269–282.

Rosenblum, L., Buehler, J. W., Morgan, W. M., Costa, S., Hidalgo, J., Holmes, R., Lieb, L., Shields, A., and Whyte, B. M. (1992). The completeness of AIDS case reporting, 1988: a multisite collaborative surveillance project. *Amer. J. Pub. Health* 82:1495–1499.

Stoneburner, R. L., Des Jarlais, D. C., Benezra, D., Gorelkin, L., Soteran, J. L., Friedman, S. R., Schultz, S., Marmor, M., Mildvan, D., and Maslansky, R. (1988). A larger spectrum of severe HIV-1–related disease in intravenous drug users in New York City. *Science* 242:916–919.

9

Analytic Methods for Estimating HIV-Treatment and Cofactor Effects

James M. Robins

1. INTRODUCTION

This chapter describes new statistical methods developed by the author and co-workers for analyzing randomized trials and observational data bases of HIV-infected persons (Robins, 1986, 1987a,b, 1989a,b, 1992, 1993a,b; Robins and Tsiatis, 1991, 1992, 1993; Robins and Greenland, 1992; Robins and Rotnitzky, 1992; Robins *et al.,* 1992; Mark and Robins, 1993a,b). Each of the proposed approaches is based to a large extent on the estimation of the parameters of a new class of causal models, the structural nested models, using a new class of estimators—the G-estimators. Most of the new methods are fundamentally "epidemiologic" or "observational" in that they require data on time-independent and time-dependent confounding factors, that is, risk factors for the outcome of interest that also predict subsequent treatment with or exposure to the drug or cofactor under study. The proposed methods of analysis improve upon previous methods in the following ways:

1. The new methods are the best methods available to adjust for non-random noncompliance and dependent censoring in randomized clinical trials. In Section 3, we shall use these methods to adjust for the concurrent effect of an additional nonrandomized treatment in a randomized clinical trial. Specifically, in the AIDS Clinical Trial Group (ACTG) trial 002 of the effect of high-dose versus low-dose AZT on the survival of AIDS patients, patients in the low-dose AZT

James M. Robins • Departments of Epidemiology and Biostatistics, Harvard School of Public Health, Boston, Massachusetts 02115.

Methodological Issues in AIDS Behavioral Research, edited by David G. Ostrow and Ronald C. Kessler. Plenum Press, New York, 1993.

arm had improved survival, but they also took more prophylactic
therapy for pneumocystis carinii pneumonia (PCP) such as aerosolized
pentamidine (a nonrandomized concurrent treatment) (Fischl
et al., 1990).

2. The new methods are the best methods available to estimate the effect
   of a nonrandomized treatment (e. g., DDI, aerosolized pentamidine,
   or psychological counseling) or a cofactor (e. g., marijuana use) on
   an outcome of interest (e. g., mortality, time to AIDS, or CD4 count
   level) from data available in an observational data base or randomized
   trial, whenever symptoms of HIV disease (e. g., thrush, fever, weight
   loss) are simultaneously confounders and intermediate variables on
   the causal pathway from the treatment or cofactor under study to the
   outcome of interest. In particular, we shall, in Section 3.7.1, present
   an analysis of the effect of prophylaxis for PCP on survival in ACTG
   trial 002 and, in Section 5, the effect of marijuana on the evolution
   of CD4 counts in HIV-infected subjects in the San Francisco Men's
   Health Study (Fischl *et al.,* 1990; Lang *et al.,* 1987; Winkelstein *et
   al.,* 1987).

Randomized trials analyzed by intent-to-treat should be used to answer
any causal question that can be so studied. But the reality is that observational
(correlational) methods are used everyday in an attempt to answer, even
provisionally, pressing causal questions that cannot be or have not yet been
studied in randomized trials. For example, many investigators have used observational data to examine the effect of cofactors such as illicit drugs, continued unsafe sex, cigarette smoking, and alcohol on the progression of HIV
disease. In addition, certain "nontraditional" or "unapproved" therapies are
used in the community long before their effectiveness is tested in a randomized
trial. Thus, it is important to develop observational methods to estimate the
causal effects of these treatments on survival in order to prevent further needless suffering and death caused by hazardous therapies and to recognize potentially beneficial therapies that should be studied further in a randomized
clinical trial. As every epidemiologist and statistician is well aware, no observational analysis can produce valid causal inferences if one fails to measure
important confounding factors that predict both outcome and cofactor use.
Nonetheless, standard methods of analysis such as Cox (1972) regression and
generalized estimating equations for longitudinal data (Zeger and Liang, 1986)
are biased when risk factors predict subsequent exposure to the cofactor or
therapy under study, *even when data on all-important confounders are available*
(Robins, 1986, 1987a,b, 1989a,b, 1992, 1993a); however, in this setting, the
new methods of analysis can produce valid causal inferences. These new

methods take into account the fact that symptoms of HIV disease progression can be both confounders and intermediate variables.

Correlational analyses are also used routinely in subsidiary analyses of randomized clinical trials. In their *New England Journal of Medicine* article reporting the results of trial 002, Fischl *et al.* (1990) expressed concern that the improved survival in the low-dose AZT arm might be the result of the more frequent use of aerosolized pentamidine. Since the authors correctly recognized that an intent to treat analysis cannot test this hypothesis, the authors reported the results of a "landmark analysis," a correlational method. Below, we show that one would typically expect a landmark analysis to provide a biased estimate of the causal effect of AZT treatment on survival adjusted for differential pentamidine use even if data on important predictors of pentamidine usage were available.

The relationship of the proposed methods to the methods described by Heckman and Robb (1985) is considered in Robins (1989b).

2. THE ACTG TRIAL 002: SOME BACKGROUND

The AIDS clinical trials group's study number 002 compared the effect of high-dose AZT (3-azido-3-deoxythymidine) therapy (1500 mg/day) versus low-dose AZT therapy (1200 mg/day for 4 weeks and 600 mg/day thereafter) on the survival of 524 AIDS patients (Fischl *et al.*, 1990). The median survival was greater in the low-dose arm. Results of standard intention-to-treat tests of equality of the survival curves were $Q_L^* = 3.6$, $p = 0.07$ and $Q_W^* = 5.2$, $p = 0.02$ where Q_L^* is the χ_1^2 statistic from the log-rank test and Q_W^* is the χ_1^2 statistic from the Prentice–Wilcoxon weighted log-rank test—a censored data version of the Wilcoxon test (Kalbfleisch and Prentice, 1980).

There are at least two possible explanations for the apparent benefit on median survival time associated with the low-dose therapy:

1. *High-dose AZT is associated with greater toxicity than low-dose.* Forty percent of the high-dose group versus 25% of the low-dose group had to discontinue therapy because of toxicity under the specifications of the protocol.

2. *The low-dose group received more prophylactic drug treatment for the prevention of PCP than did the high-dose group.* Sixty-one percent of the low-dose group versus 50% of the high-dose group received prophylaxis for PCP (Fischl *et al.*, 1990). PCP is an opportunistic infection that afflicts AIDS patients. Patients may suffer repeated bouts of PCP and it can be fatal. Thus, prophylaxis might prolong survival by preventing further episodes of PCP.

The potential benefits of prophylactic treatment for PCP became known from other data sources during the course of the trial. Therefore, beginning in August of 1987 (9 months after enrollment in the trial began and 3 months before enrollment was closed), prophylaxis for subsequent PCP was allowed after one postrandomization bout of PCP. In April of 1988, it was decided that prophylaxis could be given to any study subject without regard to their PCP history. A number of different medications were used for prophylaxis, including aerosolized pentamidine, oral pentamidine, dapsone, and fansidar. Except for these general guidelines, the decision whether and when to administer prophylaxis to a particular patient was left up to the treating physicians. *Thus, embedded within this randomized trial of high versus low-dose AZT was an observational study of prophylaxis.* A possible contribution to the higher rate of prophylaxis in the low-dose group was a slightly higher, although not statistically significant, incidence of PCP pneumonia prior to the initiation of prophylaxis. The p value for a log-rank test comparing the low- to high-dose arm's time to first postrandomization PCP episode was 0.15 when death, end of follow-up, and initiation of prophylaxis are treated as censoring events.

With regard to AZT treatment, the public health question raised by trial 002 was whether the high- and low-dose AZT arms would have had identical survival curves had all subjects received the same prophylaxis treatment. We shall call this the hypothesis of no direct effect of treatment arm on survival. Since the low-dose arm received more prophylaxis than the high-dose arm, this hypothesis cannot be tested using a standard intention-to-treat analysis if prophylaxis itself affects survival.

Before we proceed to describe our methods for testing the null hypothesis of no direct treatment arm effect, we motivate the need for our methods by reviewing three previously proposed methods for testing this null hypothesis. We demonstrate that the true α-level of tests based on these methods will typically differ from their nominal α-level even if neither treatment arm nor prophylaxis influences survival.

Bias of Previously Proposed Methods

A landmark analysis is a commonly used method to test for a direct treatment arm effect controlling for a posttreatment variable such as prophylaxis. In a landmark analysis, one tests whether treatment arm is a predictor of subsequent survival among subjects surviving to the "landmark time," say 6 months postrandomization, stratified by prophylaxis status at the landmark time (Fischl *et al.*, 1990). In a generalized landmark analysis, stratification is based not only on prophylaxis status but also on the postrandomization but "prelandmark time" history of all other covariates (such as PCP history) that predict both prophylaxis status at the landmark time and subsequent survival. Below, we demonstrate, using a highly simplified but not implausible hypothetical example, that the true α-level of either a landmark or generalized landmark analysis is not guaranteed to equal the nominal level even if neither treatment arm nor prophylaxis influences survival.

A second common approach to testing for a direct treatment arm effect would be to compare the relative hazard for death at each time t in the high-dose with that in the low-dose arm, when controlling for prophylaxis and PCP history up to t using a (correctly specified) time-dependent Cox proportional hazards model. Below, we show that the relative hazard at t could be greater in the high-dose than low-dose arm even if neither treatment arm nor prophylaxis influences survival.

A third commonly used method that tests for a direct treatment effect is to regard, for purposes of analysis, subjects as censored at the time of initiation of prophylaxis therapy for PCP when computing the standard intention-to-treat log-rank test. Below, we show that, even if neither treatment arm nor prophylaxis influences survival, the true α-level of the log-rank test might fail to equal its nominal α-level (Lagakos *et al.,* 1990), because censoring based on initiation of prophylaxis and survival may be dependent.

The problem with all three methods is that bias can be introduced into the analysis by stratification on or adjustment for the posttreatment variables, prophylaxis and PCP history.

Hypothetical Example. Suppose the high- and low-dose treatment arms had 300 subjects. In each arm, 100 are poor-prognosis subjects who are destined to die at 10 months, 100 are moderate-prognosis subjects who will die at 20 months, and 100 are good-prognosis subjects who will die at 30 months. We assume that neither AZT treatment arm nor prophylaxis has any causal effect on survival. Next we suppose that, although AZT treatment arm has no effect on survival, high-dose AZT prevents postrandomization PCP from developing in moderate prognosis patients. Indeed, for simplicity, we shall assume that all moderate prognosis patients would develop PCP and be placed on prophylaxis by the landmark time of 6 months if on the low-dose arm while none would develop PCP or be given prophylaxis if on the high-dose AZT arm. Further we assume all poor-prognosis patients would both develop PCP and receive prophylaxis by the landmark time, irrespective of their treatment arm. Finally, we assume no good-prognosis patient would develop PCP or receive prophylaxis by the landmark time, on either treatment arm. Under these assumptions, the landmark analysis would be based on the data shown in Table 1.

In Table 1, within each stratum defined by PCP and prophylaxis status at the landmark time, the low-dose AZT arm has a greater mean survival

Table 1. Data of Hypothetical Example for Landmark Analysis

PCP and prophylaxis by 6 months postrandomization				No PCP and no prophylaxis by 6 months postrandomization			
	Time to death				Time to death		
Treatment arm	10	20	30	Treatment arm	10	20	30
High	100^a	0	0	High	0	100^b	100^c
Low	100^a	100^b	0	Low	0	0	100^c

[a] Poor-prognosis patients.
[b] Moderate-prognosis subjects.
[c] Good-prognosis subjects.

than the high-dose AZT arm. Thus, the landmark analysis would cause one to falsely reject the null hypothesis of no direct AZT effect.

Now suppose, for pedagogic purposes, that no subject develops PCP or initiates prophylaxis subsequent to 6 months and that the above data are analyzed using a stratified Cox proportional hazards model with time-dependent strata defined by past PCP and prophylaxis history. The treatment arm indicator enters the model as a time-independent covariate, say $\exp(\beta R_i)$ with $R_i = 1$ if subject i is assigned to the high-dose arm. Note within the stratum of subjects with PCP and prophylaxis prior to month 10, the (discrete) hazard at time 10 among subjects in the high-dose treatment arm is greater than that among subjects in the low-dose arm, and, in the strata of subjects with no PCP or prophylaxis, the hazard at time 20 is greater in the high-dose arm than in the low-dose arm. It follows that the estimate of β will be positive, falsely suggesting an adverse direct effect in the high-dose arm.

Finally, when the above data are analyzed using a log-rank test that treats subjects as censored at the time of initiation of prophylaxis therapy, the resulting test statistic is precisely the log-rank test applied to the stratum of subjects without prophylaxis or postrandomization PCP. Again this log-rank test will falsely suggest an adverse direct effect of the high-dose arm since the hazard rate at time 20 is greater in the high-dose than in the low-dose arm.

3. NEW METHODS OF ANALYSIS

In this section, we present three methods of testing the null hypothesis of no direct effect of AZT treatment protocol on survival. The first two methods use different, totally unrelated assumptions. The third method uses the assumptions made under both Method 1 and Method 2. As a consequence, this method will produce more powerful tests than either of the other methods.

3.1. Method 1

3.1.1. The Assumption of No Unmeasured Confounders for Prophylaxis Therapy

Method 1 is based on the assumption that there are no unmeasured confounders for prophylaxis therapy. Specifically, let $T_{p^-,i}$ be the death time of subject i if the subject were randomized to his observed AZT protocol but, possibly contrary to fact, prophylaxis was withheld at all times. Time is measured as days from start of follow-up, i. e., from enrollment in trial 002. $T_{p^-,i}$ is a counterfactual variable since it represents outcomes under circumstances that may not have actually occurred. See Rubin (1978), Holland (1986), Greenland and Robins (1986), and Robins (1986, 1987a,b, 1989a,b, 1992) for discussion of the utility of counterfactual variables in causal inference.

We pause to briefly comment on the definition and nature of a counterfactual random variable. Consider a subject i who, in the observed trial, was assigned to the high-dose AZT arm, received prophylaxis from week 10 to 40, took 1500 mg of AZT daily until week 12 and none thereafter, and died in week 40. If prophylaxis had always been withheld, it is quite conceivable that subject i would have continued to take 1500 mg of AZT daily past week 12 if either (1) prophylactic drugs potentiated the toxic effects of AZT precipitating a life-threatening toxic episode in week 12 or (2) the subject, although nontoxic, had stopped AZT at week 12 because he felt himself to be adequately protected by the prophylactic drugs. To be concrete, say subject i would have continued to take 1500 mg AZT daily through week 14 and none thereafter if prophylaxis had been withheld. Then, by its definition, $T_{p^-,i}$ would be equal to subject i's failure time when the subject was assigned to the high-dose arm, never received prophylaxis, and took AZT daily through week 14 (rather than through week 12). The above example should make it clear that the assumption of the existence of a counterfactual variable raises a number of interesting philosophical and scientific questions that we will not consider further here.

Definition. There is no unmeasured confounding for prophylaxis therapy if, at each time t, among a subset of subjects with the same treatment and measured covariate history up to t, the probability of treatment at t does not further depend on either $T_{p^-,i}$.

Since physicians tend to initiate prophylaxis in subjects who have had recurrent bouts of PCP and recurrent PCP signifies poor-prognosis patients (i. e., patients with small values of $T_{p-,i}$), it follows that our assumption of no unmeasured confounders would be false if we had neglected to measure PCP history.

We suppose throughout that once prophylaxis for PCP is initiated, a subject remains on prophylaxis thereafter. We have made this assumption because, in the available data base, there is essentially no information about termination of prophylaxis. Our assumption of no unmeasured confounding factors then states that we have available, at each time t, data on the history of all time-independent and time-dependent covariates that simultaneously (1) predict $T_{p-,i}$ and (2) predict which study subjects will initiate prophylaxis at t. It is a primary goal of epidemiologists conducting an observational study to collect data on a sufficient number of covariates to ensure that the assumption of no unmeasured confounders will be true. We shall assume that this goal has been realized while recognizing that in practice, this would never be precisely true and may, on occasion, not even be approximately true.

To give our assumption of no unmeasured confounders explicit mathematical content, let P record time to initiation of prophylaxis and T record a subject's actual survival time. Further define $\bar{L}(t)$ to be the time-dependent covariate vector with components:

R = the dichotomous (0, 1) treatment arm indicator
C = end of follow-up date (10/25/89) minus date of randomization
$\overline{PCP}(t)$ = PCP history up to t
$\overline{T4}(t)$ = T4-count history up to t
$\overline{AZT}(t)$ = AZT treatment history up to t

(Overbars will be used to denote histories of time-dependent covariates. We have temporarily suppressed the subscript i indexing study subjects.) C is a subject's potential censoring time. $\overline{AZT}(t)$ is a subject's actual history of AZT treatment through t recorded on the drug history form available in the 002 trial data base. $\overline{T4}(t)$ is the history of a subject's T4 (or equivalently CD4) lymphocyte count history recorded on a hematology form.

Then, formally, our assumption of "no unmeasured confounders" is that

$$\lambda_P[t|\bar{L}(t), T_{p-}] = \lambda_P[t|\bar{L}(t)] \tag{1}$$

where

$$\lambda_P[t|\bar{L}(t)] = \lim_{\Delta t \to 0} \text{pr}[t < P \le t + \Delta t | P > t, T > t, \bar{L}(t)]/\Delta t$$

is the hazard rate for the initiation for prophylaxis at t for subjects alive at t given covariate history $\bar{L}(t)$. Since $\lambda_P[t \mid \bar{L}(t), T_p-]\Delta t$ is the probability of initiating prophylaxis therapy in the interval $(t, t + \Delta t)$ given both past covariate history $\bar{L}(t)$ and T_p-, Eq. (1) says that, conditional on the past history $\bar{L}(t)$ of confounding factors, T_p- does not further predict which study subjects will initiate prophylaxis in the interval $(t, t + \Delta t)$. If (1) is true but $\lambda_P[t \mid T_p-, R] \neq \lambda_P[t \mid R]$, we say there is *dependent censoring by prophylaxis for T_p- given R but independent censoring given $\bar{L}(t)$*. To implement Method 1, we shall also need to assume we have correctly specified a stratified time-dependent Cox proportional hazards model for $\lambda_P[t \mid \bar{L}(t)]$. Specifically, we assume

$$\lambda_P[t \mid \bar{L}(t)] = \lambda_{0,R}(t)\exp[\alpha^{*\prime}W(t)] \tag{2}$$

where

$$\alpha^{*\prime}W(t) = \alpha^*_{1,0}I_C(1 - R) + \alpha^*_{2,0}I_{PCP1}(t)(1 - R) + \alpha^*_{3,0}I_{PCP2}(t)(1 - R)$$

$$+ \alpha^*_{4,0}I_{AZT}(t)(1 - R) + \alpha^*_{5,0}I_{T4<20}(t)(1 - R) + \alpha^*_{1,1}I_C R$$

$$+ \alpha^*_{2,1}I_{PCP1}(t)R + \alpha^*_{3,1}I_{PCP2}(t)R$$

$$+ \alpha^*_{4,1}I_{AZT}(t)R + \alpha^*_{5,1}I_{T4<20}(t)R;$$

$I_C = 1$ if $C > 886$ days and $I_C = 0$ otherwise (886 was the median value of C), $I_{PCP1}(t)$ takes the value 1 if the subject had one or more postrandomization episode of PCP prior to t and is zero otherwise, $I_{PCP2}(t)$ takes the value 1 if the subject has had two or more episodes of postrandomization PCP prior to t and is zero otherwise, $I_{AZT}(t)$ takes the value 1 if the subject is no longer receiving AZT at time t (usually because of toxicity) and is zero otherwise, $I_{T4<20}(t)$ takes the value 1 if a subject's T4 count at t is less than 20 and zero otherwise. α^* is a vector of unknown parameters to be estimated, and $\lambda_{0,R}(t)$ is an unspecified baseline hazard for the initiation of prophylaxis in stratum R.

Estimates $\hat{\alpha}$ of α^* and their standard errors (in parentheses) based on maximization of the Cox partial likelihood are given in Table 2. The indicators for past bouts of PCP and the indicator for discontinued AZT treatment are positive predictors and the potential censoring date indicator I_C is a negative predictor for the initiation of prophylaxis. These results are not surprising, since previous bouts of postrandomization PCP serve as a medical indication for physicians to initiate prophylaxis. Further, physicians might feel a subject needs prophylaxis if AZT therapy has had to be discontinued. In addition, since prophylaxis therapy was not allowed until August of 1987, it is plausible

Table 2. Fit of Cox Model (2)

Covariate	$\hat{\alpha}_{k,0}$	$\hat{\alpha}_{k,1}$
I_C	−0.64 (0.16)	−0.32 (0.16)
I_{PCP1}	0.88 (0.18)	0.46 (0.20)
I_{PCP2}	0.65 (0.30)	0.80 (0.30)
I_{AZT}	0.16 (0.18)	0.52 (0.19)
$I_{T4<20}$	−0.44 (0.18)	−0.26 (0.19)

that subjects randomized at later calendar dates (i. e., subjects with small values of C) will be more likely to receive prophylaxis soon after randomization. It is unclear why subjects with low T4 counts were less likely to receive prophylaxis.

3.1.2. Details of Method 1

With this background we are now ready to motivate the first method of testing the null hypothesis of no treatment arm effect. Suppose for the moment that, contrary to fact, prophylaxis was known *a priori* not to affect survival and that all subjects die by end of follow-up. Then T_i would equal $T_{p-,i}$, for all i, which we shall abbreviate to $T = T_{p-}$, and further if we define $X_i = \min(T_i, C_i)$, then $X_i = T_i$ for all i. We could then test the hypothesis of no direct effect of treatment arm on survival by defining the test statistic ψ to be the square of

$$\sum_{\text{all subjects}} T_i(R_i - R^{av}) \tag{3}$$

divided by its estimated variance and comparing ψ with a χ_1^2 distribution. That is, we would reject the null hypothesis of no treatment arm effect at the $\alpha = 0.05$ level if $\psi > 3.84$. Here $R^{av} = \sum_{i=1}^n R_i/n$ is the average of R_i over the entire study population. ψ is precisely the two-sample t test. Now, if prophylaxis influences survival, T_i may not equal $T_{p-,i}$ for subjects who received prophylaxis. Hence, continuing to assume $X_i = T_i$ for all i, we shall redefine ψ to be the square of

$$\sum_{\text{no prophylaxis}} T_i(R_i - R^{av})/\hat{K}_i^w(X_i) \tag{4}$$

divided by the variance estimate provided in Robins and Rotnitzky (1992) and Appendix 4 and again compare ψ with a χ_1^2 distribution. Here R^{av} remains the average of R_i over the entire study population; in contrast, the sum in (4) is only over subjects who never initiated prophylaxis. $\hat{K}_i^w(X_i)$ is the estimate of the probability that subject i survived to time X_i without initiating prophylaxis based on Cox model (2) with covariates $W(t)$.

For example, if $\hat{K}_i^w(X_i)$ is 0.1, and subject i never initiated prophylaxis, subject i then needs to count not only for himself but for nine others similar subjects for whom T_{p-i} could not be observed because they initiated prophylaxis prior to X_i. Hence, we divide the contribution of subject i by $\hat{K}_i^w(T_i)$ $= \hat{K}_i^w(X_i)$. To be more specific we shall require the following definitions.

Definitions. $V_i = \min(P_i, X_i) \equiv \min(P_i, T_i, C_i)$, $X_i \equiv \min(T_i, C_i)$, and $\tau_i = 1$ if $V_i = X_i$ and $\tau_i = 0$ otherwise (so that τ_i is 1 if and only if subject i never initiates prophylaxis); $\Delta_i = 1$ if $T_i = X_i$, $\Delta_i = 0$ otherwise [so Δ_i is 1 only if a subject is *observed* to die before EOF (end of follow-up)], $\sigma_i = 1$ if $V_i = T_i$ and $\sigma_i = 0$ otherwise (so $\sigma_i = \Delta_i\tau_i$ is one only if a subject is *observed* to die before initiating prophylaxis).

Then

$$\hat{K}_i^w(u) = \prod_{\{j;V_j \leq u, \tau_j = 0, R_j = R_i\}} \{1 - \hat{\lambda}_{R_j}^w(V_j)\exp[\hat{\alpha}'W_i(V_j)]\}$$

with

$$\hat{\lambda}_{R_j}^w(V_j) \equiv (1 - \tau_j)[\sum_{\{i;R_i = R_j, V_i \geq V_j\}} \exp[\hat{\alpha}'W_i(V_j)]]^{-1}$$

being the Cox baseline hazard for initiation of prophylaxis at V_j in treatment arm R_j. For later reference, we also define

$$\hat{K}_i^0(u) = \prod_{\{j;V_j \leq u, \tau_j = 0, R_j = R_i\}} \{1 - \hat{\lambda}_{R_j}^0(V_j)\}$$

with

$$\hat{\lambda}_{R_j}^0(V_j) \equiv (1 - \tau_j)[\sum_{\{i;R_i = R_j, V_i \geq V_j\}} 1]^{-1}$$

$\hat{K}_i^0(u)$ is the treatment-arm-specific Kaplan–Meier estimator for time to prophylaxis evaluated at u in treatment arm R_i.

Specifically, Robins and Rotnitzky (1992) prove

Theorem 3.1. If Eqs. (1) and (2) hold, the ψ is asymptotically distributed χ_1^2 under the null hypothesis

$$\mathrm{pr}[T_{\mathrm{p}^-} > t \,|\, R = 1] = \mathrm{pr}[T_{\mathrm{p}^-} > t \,|\, R = 0] \tag{5}$$

that T_{p^-} has the same distribution in the two treatment arms. Since, as discussed below, the null hypothesis of no direct treatment arm effect implies (5), a test of (5) is a test of that hypothesis.

We shall later wish to compare the efficiency (power) of our three methods, which we shall accomplish by comparing the lengths of confidence intervals for a parameter β_r that quantifies the direct treatment arm effect. To accomplish this goal, we shall specify a causal model for the direct treatment arm effect. A simple model is to assume

$$T_{\mathrm{r}^-\mathrm{p}^-,\mathrm{i}} = e^{\beta_r^* R_\mathrm{i}} T_{\mathrm{p}^-,\mathrm{i}} \tag{6}$$

where β_r^* is an unknown parameter to be estimated, and $T_{\mathrm{r}^-\mathrm{p}^-,\mathrm{i}}$ is the time a subject would have died if he had never received prophylaxis and had been assigned to the low-dose AZT protocol. That is, once we have removed the effect of prophylaxis on survival and are left with $T_{\mathrm{p}^-,\mathrm{i}}$, the further effect of AZT treatment protocol follows an accelerated failure time model with parameter β_r^*. $T_{\mathrm{r}^-\mathrm{p}^-,\mathrm{i}}$ is a pretreatment variable, in the sense that, like eye color, its value does not depend on a subject's actual prophylaxis therapy or treatment arm. In a completely randomized trial, R_i is jointly independent of all pretreatment variables. Thus,

$$R \amalg T_{\mathrm{r}^-\mathrm{p}^-} \tag{7a}$$

and

$$R \amalg (T_{\mathrm{r}^-\mathrm{p}^-}, C) \tag{7b}$$

since C is also a pretreatment variable. Equation (7b) is read as "R is jointly independent of $T_{\mathrm{r}^-\mathrm{p}^-}$ and C" and implies (7a). We shall call (7b) the physical randomization condition. By definition, the (sharp) null hypothesis of no direct treatment arm effect implies

$$\beta_r^* = 0 \tag{8a}$$

or equivalently,

$$T_{\mathrm{p}^-} = T_{\mathrm{r}^-\mathrm{p}^-} \tag{8b}$$

(7a) and (8b) imply (5) and, thus as discussed above, a test of (5) is a test of the no direct treatment arm effect hypothesis. *If, in the absence of prophylaxis therapy, survival in the low-dose AZT arm exceeds that in the high-dose arm, β_r^* will be positive.*

We can test the hypothesis that the true value of β_r^* equals a particular value β_r by replacing T_i in Eq. (4) by $e^{\beta_r R_i} T_i$. We shall call the resulting test statistic $\psi(\beta_r)$.

A 95% confidence interval for β_r^* would then be the set of test values β_r for which $\psi(\beta_r)$ is less than 3.84, the upper 95th percentile of a χ_1^2 distribution. That is, we shall invert the test $\psi(\beta_r)$ to obtain a confidence interval. A point estimate $\hat{\beta}_r$ of β_r^* is the value of β_r for which $\psi(\beta_r) = 0$. We next note that Theorem 3.1 remains true if we replace T_i in (4) by any fixed function $m(T_i)$ such as $\ln(T_i)$ where ln is the natural logarithm. Similarly, we obtain large sample confidence intervals for β_r^* if we use $m(e^{\beta_r^* R_i} T_i)$ rather than $e^{\beta_r^* R_i} T_i$ in the confidence procedure described previously.

In order to calculate the statistic (4), the survival time T_i must be observed for each subject who fails to initiate prophylaxis. But in trial 002, there were subjects who have neither initiated prophylaxis nor died by end of follow-up on 10/15/89, so that T_i is not always less than C_i. Thus, (4) cannot be computed. In order to overcome this limitation we replace T_i in the numerator of (4) by $M_i = m(\Delta_i, X_i, C_i) \equiv \Delta_i m_1(X_i, C_i) + (1 - \Delta_i) m_2(X_i, C_i) \equiv \Delta_i m_1(T_i, C_i) + (1 - \Delta_i) m_2(C_i, C_i)$. Δ_i is the indicator of censoring by end of follow-up (i. e., $\Delta_i = 1$ if $T_i < C_i$ and $\Delta_i = 0$ otherwise). Here $m_1(\cdot, \cdot)$ and $m_2(\cdot, \cdot)$ are fixed functions chosen by the data analyst. Note X_i and Δ_i are always observed for subjects who do not initiate prophylaxis. Simple choices for M_i include $M_i = \Delta_i T_i$, $M_i = X_i \equiv \Delta_i T_i + (1 - \Delta_i) C_i$ and $M_i = \Delta_i \ln T_i$.

We shall write the test statistic ψ with T_i replaced by M_i as $\psi(m)$. $\psi(m)$ is asymptotically χ_1^2 under (1) and (2) when the randomization condition (7b) and (8) are true. Hence, $\psi(m)$ can be used to test the null hypothesis of no direct treatment arm effect when (1) and (2) hold.

When (1), (2), and (7b) hold, we can test the hypothesis that the true value of β_r^* equals a particular β_r if we replace M_i in $\psi(m)$ by $M_i(\beta_r)$ and compare the resulting statistic $\psi(m, \beta_r)$ to a χ_1^2 distribution where $M_i(\beta_r) = \Delta_i(\beta_r) m_1\{X_i(\beta_r), C_i\} + [1 - \Delta_i(\beta_r)] m_2\{X_i(\beta_r), C_i\}$, $X_i(\beta_r) = \min(T_i(\beta_r), C_i(\beta_r))$; $C_i(\beta_r) = \min(C_i e^{\beta_r}, C_i)$; $T_i(\beta_r) = e^{\beta_r R_i} T_i$; $\Delta_i(\beta_r) = 1$ if $T_i(\beta_r) < C_i(\beta_r)$ and $\Delta_i(\beta_r) = 0$ otherwise (Robins & Rotnitzky, 1992; Appendix 4). Note $\Delta_i(0) = \Delta_i$ and $X_i(0) = X_i$. We call $\Delta_i(\beta_r)$ an artificial censoring (by end of follow-up) indicator since if either $\beta_r < 0$ and $R = 0$, or $\beta_r > 0$ and $R = 1$, $\Delta(\beta_r)$ need not equal the true censoring indicator Δ.

The length of our confidence intervals for β_r^* will depend on the choice of the function $m(\cdot,\cdot) \equiv [m_1(\cdot,\cdot), m_2(\cdot,\cdot)]$. A 95% confidence interval based on $m_j(x, C) = x, j = 1, 2$, [so that $M(\beta_r) = X(\beta_r)$] of $(-0.16, 0.95)$ for β_r^* is reported in row 1 of Table 3. The choice $M(\beta_r) = X(\beta_r)$ is quite inefficient leading to excessively wide intervals for two reasons. First, in small to moderate samples, the test statistic $\psi(m, \beta_r)$ will have a nonnormal heavy-tailed distribution since the contribution of subjects with large values of X_i can be excessive [because we are dividing by $\hat{K}_i(X_i)$ which can be small if X_i is large]. Second, the choice $M(\beta_r) = X(\beta_r)$ gives equal weight to subjects censored by end of follow-up $(X_i = C_i)$ and to failures $(X_i = T_i)$ which may be inefficient. Thus, it would be important to choose $m(\cdot,\cdot)$ optimally. However, in general, the optimal $m(\cdot,\cdot)$ is the solution to an integral equation without a closed form solution. However, Robins and Rotnitzky (1992) derive a closed form expression for the optimal $m(\cdot,\cdot)$ say $m^*(\cdot,\cdot)$, when

$$\lambda_T(t \mid \bar{L}(t), P > t) = \lambda_T(t \mid C, R, P > t) \tag{9}$$

$\lambda_P[t \mid C, R] = \lambda_P[t \mid C]$ and β_r^* is near zero. Equation (9) states that the time-dependent covariates in $\bar{L}(t)$ are not independent risk factors for death. Equation (9) is false in the 002 data. Specifically, we used a time-dependent Cox model for death to show that subjects who had a recurrent episode of PCP by time t had a rate ratio (for death) at t of 1.9 compared with subjects without a recurrence by t when controlling for R, C, and prophylaxis history. In addition, the assumption that censoring by prophylaxis is independent of treatment arm given C is false. Nonetheless, we expect that using $m^*(\cdot,\cdot)$ should give relatively good efficiency without requiring us to solve an integral equation. Robins and Rotnitzky (1992) show that $m_2^*(u, C) = K(u \mid C)g(u, C) + \int_0^u g(x \mid C)\lambda_P(x \mid C)K(x \mid C)dx$ and $m_1^*(u, C) = K(u \mid C)\partial \ln\lambda_{\ln T}(x \mid C)/\partial x|_{x=\ln u} + m_2^*(u, C)$, where $g(u, C) = -\lambda_{\ln T}(x \mid C)|_{x=\ln u}$ and $\lambda_{\ln T}$ is the hazard of $\ln T$ and $K(x \mid C) = \exp[-\int_0^x \lambda_P(u \mid C)du]$. Since $\lambda_P(x \mid C)$ and $\lambda_{\ln T}(X \mid C)$ were unknown, we estimated them from the data under the further (false) assumptions that (i) $\lambda_P(x \mid C) = \lambda_P(x)$ and (ii) $\lambda_{\ln T}(x \mid C) = \lambda_{\ln T}(x)$ with T distributed Weibull with hazard $\lambda_T(t) = at^b$. Specifically, $\hat{\lambda}_P(x)$ and $\hat{\lambda}_{\ln T}(x)$ were respectively the Nelson estimator of $\lambda_P(x)$ and the maximum likelihood estimator of $\lambda_{\ln T}(x)$ under our Weibull assumption based on all the data under the assumption of independent censoring. The fact that the assumptions used in estimating $m^*(\cdot,\cdot)$ are incorrect will lead to some additional loss of efficiency. However, the confidence interval of $(-0.16, 0.38)$ provided in row 2 of Table 3 based on inverting the test $\psi(\hat{m}^*, \beta_r)$ that uses $\hat{M}^*(\beta_r)$ will still have its stated coverage properties under assumptions (1), (2), and (7b)

Table 3. Estimation of β_r^* Using a Variety of Methods and Assumptions

Row	Procedure	Comments	Assumptions	$\hat{\beta}_r$	Nominal 95% confidence interval	χ_1^2 statistic at $\beta_r = 0$
1	Method 1	$M(\beta_r) = X(\beta_r)$	Eqs. (1)–(2)	0.10	(−0.65, 0.95)	0.4
2	Method 1	$\hat{m}^*$	Eqs. (1)–(2)	0.12	(−0.16, 0.38)	0.7
3	$Q_L^*(\beta_r)$		Prophylaxis has no effect Independent censoring by EOF	0.11	(−0.01, 0.23)	3.6
4	$Q_W^*(\beta_r)$		Prophylaxis has no effect Independent censoring by EOF	0.13	(0.02, 0.25)	5.2
5	$Q_L^{**}(\beta_r)$		Independent censoring by prophylaxis and EOF	0.17	(−0.08, 0.42)	1.6
6	Log-rank test		Treat prophylaxis as death Independent censoring by EOF	−0.025	(−0.17, 0.12)	0.3
7	$Q_L(\beta_r)$		Prophylaxis has no effect Dependent censoring by EOF	0.11	(−0.01, 0.24)	3.6
8	$Q_W(\beta_r)$		Prophylaxis has no effect Dependent censoring by EOF	0.13	(0.02, 0.25)	5.2
9	Method 2		Eq. (12)	0.25	(−0.03, 0.51)	3.2
10	Method 3	Prentice–Wilcoxon	Eqs. (1), (2), (12)	0.14	(0.03, 0.26)	5.0
11	Method 3	Log rank	Eqs. (1), (2), (12)	0.12	(0.0, 0.25)	3.9
12	$Q_L^W(\beta_r)$		Eqs. (1), (2) Independent censoring by EOF	0.12	(−0.16, 0.35)	0.5

where $\hat{m}^*(\cdot,\cdot)$ is our estimate of $m^*(\cdot,\cdot)$ (Robins and Rotnitzky, 1992). Further, it is much narrower than the interval in row 1 based on $M(\beta_r) = X(\beta_r)$.

3.2. Comparison of Method 1 with Weighted Log-Rank Estimates of β_r^*

The standard approach to analyzing the 002 data would be to ignore prophylaxis entirely and apply a weighted log-rank test to the data $X_i = \min(T_i, C_i)$, Δ_i, R_i. Specifically, in Section 2, we noted that standard log-rank test Q_L^* and the Prentice–Wilcoxon weighted log-rank test Q_W^* gave p values of 0.07 and 0.02, respectively. But, as discussed previously, Q_L^* and Q_W^* are appropriate α-level tests of the hypothesis $\beta_r^* = 0$ and thus of the hypothesis of no direct treatment arm effect only if it were known *a priori* that prophylaxis had no effect on survival, i. e., $T = T_{p^-}$. Were it known that prophylaxis had no effect on survival, Louis (1981) and Tsiatis (1990) show how one can use a weighted log-rank test to estimate β_r^* of model (6) under the additional assumption that censoring by end of follow-up (EOF) and failure are independent given R, i. e.,

$$C \amalg T \,|\, R \tag{10a}$$

To explain the Louis–Tsiatis procedure, we need to define a generic weighted log-rank test.

A weighted log-rank test $Q^\dagger(\omega)$ is generically defined as follows. Let $T_i^\dagger$ be a generic continuous failure time variable, $C_i^\dagger$ a generic censoring variable, and $X_i^\dagger = \min(T_i^\dagger, C_i^\dagger)$. Suppose we can observe $\{X_i^\dagger, \Delta_i^\dagger, R_i\}$, $i = 1, \ldots, n$, where $\Delta_i^\dagger = 1$ if $X_i^\dagger = T_i^\dagger = 0$ otherwise. Here R_i is a dichotomous $(0, 1)$ variable. Let $Y_i^\dagger(t) = 1$ if $X_i^\dagger \geq t$ so $Y_i^\dagger(t)$ is 1 if a subject is at risk at t. Then, by definition, a weighted log-rank test $Q^\dagger(\omega)$ with weight function $\omega(\cdot)$ applied to the data $\{R_i, X_i^\dagger, \Delta_i^\dagger\}$, $i = 1, \ldots, n$ equals $S^2(\omega)/\Sigma(\omega)$, where

$$S(\omega) = \sum_{i=1}^{n} \Delta_i^\dagger \omega(X_i^\dagger)\{R_i - E_i\}, \quad E_i \equiv \sum_{j=1}^{n} Y_j^\dagger(X_i^\dagger)R_j \Big/ \sum_{j=1}^{n} Y_j^\dagger(X_i^\dagger)$$

is the proportion of subjects at risk at $X_i^\dagger$ with $R = 1$, and $\Sigma = \Sigma_{i=1}^{n} \Delta_i^\dagger \omega^2(X_i^\dagger)E_i(1 - E_i)$. $\omega(\cdot)$ can depend on the failure and censoring history up to $X_i^\dagger$. The standard log-rank test $Q_L^\dagger$ has $\omega(X_i^\dagger)$ identically equal to one. The Prentice–Wilcoxon test $Q_W^\dagger$ has

$$\omega(X_i^\dagger) = \prod_{\{j; \Delta_j^\dagger = 1, X_j^\dagger < X_i^\dagger\}} [1 - 1/\sum_{i=1}^{n} Y_i^\dagger(X_j^\dagger)]$$

equal to the Kaplan–Meier survival curve for failure.

If prophylaxis therapy was known *a priori* not to influence survival, i. e., $T = T_{p-}$, then under (7) and (10a) we can validly test the hypothesis that the true value of β_r^* equals a particular value β_r by applying any weighted log-rank test $Q^\dagger(\omega)$ to the data $\{R_i,\ X_i^*(\beta_r),\ \Delta_i\}$, $i = 1, \ldots, n$ where $X_i^*(\beta_r) = \min[T_i(\beta_r),\ C_i e^{\beta_r R_i}]$ and $T_i(\beta_r) = T_i e^{\beta_r R_i}$ (Louis, 1981; Tsiatis, 1990). We denote this test by $Q^*(\omega, \beta_r)$. A 95% confidence interval for β_r^* would then be the set of test values β_r for which $Q^*(\omega, \beta_r)$ is less than 3.84, the upper 95th percentile of a χ_1^2 distribution. A point estimate $\hat\beta_r$ of β_r^* is the value of β_r for which $Q^*(\omega, \beta_r) = 0$.

Point estimates and confidence intervals for the log-rank test $Q_L^*(\beta_r)$ and the Prentice–Wilcoxon test $Q_W^*(\beta_r)$ are given in rows 3 and 4 of Table 3. (Note that at $\beta_r = 0$, these test statistics are precisely the tests Q_L^* and Q_W^* discussed previously.) It is of interest to note that the point estimate $\hat\beta_r = 0.13$ under Method 1 is essentially equal to the point estimates of 0.11 and 0.13 based on $Q_L^*(\beta_r)$ and $Q_W^*(\beta_r)$. This suggests that prophylaxis may have little effect on survival. However, the confidence interval of $(-0.16, 0.38)$ based on Method 1 is much wider than intervals of $(-0.01, 0.23)$ and $(0.02, 0.25)$ based on $Q_L^*(\beta_r)$ and $Q_W^*(\beta_r)$, since Method 1 does not use the information contained in the actual death times of the 252 subjects who died after initiating prophylaxis but before EOF.

Suppose that one was not willing to assume that prophylaxis had no effect on survival, but one was willing to assume that censoring by both prophylaxis and EOF was independent of T_{p-} given R, i. e.,

$$T_{p-} \amalg (C, P) \mid R \tag{10b}$$

Then one could obtain valid tests and estimates for β_r^* by applying any weighted log-rank test $Q^\dagger(\omega)$ to the data $(R_i,\ V_i(\beta_r),\ \sigma_i)$ where $V_i(\beta_r) = V_i e^{\beta_r R_i}$, $V_i = \min(T_i, P_i, C_i)$, $\sigma_i = 1$ if and only if $V_i = T_i$. That is, we apply a weighted log-rank test that treats both censoring by end of follow-up C and initiation of prophylaxis P as independent censoring. In row 5 of Table 3, we report results based on the log-rank version of this test, $Q_L^{**}(\beta_r)$ say. Note the point estimate $\hat\beta_r = 0.17$ is somewhat greater than the estimate $\hat\beta_r = 0.11$ based on $Q_L^*(\beta_r)$ and the estimate of 0.12 based on Method 1. This presumably reflects the fact that (10b) is false because (i), as we have demonstrated by our fit of Cox model (2), recurrent PCP is a predictor of time to prophylaxis P and (ii), as noted above, recurrent PCP also independently predicts failure (rate ratio 1.9). Thus, subjects initiating prophylaxis at t have poorer prognosis (i. e., smaller T_{p-}) than others. Hence, censoring by prophylaxis will be dependent and (10b) will be false. Since more subjects in the low- than high-dose AZT arm initiate prophylaxis, it may be that the selection bias relating to dependent censoring by prophylaxis is greater in the low- than high-dose arm, leading to an artifactually higher estimate of β_r^* based on $Q_L^{**}(\beta_r)$.

Of course, if, as we have assumed, Eqs. (1) and (2) are true, Method 1 appropriately adjusts for dependent censoring by prophylaxis.

An extreme (unrealistic) assumption concerning dependent censoring by prophylaxis would be to assume, not that Eqs. (1) and (2) were true, but rather than any subject i observed to initiate prophylaxis does so only seconds before the subject would have died in the absence of prophylaxis therapy, i. e.,

$$P_i < \min(T_i, C_i) \quad \text{implies} \quad P_i = T_{p-,i} \tag{10c}$$

Under (10c), for subjects with $T_i > P_i$, $T_i - P_i$ would reflect the beneficial causal effect of prophylaxis on survival. As a sensitivity analysis, in row 6 of Table 3 we estimated β_r^* under assumption (10c) by regarding any subject observed to initiate prophylaxis at t as a failure at t. That is, we applied the generic log-rank test $Q_L^\dagger$ to the data $(R_i, V_i(\beta_r), \sigma_i^*)$ where $\sigma_i^* = 1$ if V_i is either T_i or P_i and $\sigma_i^* = 0$ if $V_i = C_i$. We obtained a point estimate $\hat\beta_r$ of -0.025 and a 95% confidence interval of $(-0.17, 0.12)$. Our point estimate of -0.025 suggests that, were (10c) true, the improved survival in the low-dose arm would be fully attributable to differential prophylaxis usage.

Rather than simply testing the null hypothesis (5) [or equivalently Eq. (8)] that T_{p-} has the same distribution in the two treatment arms, it is of interest to actually estimate the treatment-arm-specific survival curves $F(u|r) = \text{pr}[T_{p-} > u | R = r]$, $r = 0, 1$, by calculating Kaplan–Meier (KM) survival curve estimates.

Hence, for generic variables $X_i^\dagger$, $\Delta_i^\dagger$ define the group-specific KM survival estimator at time u to be $\hat F^\dagger(u) = \prod_i \Delta_i^\dagger [1 - \{\sum_j Y_j^\dagger(X_i^\dagger)\}^{-1}] I[X_i^\dagger < u]$ where the product and sum are over a specified group of subjects and $I[A] = 1$ if A is true and $I[A] = 0$ otherwise.

Figure 1a shows the treatment-arm-specific KM curves for T_{p-} obtained by ignoring prophylaxis and applying $\hat F^\dagger(u)$ to the data (X_i, Δ_i) in treatment arm r for $r = 0, 1$. This will be consistent for $F(u|r)$ if $T = T_{p-}$ and (10a) holds.

Figure 1b shows the KM survival curves for T_{p-} calculated by treating both EOF and initiation of prophylaxis as independent censoring, and thus, applying $\hat F^\dagger(u)$ to the data (V_i, σ_i) in treatment arm r. This will be consistent for $F(u|r)$ if (10b) holds.

The treatment-arm-specific KM curves in Fig. 1b are algebraically equivalent to the treatment-arm-specific curves

$$\hat F^0(u) = \prod_i I(X_i < u)\sigma_i\{1 - [\hat K_i^0(X_i)]^{-1}/[\sum_j \tau_j I(X_j \geq X_i)/\hat K_j^0(X_j)]\}$$

provided that the subject with the largest value of V in each treatment arm r has $\tau = 1$, a condition that is fulfilled in the 002 data. Here the product and the sum are over subjects in a given treatment arm r, and for any u, $\hat{K}_i^0(u)$ is the treatment-arm-specific KM survival curve for time to prophylaxis for subject i evaluated at u obtained by applying $\hat{F}^\dagger(u)$ to the data $\{V_j, (1 - \tau_j)\}$ in treatment arm R_i.

Figure 1c plots the treatment-arm-specific curves $\hat{F}^w(u)$ obtained by replacing $\hat{K}^0$ by $\hat{K}^w$ in the definition of $\hat{F}^0(u)$. $\hat{F}^w(u)$, for treatment arm r, will be consistent for $F(u|r)$ provided that Eqs. (1), (2), and (10a) are true since $\hat{F}^w(u)$ appropriately adjusts for dependent censoring of T_{p^-} by prophylaxis (Robins and Rotnitzky, 1992). Thus, we would tend to rely on the curves in Fig. 1c, if we are not willing to assume a priori either that prophylaxis has no effect on survival or that (10b) is true. A modification of $\hat{F}^w(u)$ that is always at least as efficient as the unmodified $\hat{F}^w(u)$ is obtained by replacing $\tau_j/\hat{K}_j^0(X_j)$ by $1/\hat{K}_j^w(X_i)$ in $\hat{F}^0(u)$. This modification and its properties are discussed in unpublished manuscripts by Malani; Robins, Rotnitzky, and Zhao; and Robins.

3.3. Dependent versus Independent Censoring by End of Follow-up

Even if prophylaxis has no effect on survival, i. e., $T = T_{p^-}$, the confidence intervals for β_r^* based on $Q_L^*(\beta_r)$ and $Q_W^*(\beta_r)$ are valid only if

$$\lambda_T[t|R] = \lambda_T[t|R, C > t] \qquad (10d)$$

[This follows from the fact that if (10d) is false, the cause-specific hazard for $X^*(\beta_r^*)$ corresponding to $\Delta = 1$ need not be equal in the two treatment arms if $\beta_r^* \neq 0$.]. Equation (10d) is the standard assumption made in analyzing censored survival data in a randomized trial. Clearly (10d) cannot be tested based on the observed data. Although (10a) implies (10d), the converse is false. Nonetheless, if (10a) were false, it seems highly probable that (10d) would be false as well based on smoothness considerations. However, since the potential censoring time C is observed even for subjects failing prior to C, we are able to test (10a) in our data by fitting the proportional hazard model for T given by $\lambda_T[t|R, C] = \lambda_0(t)\exp\{\gamma_0 R + \gamma_1 C\}$. We obtained a point estimate $\hat{\gamma}_1$ of 0.68×10^{-3} and a 95% confidence interval of $(0.12 \times 10^{-3}, 1.36 \times 10^{-3})$ for γ_1 and thus we rejected (10a) [since (10a) implies $\gamma_1 = 0$]. $\hat{\gamma}_1$ corresponds to a rate ratio comparing an early enrollee ($C = 1100$ days) and a late enrollee ($C = 700$) of about 1.3.

Hence, it is important to develop methods that do not require (10d) to be true. It follows from Robins and Tsiatis (1991) and Robins and Rotnitzky (1992) that, when the randomization condition (7b) holds and $T = T_{p^-}$, valid confidence intervals for β_r^* can be obtained by inverting any weighted log-rank test $Q(\omega, \beta_r)$ even if (10d) is false where $Q(\omega, \beta_r)$ is the generic $Q^\dagger(\omega)$ applied to data $(R_i, X_i(\beta_r), \Delta_i(\beta_r))$, $i = 1, \ldots, n$, and $X_i(\beta_r)$ and $\Delta_i(\beta_r)$ are as defined in Section 3.1. [This reflects the fact that $\{X(\beta_r^*),$ $\Delta(\beta_r^*)\}$ are functions only of C and $T(\beta_r^*)$ and thus are jointly independent of R when (7b) holds and $T = T_{p^-}$, since (6) then implies $T(\beta_r^*) = T_{r^-p^-}$. Hence, the cause-specific hazard of $X(\beta_r^*)$ corresponding to $\Delta(\beta_r^*) = 1$ will be the same in the two treatment arms.] Results for $Q_L(\beta_r)$ and $Q_W(\beta_r)$, the log-rank and Prentice–Wilcoxon version of $Q(\omega, \beta_r)$, are given in rows 7 and 8 of Table 3.

$Q_L^*(0)$ is algebraically equal to $Q_L(0)$, so the χ_1^2 statistics in rows 4 and 7 of Table 3 are exactly equal. Further, the confidence interval of $(-0.01, 0.23)$ based on $Q_L^*(\beta_r)$ and that of $(-0.01, 0.24)$ based on $Q_L(\beta_r)$ are almost exactly equal, demonstrating that, although (10a) is false [and thus most likely (10d) is false as well], little bias is introduced by supposing it to be true. Indeed, results based on $Q_W^*(\beta_r)$ and $Q_W(\beta_r)$ are identical to two significant digits.

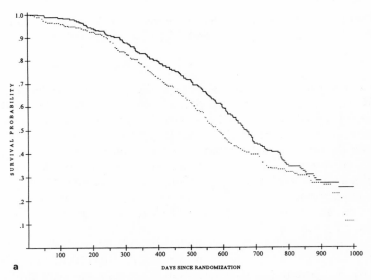

Figure 1. Treatment-arm-specific survival curve estimates for T_{p^-} under various assumptions. (a) Assumes prophylaxis has no effect on survival, $T = T_{p^-}$; (b) assumes independent censoring by prophylaxis conditional on treatment arm; (c) assumes dependent censoring by prophylaxis conditional on treatment but independent censoring conditional on the covariates $\bar{L}(t)$. (a–c) All assume independent censoring by end of follow-up conditional on treatment arm. Solid curve, low-dose AZT arm; dotted curve, high-dose AZT arm.

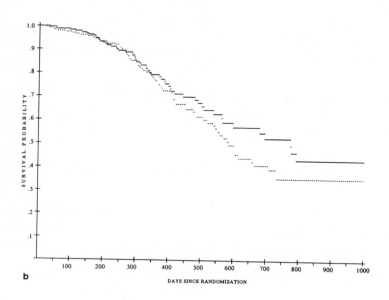

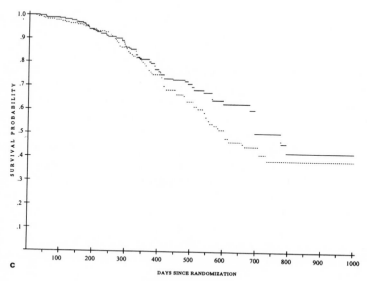

Figure 1. (*continued*)

Of course, in general, we are not willing to assume that $T = T_{p^-}$. Importantly, therefore, given (1), (2), and (7b) hold, *the confidence intervals for β_r^* based on Method 1 are valid even if (10d) is false.*

The following remark as well as Sections 3.4 and 3.5 may be bypassed in a first reading without losing the thread of the argument.

Remark. In contrast, the treatment-arm-specific estimator $\hat{F}^w(u)$ will no longer be consistent for $F(u|r)$ if (10d) is false. However, suppose, with $X^* \equiv \min(P, C)$, that

$$\lambda_{X^*}[t|\bar{L}^*(t), T > t, T_{p^-}] = \lambda_{X^*}[t|\bar{L}^*(t), T > t] \qquad (10e)$$

where $\bar{L}^*(t)$ is $\bar{L}(t)$ less the variable C. If (10e) is true, but (10b) is false, we say we have dependent censoring by (C, P) jointly given treatment arm R but independent censoring given $\bar{L}^*(t)$. If (10e) is true, a consistent estimator of

$F(u|r)$ is $\hat{F}^{*w}(u)$

$$= \prod_i \sigma_i I(T_i < u)\{1 - [\hat{K}_i^{*w}(V_i)]^{-1}[\sum_j \sigma_j^* I(V_j > V_i)/\hat{K}_j^{*w}(V_j)]^{-1}\}$$

where the sum and product are over subjects in arm r, $\sigma_j^* = 1$ if either $\sigma_j = 1$ or subject j has the largest value of V in his arm R_j and $\bar{K}^{*w}(u)$ is an estimate of $K^*(u) \equiv \exp\{-\int_0^u \lambda_{X^*}[t|\bar{L}^*(t), T > t]dt\}$ based on a correctly specified Cox model for $\lambda_{X^*}[t|\bar{L}^*(t), T > t]$. (In fitting this Cox model it is necessary to artificially treat any subject with $\sigma^* = 1$ as having $V = T$. That is, if, as in the 002 data, the subject with the largest value of V in a given treatment arm has $V = C$, we artificially set that subject's V to T prior to fitting the above Cox model.) In practice, to avoid specification bias, we would specify two separate time-dependent Cox models for the cause-specific hazards $\lambda_{X^* \cdot k}[t|\bar{L}^*(t), T > t]$, $k = 1, 2$ (each model stratified on treatment arm) corresponding to the causes "prophylaxis initiation" and "EOF" and define $\hat{K}^{*w}(u) = \hat{K}_1^{*w}(u)\hat{K}_2^{*w}(u)$, where $\hat{K}_k^{*w}(u) = \exp\{-\int_0^u \hat{\lambda}_{X,k}^{*w}[t|\bar{L}^*(t), T > t]dt\}$, and $\hat{\lambda}_{X,k}^{*w}[t|\bar{L}^*(t), T > t]$ is the Cox hazard estimate for cause k given $\bar{L}^*(t)$. The "w" in $\hat{K}^{*w}$ refers to the covariates $W(t)$ [depending on $\bar{L}^*(t)$] that were used in the Cox models for $\lambda_{X^* \cdot k}[t|\bar{L}^*(t), T > t]$. (Of course, if T_{p^-} and C are correlated, there may be little substantive interest in the marginal distribution of T_{p^-}.)

3.4. Remarks on Efficiency

In Appendix 4, we show that when (7b) and (10d) holds and $T = T_{p^-}$ [so intervals based on either $Q(\omega, \beta_r)$ or $Q^*(\omega, \beta_r)$ are valid], (i) for fixed $\omega(\cdot)$, intervals based on $Q^*(\omega, \beta_r)$ are always (asymptotically) strictly narrower than those based on $Q(\omega, \beta_r)$ except if $\beta_r^* = 0$ in which case they are (asymptotically) of equal width; (ii) if (the distribution of) T given R is Weibull, (a) the intervals based on $Q_L^*(\beta_r)$ are the narrowest possible (Ritov and Wellner, 1988), and (b) the intervals based on $Q_L(\beta_r)$ are the narrowest among all confidence procedures that [like $Q_L(\beta_r)$ but unlike $Q_L^*(\beta_r)$] are guaranteed to yield valid large sample confidence intervals even were (10a) false.

Further, Robins and Rotnitzky (1992, Appendix 4) showed that, given (7b), when (10a) and (10d) are false, the interval based on $Q_L(\beta_r)$ is no longer the narrowest possible confidence interval for β_r^* of model (6) that is guaranteed to cover at its nominal rate under the restriction $T = T_{p^-}$. Rather, the narrowest interval is obtained by inverting the test $\psi(m, \beta_r)$ when (i) $m_2(u, C) \equiv g(u, C)$, $m_1(u, C) \equiv g(\omega, C) + \partial \ln\lambda_{\ln T}(x|C)/\partial x|_{x=\ln u}$, $g(u, C)$ is as defined following Eq. (9) and (ii) τ_i and $\hat{K}_i^w(X_i)$ are (artificially) set to 1 for all i. This interval (i) will be strictly narrower than the interval based on inverting $Q_L(\beta_r)$ except if both (10d) holds and T given R is Weibull in which case they are equal in length and (ii), when (10d) holds and T given R is Weibull, will be strictly longer than that based on $Q_L^*(\beta_r)$ except at $\beta_r^* = 0$ where they are equal.

3.5. An Improvement on the Log-Rank Test with Independent Censoring by Using Surrogate Markers

Suppose (10b) were true, so we could obtain valid confidence intervals for β_r^* by inverting the log-rank test $Q_L^{**}(\beta_r)$ that treats both EOF and initiation of prophlaxis as independent censoring. Write $\bar{L}^{\cdot}(t) = (\bar{L}^*(t), R)$. The covariates $\bar{L}^*(t)$ are the posttreatment time-dependent covariates and are often referred to as surrogate markers. Note $Q_L^{**}(\beta_r)$ does not use data on the time-dependent covariates $\bar{L}^*(t)$ such as PCP history. We will show how to construct valid confidence intervals that are guaranteed to be narrower than those based on $Q_L^{**}(\beta_r)$ by incorporating surrogate marker data $\bar{L}^*(t)$ provided $\bar{L}^*(t)$ is an independent predictor of mortality, i. e., provided $\lambda_T[t|\bar{L}^*(t), R] \neq \lambda_T[t|R]$ and that (10e) holds. [One would often be unwilling to assume (10b) held unless one assumed that (10e) also held.] To do so, we first note that the numerator, $S_L^{**}(\beta_r)$ say, of the usual log-rank test $Q_L^{**}(\beta_r)$ is algebraically equivalent to $S_L^{\cdot 0}(\beta_r) = \sum_{i=1}^n \sigma_i[R_i - E_i^{\cdot 0}(\beta_r)]$, where

$$E_i^{\cdot 0}(\beta_r) = [\sum_{j=1}^{n} \sigma_j^* R_j I[V_j(\beta_r) > V_i(\beta_r)]$$

$$\times \hat{K}_j^{\cdot 0}[V_i(\beta_r)e^{-\beta_r R_j}]/\{\hat{K}_j^{\cdot 0}(V_j)\}]/\sum_{j=1}^{n} \sigma_j^* I[V_j(\beta_r) > V_i(\beta_r)]$$

$$\times \hat{K}_j^{\cdot 0}[V_i(\beta_r)e^{-\beta_r R_j}]/\{\hat{K}_j^{\cdot 0}(V_j)\}$$

and, for each subject j, $\hat{K}_j^{\cdot 0}(u)$ is the KM curve for censoring by either C or P, except that the subject with the largest value of V in each treatment arm is treated as a failure. That is, $\hat{K}_j^{\cdot 0}(u)$ is the generic KM estimator $\hat{F}^\dagger(u)$ applied to data $\{V_i, 1 - \sigma_i^*\}$ in treatment arm R_j.

$S_L^{\cdot 0}(\beta_r)$ can be rewritten as $S_L^{\cdot 0}(\beta_r) = \sum_{i=1}^{n} \{\hat{K}_i^{\cdot 0}(V_i)\}^{-1}\sigma_i\hat{K}_i^{\cdot 0}(V_i)[R_i - E_i^{\cdot 0}(\beta_r)]$. Now define $E_i^{\cdot w}(\beta_r)$ like $E_i^{\cdot 0}(\beta_r)$ except replace the $\hat{K}_j^{\cdot 0}(V_j)$ in set braces by $\hat{K}_j^{\cdot w}(V_j)$. Set $S_L^{\cdot w}(\beta_r) = \sum_{i=1}^{n} \{\hat{K}_i^{\cdot w}(V_i)\}^{-1}\sigma_i\hat{K}_i^{\cdot 0}(V_i)[R_i - E_i^{\cdot w}(\beta_r)]$. Let $Q_L^{\cdot w}(\beta_r)$ be $\{S_L^{\cdot w}(\beta_r)\}^2$ divided by the variance estimate given in Appendix 4.2. In Appendix 4.3, we prove that, if $\hat{K}_j^{\cdot w}(u)$ is computed based on a correctly specified model, intervals based on inverting $Q_L^{\cdot w}(\beta_r)$ will be strictly narrower than those based on the log-rank test $Q_L^{**}(\beta_r)$ when (10e) and (10b) are true. Further, when (10b) is false, but (10e) is true, intervals based on $Q_L^{\cdot w}(\beta_r)$ in contrast to those based on $Q_L^{**}(\beta_r)$ will continue to cover at their nominal rate.

Now define $E_i^0(\beta_r)$ and $E_i^w(\beta_r)$ like $E_i^{\cdot 0}(\beta_r)$ and $E_i^{\cdot w}(\beta_r)$ except τ_j replaces σ_j^* and $\hat{K}^0$ and $\hat{K}^w$ (defined previously) replace $\hat{K}^{\cdot 0}$ and $\hat{K}^{\cdot w}$. Let $S_L^0(\beta_r)$, $S_L^w(\beta_r)$, and $Q_L^w(\beta_r)$ be defined like their "$\cdot$" counterparts but with $\hat{K}^w$, $\hat{K}^0$, E^w, E^0 replacing their "$\cdot$" counterparts. Then (i) $S_L^0(\beta_r) = S_L^{\cdot 0}(\beta_r)$, (ii) intervals based on inverting $Q_L^w(\beta_r)$ will be valid when (1), (2), and (10a) hold, and will be strictly narrower than the (now valid) intervals based on $Q_L^{**}(\beta_r)$ when (10b) holds as well. In the 002 data, a 95% confidence interval based on inverting $Q_L^w(\beta_r)$ was $(-0.16, 0.35)$ with a point estimate $\hat{\beta}_r$ of 0.125. See row 12 of Table 3. When assumptions justifying both methods are satisfied, intervals based on $Q_L^{\cdot w}(\beta_r)$ will be narrower than those based on $Q_L^w(\beta_r)$. Intervals that are at least as narrow as those based on $Q_L^{\cdot w}(\beta_r)$ can be obtained upon modifying $Q_L^{\cdot w}(\beta_r)$ by redefining $E_i^{\cdot w}(\beta_r)$ to be $E_i^{\cdot 0}(\beta_r)$ with $\sigma_j/\hat{K}_j^{\cdot 0}(V_j)$ replaced by $1/\hat{K}_j^{\cdot w}(V_i)$ in the numerator and denominator. This modification and its properties are considered in unpublished manuscripts by Malani; Robins, Rotnitzky, and Zhao; and Robins.

3.6. Method 2

In Method 2, as with Method 1, we shall assume the randomization condition (7b) holds and test the null hypothesis of no direct treatment arm effect by testing whether Eq. (8) holds. In contrast to Method 1, we shall not assume that either Eq. (1) or (2) is correct. Rather, we shall assume that the causal effect of prophylaxis treatment on survival can be described by a particular SNFTM. Let $T_{p+,i}$ represent subject i's death time if continuous prophylaxis therapy was begun at start of follow-up.

One simple SNFTM assumes that, under continuous prophylaxis therapy, a subject's life is expanded or contracted by the factor $e^{-\beta_p^*}$, where β_p^* is an unknown parameter that we will later estimate. That is,

$$T_{p-,i}e^{-\beta_p^*} = T_{p+,i}$$

In particular, if $\beta_p^* < 0$, then $T_{p-,i} < T_{p+,i}$ and prophylaxis therapy is beneficial. If $\beta_p^* = 0$, then $T_{p-,i} = T_{p+,i}$, and there is no effect of prophylaxis on survival. Finally, if $\beta_p^* > 0$, then prophylaxis decreases survival. We note that the expansion factor $e^{-\beta_p^*}$ is related to a parameter of public health interest. Specifically, $(T_{p+,i} - T_{p-,i})/T_{p-,i} = e^{-\beta_p^*} - 1$ is the fractional increase in life expectancy because of continuous prophylaxis therapy.

We next extend our causal model to incorporate other counterfactual prophylaxis histories. Let $T_{p=(v),i}$ represent subject i's death time if prophylaxis therapy were to begin at time v after enrollment and continued thereafter. If, in the absence of prophylaxis, a subject would die prior to v, then $T_{p=(v),i}$ equals $T_{p-,i}$. Note that we can write $T_{p+,i}$ as $T_{p=(0),i}$ and $T_{p-,i}$ as $T_{p=(\infty),i}$. In our extended causal model, $e^{-\beta_p^*}$ is the factor by which a subject's remaining life ($T_{p-,i} - v$) is expanded or contracted by initiating prophylaxis therapy at time v (Cox and Oakes, 1984). That is, for each v,

$$e^{-\beta_p^*}(T_{p-,i} - v) = (T_{p=(v),i} - v) \qquad \text{if } T_{p=(v),i} > v \qquad (11a)$$

$$T_{p-,i} = T_{p=(v),i} \qquad \text{otherwise} \qquad (11b)$$

When we substitute $v = 0$ into (11a), we recover our previous SNFTM linking $T_{p+,i}$ and $T_{p-,i}$.

Let P_i be the time, if any, subject i was observed to initiate prophylaxis in the actual study. Then a subject's observed death time T_i must be $T_{p=(v),i}$ with $v = P_i$ and thus, by (11a), $e^{-\beta_p^*}(T_{p-,i} - P_i) = (T_i - P_i)$. On the other hand, if a subject never initiates prophylaxis, his observed death time T_i obviously equals $T_{p-,i}$. Thus, on solving for $T_{p-,i}$, the SNFTM (11) implies that $T_{p-,i}$ is linked to the observed death time and prophylaxis history by

$$T_{p-,i} = P_i + (T_i - P_i)e^{\beta_p^*} \qquad \text{if } P_i < T_i \qquad (12a)$$

and

$$T_{p^-,i} = T_i \qquad \text{otherwise} \qquad (12b)$$

Note $\beta_p^* = 0$ implies $T = T_{p^-,i}$.

(12a) and (12b) are the only assumptions beyond the randomization condition (7b) that are used in Method 2 to test the null hypothesis (8). To estimate the magnitude of the direct treatment arm effect, we shall also assume (6) holds. We shall now describe how we can test the hypothesis that a particular value β_r equals the true value β_r^* in (6) under Method 2. The choice $\beta_r = 0$ will give a test of the null hypothesis (8). We first describe how to construct a test for the *joint hypothesis* that (β_r, β_p) equals the true parameter values (β_r^*, β_p^*). We then show how to use our *joint hypothesis test* to construct a test of the univariate hypothesis $\beta_r = \beta_r^*$ of interest.

Define $T_{p^-,i}(\beta_p)$ by (12a) and (12b) except with β_p substituted for the true β_p^*. Define $T_i(\beta_r, \beta_p) = e^{\beta_r R_i} T_{p^-,i}(\beta_p)$ so that $T_i(0, \beta_p) = T_{p^-,i}(\beta_p)$ and $T_i(\beta_r, 0) = T_i(\beta_r)$, where $T_i(\beta_r)$ is as defined previously. Note that for each (β_r, β_p), $T_i(\beta_r, \beta_p)$ is an observable random variable. Further, at the true but unknown (β_r^*, β_p^*), $T_i(\beta_r^*, \beta_p^*) = T_{r^-p^-,i}$. Since, by (7b), $T_{r^-p^-,i}$ is independent of R_i, it immediately follows that for any given (β_r, β_p), we obtain an asymptotic α-level test of the hypothesis $(\beta_r^*, \beta_p^*) = (\beta_r, \beta_p)$ by the following procedure. Choose two weighted log-rank tests. We shall use the log-rank test itself and the Prentice–Wilcoxon test. Let $S_L(\beta_r, \beta_p)$, $S_W(\beta_r, \beta_p)$, and $\Sigma_{LW}(\beta_r, \beta_p)$ be respectively the numerators of the generic log-rank test $Q_L^\dagger$ and Prentice–Wilcoxon test $Q_W^\dagger$ and their joint estimated covariance matrix applied to the data $\{R_i, T_i(\beta_r, \beta_p)\}; i = (1, \ldots, n)\}$. [The 2×2 estimated covariance matrix Σ_{12} of a bivariate generic weighted log-rank test with numerators $(S_1^\dagger, S_2^\dagger)$ based on weight functions $\omega_1(\cdot)$ and $\omega_2(\cdot)$ respectively has (m, k) entry equal to $\sum_{i=1}^n \Delta_i^\dagger \omega_m(X_i^\dagger) \omega_k(X_i^\dagger) E_i(1 - E_i)$.]

We compare $Q_{LW}(\beta_r, \beta_p) \equiv (S_L(\beta_r, \beta_p), S_W(\beta_r, \beta_p)) \Sigma_{LW}(\beta_r, \beta_p)^{-1}(S_L(\beta_r, \beta_p), S_W(\beta_r, \beta_p))'$ to 5.99, the 95th percentile of a χ_2^2 distribution. If $Q_{LW}(\beta_r, \beta_p)$ exceeds 5.99, we reject the hypothesis $(\beta_r, \beta_p) = (\beta_r^*, \beta_p^*)$ at the 5% level. Robins and Tsiatis (1991) provide a formal proof.

In order to compute $Q_{LW}(\beta_r, \beta_p)$, we need to have observed T_i for all subjects. In fact, as discussed previously, we actually observed only (X_i, Δ_i, C_i) because of censoring by end of follow-up. Robins and Tsiatis (1991) show that the test of joint null hypothesis $(\beta_r, \beta_p) = (\beta_r^*, \beta_p^*)$ given above is still valid in the presence of censoring by end of follow-up if (12a), (12b), and (6) are true when we modify $Q_{LW}(\beta_r, \beta_p)$ as follows. Define $X_i(\beta_r, \beta_p) \equiv \min[C_i(\beta_r, \beta_p), T_i(\beta_r, \beta_p)]$ where $C_i(\beta_r, \beta_p) = \min(C_i, e^{\beta_p} C_i, e^{\beta_r} C_i, e^{\beta_r \beta_p} C_i)$ and $\Delta_i(\beta_r, \beta_p) = 1$ if $X_i(\beta_r, \beta_p) = T_i(\beta_r, \beta_p)$ and $\Delta_i(\beta_r, \beta_p) = 0$

otherwise. Then $Q_{LW}(\beta_r, \beta_p)$ is as defined above except we apply the generic log-rank and Prentice–Wilcoxon tests to the data $\{R_i, X_i(\beta_r, \beta_p), \Delta_i(\beta_r, \beta_p)\}$, $i = (1, \ldots, n)$, treating $\Delta_i(\beta_r, \beta_p)$ as a censoring indicator.

We used Newton's method to solve the equation $Q_{LW}(\beta_r, \beta_p) = 0$ using "numerical derivatives" of the step function $Q_{LW}(\beta_r, \beta_p)$. Using a large number of starting values, we found a unique "solution" $(\tilde{\beta}_r, \tilde{\beta}_p)$ of $(0.25, 0.61)$. Although these values of β_r and β_p are most compatible with the data based on $Q_{LW}(\beta_r, \beta_p)$, we still cannot rule out the hypothesis that both β_r and β_p are 0 since $Q_{LW}(0, 0) < 5.99$. Indeed, we cannot rule out the hypothesis that $\beta_r = 0$ and $\beta_p = -0.5$.

Wei et al. (1990) show that the following procedure produces a univariate asymptotic 0.05-level test of the univariate hypothesis $\beta_r = \beta_r^*$ based on $Q_{LW}(\beta_r, \beta_p)$. Given a test value β_r, find β_p for which $Q_{LW}(\beta_r, \beta_p)$ attains a local minimum. Call this value of β_p, $\beta_p^{(\min)}(\beta_r)$. Compare $Q_{LW}(\beta_r, \beta_p^{(\min)}(\beta_r))$ to 3.84, the 95th percentile of a χ_1^2 distribution. In our case, with $\beta_r = 0$, $\beta_p^{(\min)}(0) = -0.48$ and $Q_{LW}(0, \beta_p^{(\min)}(0)) = 3.2$ was both a global and local minimum. Thus, we cannot reject the hypothesis that $\beta_r^* = 0$ of no direct treatment effect based on Method 2. Confidence intervals for β_r^* (defined as the set of β_r for which our test fails to reject) are given in row 9 of Table 3.

If $\beta_p^* = 0$, i. e., $T = T_{p^-}$, then interval estimates based on $Q_L(\beta_r)$, $Q_W(\beta_r)$, and $Q_{LW}(\beta_r, \beta_p^{(\min)}(\beta_r))$ are all valid 95% large sample confidence intervals for β_r^* under the randomization condition (7b). The interval $(-0.03, 0.51)$ based on $Q_{LW}(\beta_r, \beta_p^{(\min)}(\beta_r))$ is wider than the intervals $(0.02, 0.25)$ and $(-0.01, 0.24)$ based on $Q_W(\beta_r)$, and $Q_L(\beta_r)$, since it incorporates uncertainty concerning β_p^* and thus sacrifices power. On the other hand, if prophylaxis has an effect on survival, i. e., $\beta_p^* \neq 0$, then $Q_W(\beta_r)$ and $Q_L(\beta_r)$ fail to provide valid tests and confidence intervals for β_r^*. In contrast, the statistic $Q_{LW}(\beta_r, \beta_p^{(\min)}(\beta_r))$ provides asymptotically valid tests for β_r^* if our two-stage causal model given by Eqs. (6) and (12) is correctly specified. Further, it provides an asymptotically valid test of $\beta_r^* = 0$ under the sole assumption that the prophylaxis part of the causal model, i. e., Eq. (12), is correctly specified.

The excessive width of the interval based on $Q_{LW}(\beta_r, \beta_p^{(\min)}(\beta_r))$ may also result in part from our choice of weighted log-rank tests. That is, choosing the ordinary log-rank test and the Prentice–Wilcoxon test may have been an inefficient choice. Thus, we replaced the log-rank and Prentice–Wilcoxon test by alternative-weighted log-rank tests, say A and B, such that a test of $\beta_r^* = 0$ based on comparing $Q_{AB}(\beta_r, \beta_p^{(\min)}(\beta_r))$ has greater power than the test based on $Q_{LW}(\beta_r, \beta_p^{(\min)}(\beta_r))$. To find such weighted log-rank tests, A and B, one can use the results of Robins and Tsiatis (1991) to derive the form of the asymptotically optimal weighted log-rank test for testing the univariate hypothesis $\beta_r^* = 0$ against alternatives specified by our causal model (4). The asymptotically optimal test is not feasible because it depends on unknown population parameters. Therefore, we constructed adaptive weighted log-rank test statistics A and B as described in Robins and Tsiatis (1991) such that the power of the test based on $Q_{AB}(\beta_r, \beta_p^{(min)}(\beta_r))$ would approach that of the optimal but infeasible test. Unfortunately, the confidence interval for β_r^* based on these approximately optimal weighted log-rank tests A and B were, in our data set, of essentially the same width as those based on the log-rank and Prentice–Wilcoxon test. Because this approach was not useful for these data, we refer the reader to Robins and Tsiatis (1991) for details of our approach to constructing nearly optimal adaptive tests.

3.7. Method 3

The interval estimates of $(-0.16, 0.38)$ for β_r^* based on $\psi(\hat{m}^*, \beta_r)$ under Method 1 were wide [in comparison to the potentially biased intent-to-treat intervals of $(-0.01, 0.24)$ and $(0.02, 0.25)$ based on $Q_L(\beta_r)$ and $Q_W(\beta_r)$] because Method 1 censors all subjects who initiate prophylaxis and thus disregards any information concerning β_r^* that may be contained in the observed failure times of such subjects. In contrast, the interval estimates based on $Q_{LW}(\beta_r, \beta_p^{(min)}(\beta_r))$ can potentially extract information concerning β_r^* from the observed failure times of subjects receiving prophylaxis therapy by specifying the causal model (12) for the prophylaxis effect. However, the causal model (12) can be used to efficiently extract additional information concerning β_r^* only if relatively precise estimates of the parameter β_p^* of (12) are available. Thus, the interval estimates of $(-0.03, 0.51)$ based on $Q_{LW}(\beta_r, \beta_p^{(min)}(\beta_r))$ were quite wide since the only restriction used to estimate β_p^* and β_r^* was that R_i was independent of $(T_{r^-p^-,i}, C_i)$ by physical randomization of R_i. This resulted in highly imprecise estimates of β_p^*. In Method 3, we will obtain independent, relatively precise estimates of β_p^* using the observational study assumptions (1) and (2) of Method 1. These estimates of β_p^* are "observational" in that they do not use the information that R_i was assigned by physical randomization. We first describe how we computed our observational estimates of β_p^*. We then describe Method 3.

3.7.1. Observational Estimation of β_p^* under Assumptions (1) and (2)

Based on the maximum partial likelihood estimates $\hat{\alpha}$ of α in model (2) given in Section 3.1, we can proceed to estimate the parameter of interest β_p^* as follows. Separately, for each of the 41 values of β_p in the set $\{-1, -0.95, \ldots, 0, 0.05, \ldots, 1\}$, we again compute the random variable $T_{p^-,i}(\beta_p) \equiv P_i + (T_i - P_i)e^{\beta_p}$, add the term $\alpha_6^* T_{p^-}(\beta_p)$ to the expression in brackets in

Model (2), and perform a Cox partial likelihood score test of the hypothesis $\alpha_6^* = 0$. A large sample 95% confidence interval for β_p^* consists of those β_p for which the score test of the hypothesis $\alpha_6^* = 0$ fails to reject at a 5% level. This follows immediately from the observation that, provided our Cox model of Eq. (2) is correctly specified, under assumption (1) and causal model (12), the hypothesis $\beta_p^* = \beta_p$ is equivalent to the hypothesis that the coefficient α_6^* of the random variable $T_{p^-}(\beta_p)$ is zero. Note for each of the 41 random variables $T_{p^-}(\beta_p)$, the score test of $\alpha_6^* = 0$ can be obtained without refitting the Cox model (2).

Of course, $T_{p^-,i}(\beta_p)$ is not observed for subjects censored by end of follow-up. Hence, in practice, we estimated β_p^* by the above procedure except we substituted $X_{p^-,i}(\beta_p) \equiv X_i(0, \beta_p)$ for $T_{p^-,i}(\beta_p)$.

Using the above approach we obtained a 95% confidence interval of $(-0.15, 0.20)$ for β_p^*. Interpolating, we found the score test would be 0 at $\beta_p = 0.025$ which we used as a point estimate $\hat{\beta}_p$ of β_p^* in the further calculations described below. Robins (1992) and Robins *et al.* (1992) shows that, under our assumptions, $\hat{\beta}_p$ is asymptotically normal and unbiased as an estimator of β_p^*.

3.7.2. Details of Method 3

We next consider how we can use the estimate $\hat{\beta}_p = 0.025$ to produce more powerful tests of the hypothesis (8). Recall that the randomization condition (7b) implies (8) is true only if $T_{p^-,i}$ has the same distribution in the two treatment arms. Thus, if we knew β_p^*, we could use (12) to compute $T_{p^-,i}$ and then use the standard intention-to-treat log-rank test or the Prentice–Wilcoxon test to determine whether the distribution of $T_{p^-,i}$ was the same in the two treatment arms, i. e., whether the two treatment arms would have had the same distribution of death times had prophylaxis been withheld. Of course, we do not know β_p^*, but under the assumptions that (1) and (2) hold, we previously obtained a consistent estimate $\hat{\beta}_p$ of β_p^*. Thus, we estimate $T_{p^-,i}$ using Eq. (12) based on $\hat{\beta}_p$ and then apply a standard intention-to-treat (weighted) log-rank test to the estimated $T_{p^-,i}$. In practice, we apply a generic weighted log-rank test to $\{X_{p^-,i}(\hat{\beta}_p), \Delta_{p^-,i}(\hat{\beta}_p)\} i = 1, \ldots, n$ where $\Delta_{p^-,i}(\beta_p) \equiv \Delta_i(0, \beta_p)$ to properly account for censoring by end of follow-up. Further, we have to appropriately inflate the variance of the test to reflect the fact that β_p^* has been replaced by an estimate. When we did so, we obtained the χ_1^2 value of 4.90 for the Prentice–Wilcoxon test $Q_W^\dagger$ and a value of 3.85 for the log-rank test $Q_L^\dagger$ as reported in rows 10 and 11 of Table 3. Thus, both tests rejected the null hypothesis of no direct treatment arm effect, in the direction of better survival for the low-dose treatment arm. In general, we test the hypothesis $\beta_r^* = \beta_r$ as follows. Given a weighted log-rank test, say the Prentice–Wilcoxon test, a large sample 0.05-level test of the hypothesis that $\beta_r = \beta_r^*$ is obtained by comparing $S_W(\beta_r, \hat{\beta}_p)^2 / \hat{V}ar(S_W(\beta_r, \hat{\beta}_p))$ to 3.84, the 95th percentile of a χ_1^2 distribution, where

$$\hat{V}ar(S_W(\beta_r, \hat{\beta}_p)) \equiv \sum_W (\beta_r, \hat{\beta}_p) + \{ \Delta_{W, \beta_p, k/\sqrt{n}}(\beta_r, \hat{\beta}_p) \}^2 \, \hat{V}ar(\hat{\beta}_p)$$

$S_W(\beta_r, \hat{\beta}_p)$ and $\Sigma_W(\beta_r, \hat{\beta}_p)$ refer to the numerator and estimated variance of $Q_L^\dagger$ applied to data $\{ R_i, X_i(\beta_r, \hat{\beta}_p), \Delta_i(\beta_r, \hat{\beta}_p); \ i = 1, \ldots, n \}$, k is a fixed constant, $\Delta_{W, \beta_p, u}(\beta_r, \hat{\beta}_p) \equiv [S_W(\beta_r, \hat{\beta}_p + u) - S_W(\beta_r, \hat{\beta}_p - u)]/2u$ is the symmetric "numerical partial derivative" of $S_W(\beta_r, \beta_p)$ with respect to β_p with step size u, and $\hat{V}ar(\hat{\beta}_p) = [\{0.20 - (-0.15)\} / \{(1.96)(2)\}]^2$ is the square of the estimated standard error of $\hat{\beta}_p$ defined as the length of the 95% confidence interval for β_p^*, i. e., $(0.20 + 0.15)$, divided by $[(2)(1.96)]$. The additional term $\hat{V}ar(\hat{\beta}_p)\{\Delta_{W, \beta_p, k/\sqrt{n}}(\beta_r, \hat{\beta}_p)\}^2$ represents additional uncertainty caused by estimation of the unknown β_p^* by $\hat{\beta}_p$.

In our data $\Delta_{W, \beta_p, k/\sqrt{n}}(\beta_p, \hat{\beta}_p)$ was a linear function of $k/\sqrt{n}$ for $k/\sqrt{n}$ in the interval $(0.15, 0.35)$. We therefore chose $k/\sqrt{n} = 0.25$ in our calculations. The contribution of the correction term $\{\Delta_{W, \beta_p, k/\sqrt{n}}(\beta_r, \hat{\beta}_p)\}^2 \, \hat{V}ar(\hat{\beta}_p)$ to the total variance was less than 3%, which means that our observational estimate $\hat{\beta}_p$ of β_p^* was sufficiently precise that essentially no power was lost because of residual uncertainty concerning β_p^*. We obtained 95% confidence intervals for β_r^* of $(0.03, 0.26)$ and $(0.0, 0.25)$ given in rows 10 and 11 of Table 3 by inverting the Prentice–Wilcoxon and log-rank tests.

4. EFFECTS OF INTERACTIONS

4.1. Treatment Arm–Prophylaxis Interaction

We have developed three methods to test the null hypothesis (8) that, in the absence of prophylaxis therapy, a subject's survival time does not depend on his AZT treatment protocol, i. e., his treatment arm. We shall refer to (8) as the hypothesis of no direct treatment arm effect in the absence of prophylaxis therapy. However, since it is now recommended that all AIDS patients receive prophylaxis therapy, it would be of greater public health interest to test the hypothesis of no direct treatment arm effect in the presence of continuous prophylaxis therapy (since enrollment); that is, to test the hypothesis that

$$T_{r^-p^+} = T_{r^+p^+} \tag{13}$$

where $T_{r^-p^+}$ and $T_{r^+p^+}$ are a subject's death time if prophylaxis was begun at time of enrollment, and the subject was assigned to a high- or low-AZT protocol, respectively. (13) implies that $T_{p^+,i} \equiv T_{R_ip^+,i}$ equals $T_{r^-p^+,i}$ and thus, under the randomization condition (7b), that the distribution of T_{p^+} is the same in the two treatment arms. To understand how we might test (13) using an analogue of Method 1, we note that, in applying Method 1 to test the null hypothesis (8), we treated a subject as (dependently) censored the moment he initiated prophylaxis and thus deviated from the prophylaxis history with which (8) was concerned. [We used the assumptions of Eqs. (1) and (2) to adjust for the dependent censoring.] Since we have assumed that once a subject initiates prophylaxis therapy, he continues on therapy thereafter, the analogue of Method 1 to test (13) would be to restrict the analysis to the 7 subjects who were on prophylaxis at time of randomization. Clearly this analogue of Method 1 will lack power, and will not be pursued further.

Now if we are willing to assume that model (11a) is true, then, since this model implies there is no treatment arm prophylaxis interaction, β_r^* represents the effect of AZT treatment arm both in the presence and absence of prophylaxis therapy. Here we generalize (11a) to the two-parameter model

$$e^{-(\beta_{p,1}^* + \beta_{p,2}^* R)}(T_{p^-} - v) = (T_{p=(v)} - v) \qquad \text{if } T_{p=(v)} > v \tag{11a'}$$

and thus (12a) to

$$T_{p^-} = P + (T - P)e^{\beta_{p,1}^* + \beta_{p,2}^* R} \qquad \text{if } P < T \tag{12a'}$$

while retaining model (6). $\beta_{p,2}^*$ represents a treatment arm prophylaxis interaction. β_r^* continues to represent the effect of AZT treatment in the absence of prophylaxis therapy. It follows from (11a'), (11b), and (6) that $T_{p^+} = e^{-\beta_{p,1}^*} e^{-(\beta_r^* + \beta_{p,2}^*)R} T_{r^-p^-}$ so that, under (7b), T_{p^+} will have the same distribution in the two treatment arms if and only if

$$\gamma_r^* \equiv \beta_r^* + \beta_{p,2}^* = 0 \tag{14}$$

More generally, if as suggested by this model, we assume

$$T_{r^-p^+} = e^{\gamma_r^* R} T_{p^+} \tag{15}$$

then γ_r^* represents the effect of AZT treatment arm given continuous prophylaxis therapy. We could estimate the three parameters $(\beta_r^*, \beta_p^{*\prime})'$ jointly, where $\beta_p^* = (\beta_{p,1}^*, \beta_{p,2}^*)'$, using Method 2 by using three different log-rank tests rather than two, although the power to test (14) or (8) would be quite poor. Hence, we estimated (β_r^*, β_p^*) under Method 3. We first estimated $\beta_{p,1}^*$ as -0.05 [95% CI of $(-0.4, 0.3)$] by restricting our observational estimates of β_p^* described in Section 3.1 to subjects with $R = 0$. We estimated $\beta_{p,1}^* + \beta_{p,2}^*$ as 0.075 [95% CI $(-0.25, 0.4)$] by restricting our observational analysis to subjects with $R = 1$, and thus, obtain an estimate of $\beta_{p,2}^*$ of 0.125 [95% CI $(-0.4, 0.6)$] as the difference of these treatment-arm-specific estimates of the prophylaxis effect. We then estimate β_r^* as described previously under Method 3 except now $C(\beta_r, \beta_p) = C \min(e^{\beta_r + \beta_{p,2}}, e^{\beta_r}, e^{\beta_{p,1}}, 1)$, $T(\beta_r, \beta_p)$ and $T_p(\beta_p)$ now use (12a') with β_p substituted for β_p^*, and the variance correction term in $\hat{V}ar(S_W(\beta_r, \hat{\beta}_p))$ now requires partial derivatives with respect to both $\beta_{p,1}$ and $\beta_{p,2}$. We obtain $\hat{\beta}_r = 0.05$ with a 95% confidence interval of $(-0.20, 0.30)$ based on the standard log-rank test. Comparing this interval with the confidence interval of $(0.0, 0.25)$ in row 11 of Table 3 we see that allowing for a possible treatment arm prophylaxis interaction by adding the parameter $\beta_{p,2}^*$ to our model markedly increased our uncertainty concerning β_r^*. [The variance correction term now represents 82% rather than 3% of the total variance of $\hat{V}ar(S_W(\beta_r, \hat{\beta}_p))$. Indeed, our confidence interval length of 0.5 is almost as great as the confidence interval length of $(0.38, -0.16) = 0.54$ given in row 2 of Table 3, even though this latter interval did not require us to specify a structural nested failure time model for the prophylaxis effect at all.

Given the above estimates we obtain an estimate $\hat{\gamma} = 0.17$ by calculating $\hat{\beta}_r + \hat{\beta}_{p,2}$. An alternative approach to obtaining the estimate $\hat{\gamma}$ (given our estimates of $\hat{\beta}_{p,1}$ and $\hat{\beta}_{p,2}$) that also produces a valid confidence interval for γ_r^* is as follows.

Note (6), (11a'), and (11b) imply

$$T_{p^+} = v e^{\beta_{p,1}^* + \beta_{p,2}^* R} + T_{p=(v)} - v, \qquad \text{if } v < T_{p=(v)} \tag{16a}$$

$$T_{p^+} = e^{\beta_{p,1}^* + \beta_{p,2}^* R} T_{p=(v)}, \qquad \text{otherwise} \tag{16b}$$

(16a) and (16b) imply

$$T_{p^+} = e^{+\beta_{p,1}^* + \beta_{p,2}^* R} P + T - P, \qquad \text{if } P < T \tag{17a}$$

$$T_{p^+} = e^{(+\beta_{p,1}^* + \beta_{p,2}^* R)} T, \qquad \text{otherwise} \tag{17b}$$

Given (17a), (17b), and (15), Methods 2 and 3 can be used to estimate γ_r^* with T_{p^+} now playing the role that T_{p^-} played previously. Using this approach we obtain a point estimate of 0.17 and a 95% confidence interval of $(-0.08, 0.46)$ for γ_r^*.

Note that our inferences concerning the equality of the distribution of T_{p^+} in the two arms using a model such as (11a′) will be quite sensitive to model choice and yet we will have little power to discriminate between models, since T_{p^+} was observed only for the 7 subjects who were on prophylaxis at time of enrollment.

4.2. Interactions with Unmeasured Covariates

Our simple SNFTM models assume no interaction with unmeasured factors. For example, according to model (12), if two subjects i and j have identical observed failure times, treatment arm assignment, and prophylaxis histories, they would have had an identical failure time T_{p^-} if prophylaxis had always been withheld. In certain settings, this no-interaction assumption might be considered biologically implausible. The general class of SNFTMs discussed in Appendix 1 allows the magnitude of the treatment effect to depend on unmeasured factors.

4.3. Interactions with Measured Time-Dependent Factors

We could consider adding interactions of prophylaxis with observed time-dependent factors. For example, we could have generalized (12a′) to

$$T_{p^-,i} = P_i + (T_i - P_i)e^{\beta^*_{p,1}+\beta^*_{p,2}R_i+\beta^*_{p,3}\cdot I[\text{PCP}(P_i)]} \qquad (12a'')$$

where $I[\text{PCP}(P_i)] = 1$ if a postrandomization PCP episode occurs by P_i and is 0 otherwise. Under this model, the magnitude of the prophylaxis effect on survival can depend both on the treatment arm R and on past PCP history.

Given (12a″), we can estimate the parameters $\beta^*_{p,1}$, $\beta^*_{p,2}$, $\beta^*_{p,3}$ under the assumptions of Eqs. (1) and (2) as described in Appendixes 1 and 4 and thus, using Method 3, test the null hypothesis (8) of no direct treatment arm effect in the absence of prophylaxis therapy. However, specifying model (12a″) linking a subject's observed data with $T_{p^-,i}$ will not allow us to compute $T_{p^+,i}$ or to identify the treatment-arm-specific distribution of T_{p^+} without further assumptions. In Appendix 1, we discuss further assumptions that would allow such identification. Even under these further assumptions, it is difficult to use model (12a″) to test the null hypothesis that T_{p^+} has the same distribution in both arms since, even if β^*_r and $\beta^*_{p,2}$ were zero and (7b) were true, the distribution of T_{p^+} need not be the same in the two treatment arms if $\beta^*_{p,3}$ is nonzero. Under these conditions, this null hypothesis could only be tested by further modeling probability of contracting PCP at time t as a function of past prophylaxis history and treatment arm (Robins *et al.*, 1992).

Thus, it would be prudent to specify models linking the observed data on survival time, prophylaxis, and PCP history with T_{p^+} rather than T_{p^-} if one were interested in testing the null hypothesis (13). See Section A2.12 of Robins *et al.* (1992).

4.4. Interactions with Measured Pretreatment Variables

Methods for estimating how the effect of AZT protocol or PCP prophylaxis is modified by pretreatment variables such as age or sex are considered in Appendix 1.

5. ANALYSIS OF THE EFFECT OF MARIJUANA ON CD4 COUNTS

This section describes, in an abbreviated fashion, a very preliminary analysis of the effect of marijuana usage on the evolution of CD4 counts among HIV-infected members of the San Francisco Men's Health Study (SFMHS). The SFMHS cohort is a population sample of single males in San Francisco. Every *6 months* cohort members were evaluated through interviews, physical examinations, and laboratory studies of blood specimens. Details on the study methods have been described in Lang *et al.* (1987) and Winkelstein *et al.* (1987). The analysis reported here is based on data obtained through the eighth wave of interviews. In the analysis, we first determined that symptoms of HIV infection might be simultaneously confounders and intermediate variables. Specifically, at each wave, we abstracted data on 12 symptoms of HIV-related disease—presence of thrush, worsening herpes, fever, weight loss, etc. We next created a three-level "symptom variable," coded as "0" for no symptoms, "1" for one symptom, and as "2" for 2–12 symptoms. Our symptom variable appeared to be simultaneously a confounder and an intermediate variable on the causal pathway from marijuana to a change in CD4 counts. That HIV symptoms might be an intermediate variable followed from the fact that past marijuana use predicted fewer current symptoms and an increased number of symptoms independently predicted a subsequent decrease in CD4 counts. Further, since increased symptoms also predicted a subsequent decrease in marijuana use, symptoms of HIV disease appear to be confounders as well. Therefore, we undertook an analysis based on the G-estimation of a (rank-preserving) structural nested distribution model (SNDM) described in Section A2.16 of Robins *et al.* (1992). We use a simple SNDM that assumed

$$H_{k,i} = Y_{k,i} - \beta_0 \, cum_{k,i} \tag{18}$$

where $Y_{k,i}$ is subject i's observed CD4 count at wave k, $cum_{k,i}$ is subject i's cumulative marijuana dosage from start of follow-up until wave k, $H_{k,i}$ is a counterfactual variable recording what subject i's T4 count would have been at wave k, if the subject had smoked no marijuana since start of follow-up. In analogy to our SNFTMs, a structural nested distribution model links a subject's observed CD4 count and cofactor history with the CD4 count the subject would have had in the absence of exposure to the cofactor (since start of follow-up). We then estimated the parameter β_0 of SNDM (18) from the data, under the assumption of no unmeasured confounders. Specifically, in analogy with Eq. (1), we assumed that the probability of smoking marijuana at wave k conditional on HIV symptom and CD4-count history through occasion k, and marijuana history through $k - 1$ did not further depend on a subject's future counterfactual CD4-count history, that is, on $H_{m,i}$, $m > k$. That is, we assume for $m = 1, \ldots, 8$

$$(H_{m+1}, \ldots, H_8) \amalg A_m \mid \bar{L}_m, \bar{A}_{m-1} \tag{19}$$

where A_m records marijuana smoking as 0 or 1 at wave m, $L_m = (Y_m, L_m^\dagger)$ where Y_m is observed T4 count, $L_m^\dagger$ is the symptom variable recorded at m, and, e. g., $\bar{L}_m = (L_0, L_1, \ldots, L_m)$, and L_0 are other variables recorded at baseline such as age and lifetime number of sexual partners.

Given (19), the sharp null hypothesis

$$H_{m,i} = Y_{m,i} \qquad \text{for all } i, m \tag{20}$$

which is equivalent to the hypothesis that $\beta_0 = 0$ in (18) implies

$$(Y_{m+1}, \ldots, Y_8) \amalg A_m \mid \bar{L}_m, \bar{A}_{m-1} \tag{21a}$$

and, for $k > m$,

$$E[Y_k \mid \bar{L}_m, \bar{A}_m] = E[Y_k \mid \bar{L}_m, \bar{A}_{m-1}] \tag{21b}$$

but, without further assumptions, does not imply

$$E[Y_m \mid \bar{A}_{m-1}, \bar{L}_{m-1}] = E[Y_m \mid \bar{L}_{m-1}] \tag{22}$$

or

$$E[Y_m \mid \bar{A}_{m-1}, L_0] = E[Y_m \mid L_0] \tag{23}$$

Most standard methods of longitudinal data analysis such as the generalized estimating equation approach proposed by Zeger and Liang (1986) are able to test either the hypothesis (22) or (23) but not (21a) or (21b). Hence, they are not useful for testing the causal null hypothesis (20) when we only assume (19) holds.

However, given (19), we obtain a valid test of the hypothesis $\beta_0 = 0$ and a valid confidence interval for β_0 by the following G-estimation procedure. In analogy with Eq. (2), we fit a logistic regression model for the probability $p_{k,i}$ that subject i is a marijuana smoker at wave k given the subject's baseline covariates L_0 and past marijuana, CD4 count, and symptom history. That is, we fit a model for $\mathrm{pr}[A_k = 1 \mid \bar{L}_k, \bar{A}_{k-1}]$. Then, for a range of β values, we add the covariate $\sum_{m=k+1}^{8} (Y_{m,i} - \beta \, \mathrm{cum}_{m,i})$ to the logistic model and perform a score test of the hypothesis that the added covariate's coefficient is 0. The β's for which the score test does not reject form a large sample confidence interval for β_0. Note that (18) implies the covariate $\sum_{m=k+1}^{8} (Y_{m,i} - \beta_0 \, \mathrm{cum}_{m,i})$ is what the sum of the subject's post-wave-k CD4 counts would be if the subject was unexposed to marijuana since enrollment; the sum is counter-factual unless the subject is, in fact, unexposed to marijuana.

This analysis gave a 95% confidence interval exceeding $(-30, 30)$ for β_0, which includes 0 and is exceedingly wide. The excessive width of the confidence interval is the result of two factors. First, when (a) past marijuana smoking and HIV symptom history are strong predictors of current marijuana use and (b) there is large within- and between-subject variability in CD4 counts, the information available in the data on the effect of changes in marijuana smoking on mean CD4 count can be quite small. Second, the particular G-estimator of β_0 described above may have failed to efficiently extract even the small amount of information available. As discussed in Appendix 4, there always exists an optimal G-estimator that in principle can extract all of the available information. The optimal G-estimator is complex. The preliminary analysis reported in this section is likely to be biased, because we regarded missing data as "missing completely at random." Appropriate corrections are discussed in Robins et al. (1992). Finally, we note that, although unlikely, it is not inconceivable that a subject would have a higher CD4 count if he had smoked marijuana than if he had not, since it is well established that the total white blood count is elevated in both healthy and ill cigarette smokers.

A second approach to estimating the effect of marijuana smoking on the evolution of CD4 count under an assumption similar to (19) would be to use the G-computation algorithm as in Section 13 of Robins (1989b). Limitations of estimation based on the G-computation algorithm are discussed in that section. Further, as discussed in Section A2.16 of Robins et al. (1992) and Robins (1993a), a more robust approach to estimating the effect of marijuana smoking on the evolution of CD4 count would be to use a structural nested mean model rather than either the structural nested distribution model described above or the G-computation algorithm.

APPENDIX 1. A COUNTERFACTUAL APPROACH TO CAUSAL INFERENCE IN RANDOMIZED TRIALS

A1.1. Notation

For $i = 1, \ldots, n$, let R_i taking values r in $\{0, 1, \ldots, J\}$ index the treatment arm to which a subject i was assigned in a randomized trial. Let T_i be a continuous random variable recording the survival time of subject i with time measured as time since randomization. Let $A_i(t)$ record the treatment received at t. $A_i(t)$ may be vector-valued if, for instance, we were interested in the joint effect of two treatments, say ziduvodine and PCP prophylaxis.

Remark A1.1. In the body of the paper, $A_i(t) = (A_i^{(1)}(t), A_i^{(2)}(t))$ where $A_i^{(2)}(t)$ was an indicator of prophylaxis therapy at t and, for all t, $A_i^{(1)}(t) = A_i^{(1)}(0)$ was equal to the indicator R_i of whether a subject was assigned to high- versus low-dose AZT protocol. If we had been interested in the effect of actual AZT treatment, rather than the effect of the AZT protocol, we would have set $A_i^{(1)}(t)$ to be a subject's actual AZT dose at t.

For $t > 0$, let $L_i(t)$ record the value at t of all measured time-dependent covariates other than $A_i(t)$. Let $L_i(0) = (R_i, L_i^*(0)')'$ where $L_i^*(0)$ is the vector of recorded pretreatment variables. For any time-dependent variable, let $\bar{Z}_i(t) = \{Z_i(u); 0 \le u \le t\}$ be the history of the Z-process through t.

Define $L^*(t) \equiv L(t), t > 0$, so $\bar{L}^*(t)$ is L-history up to t ignoring treatment arm R, while $\bar{L}(t)$ includes R. Henceforth, it will be convenient to discretize the times at which the data on $L_i(t)$ were recorded.

Except in Remark A1.3. below, we suppose data on the covariates $L_i(t)$ were recorded at most once per day. We shall assume the recorded covariate process jumps at and only at times k, $k = (0, 1, 2, \ldots)$, days from enrollment and the recorded treatment process, $A_i(t)$, only jumps at times k^+ where k^+ is a time just after k. Let $L_{k,i}$ be subject i's recorded value of $L_i(t)$ at k. Let $A_{k,i}$ be subject i's treatment in $(k, k + 1]$, so, by convention, $A_{k,i}$ follows $L_{k,i}$. $L_{0,i} = (L_{0,i}^*, R_i)$ where $L_{0,i}^*$ is the value of all preenrollment time-dependent and time-independent covariates. Then $\bar{L}_{k,i} \equiv (L_{0,i}, \ldots, L_{k,i})$ and $\bar{A}_{k-1,i} \equiv (A_{0,i}, \ldots, A_{k-1,i})$ are the L-history and treatment history through day k. Note $\bar{L}_i(t) = \{L_i(u); 0 \le u \le t\}$. Let $\mathrm{int}(t)$ be the largest integer k less than or equal to t so that $\bar{L}_i(t) = \bar{L}_{\mathrm{int}(t),i}$ because L-history only jumps at times k. We suppose realizations $a_{k,i}$ and $l_{k,i}$ of $A_{k,i}$ and $L_{k,i}$ lie in sets $\mathbf{A}_k$ and $\mathbf{L}_k$ of feasible a_k and l_k values. Let $\bar{\mathbf{A}}_k$ and $\bar{\mathbf{L}}_k$ be the set of all vectors $\bar{a}_k$ $\equiv (a_0, a_1, \ldots, a_k)$ and $\bar{l}_k \equiv (l_0, l_1, \ldots, l_k)$ with $a_m \epsilon \mathbf{A}_m, l_m \epsilon \mathbf{L}_m, 0 \leq m \leq k$. We shall adopt the convention that m and k will denote nonnegative integers, and, if $\bar{l}_m$ and $\bar{l}_k$ are used in the same expression with $k < m$, $\bar{l}_k$ is the initial segment of $\bar{l}_m$. Similarly, if $k < t$, $\bar{l}_k$ is the initial segment of $\bar{l}(t)$. Finally, $\bar{l} \equiv \bar{l}(\infty)$ is a covariate history defined on $[0, \infty)$. Similar remarks apply to $\bar{a}_m, \bar{a}_k, \bar{a}(t)$, and $\bar{a}$.

A1.2. Estimation of the Baseline Survival Distribution

Counterfactual Random Variables. We define a *feasible treatment regime* G to be a function $G(t_k, \bar{l}_k)$ that assigns to each possible t_k and $\bar{l}_k \epsilon \bar{\mathbf{L}}_k$, a treatment rate $a_k \epsilon \mathbf{A}_k$. If $A_i(t)$ is ziduvodine (AZT) dosage, then an example of a feasible regime is "take a dosage a_k of 1000 milligrams of ziduvodine daily in the interval $(k, k + 1]$ if the subject's hematocrit exceeds 30 at time k. Otherwise, take no ziduvodine in that interval." Let $\mathbf{G}$ be the set of all feasible regimes. Note $\mathbf{G}$ depends on the covariates recorded in l_k. Given the function $G(t_k, \bar{l}_k)$ of two arguments $(t_k, \bar{l}_k)$, we define the function $G(\bar{l}_k)$ of one argument by the relation $G(\bar{l}_k) = \{ G(t_m, \bar{l}_m); 0 \leq m \leq k \}$. Since there is a one-to-one relation between the functions $G(t_k, \bar{l}_k)$ and $G(\bar{l}_k)$, we shall identify the regime G with both functions.

For each subject i and each regime G, we shall assume there exists $T_{i,G}$ representing the time-to-death that would be observed if, possibly contrary to fact, subject i had followed a treatment history consistent with regime G in the randomized trial. This assumption will be particularly reasonable in a double-blind randomized trial (Robins, 1989b). We shall make the following consistency assumption that formalizes the idea that a subject's survival through t depends only on treatment received prior to t.

Consistency Assumption 1 (CA1). For any regime G and time k for which $G[\bar{L}_{k,i}] = \bar{A}_{k,i}$, we assume $T_{i,G} \geq t \Leftrightarrow T_i \geq t$, for $t \epsilon (k, k + 1]$.

We shall assume that the observed and counterfactual data $(t_i, \bar{l}_i(t_i),$ $\bar{a}_i(t_i), \{ t_{i,G}; G \epsilon \mathbf{G} \})$ are realizations of independent and identically distributed random vectors $(T_i, \bar{L}_i(T_i), \bar{A}_i(T_i), \{ T_{i,G}; G \epsilon \mathbf{G} \})$. Therefore, for notational convenience, we shall often drop the subscript i when referring to these random variables. $\text{pr}(T_G > t)$ is the treatment regime-specific counterfactual survival curve for regime G. To avoid identifiability difficulties, we shall suppose that, for all k, the density $f_{\bar{A}_k, \bar{L}_k}(\bar{a}_k, \bar{l}_k | T > k) \neq 0$ for all $\bar{a}_k \epsilon \bar{\mathbf{A}}_k, \bar{l}_k \epsilon \bar{\mathbf{L}}_k$ whenever $f(\bar{a}_{k-1}, \bar{l}_k | T > k) \neq 0$.

The Randomization Assumption. We shall formalize the assumption that the treatment arm indicator was assigned completely at random by

$$\{T_{i,G}; G \in \mathbf{G}\} \amalg R_i \mid L^*_{0,i} \tag{A1.1a}$$

and

$$R_i \amalg L^*_{0,i} \tag{A1.1b}$$

which together imply

$$\{T_{i,G}; G \in \mathbf{G}\} \amalg R_i \tag{A1.1c}$$

The sharp null hypothesis

$$T_{i,G} = T_i \qquad \text{for all } G \in \mathbf{G} \tag{A1.2}$$

plus (A1.1) implies the usual intention-to-treat null hypotheses

$$T_i \amalg R_i \mid L^*_{0,i} \tag{A1.3a}$$

and

$$T_i \amalg R_i \tag{A1.3b}$$

as well as the G-null hypothesis

$$T_{i,G} \amalg R_i, \qquad G \in \mathbf{G} \tag{A1.4}$$

(A1.4) implies neither (A1.3b) nor (A1.2) [even given (A1.1)]. Similarly, (A1.3) implies neither (A1.4) nor (A1.2).

Our goal is to test the sharp null hypothesis (A1.2) and to estimate the counterfactual survival curves $\mathrm{pr}(T_{i,G} > t)$, $G \in \mathbf{G}$.

Structural Nested Failure Time Models. Given any treatment history $\bar{a} = (a_0, a_1, \ldots)$ on $(0, \infty)$, let $G = (\bar{a})$ be the regime defined by $G(\bar{l}_k) = \bar{a}_k$ for all $\bar{l}_k$. Let $T_{G=(\bar{a})}$ be the corresponding counterfactual variable. Also, given $\bar{a}$ as above, adopt the convention that $(\bar{a}_m, 0)$ will be the history $\bar{a}^{(1)}$ on $(0, \infty)$ characterized by $a_k^{(1)} = a_k$ if $k \leq m$ and $a_k^{(1)} = 0$ if $k > m$. Thus, $T_{G=(0)}$ is the counterfactual survival time in the absence of treatment.

For $t > t_m$, define the "blip" function $\gamma(t, \bar{l}_m, \bar{a}_m)$ by the relation

$$\text{pr}[T_{G=(\bar{a}_m,0)} > t \,|\, \bar{l}_m, \bar{a}_m, T > m]$$
$$= \text{pr}[T_{G=(\bar{a}_{m-1},0)} > \gamma(t, \bar{l}_m, \bar{a}_m) \,|\, \bar{l}_m, \bar{a}_m, T > m]$$

To clarify the meaning of the function $\gamma(t, \bar{l}_m, \bar{a}_m)$, consider a subset with observed history $(\bar{l}_m, \bar{a}_m, T > m)$. The function $\gamma(t, \bar{l}_m, \bar{a}_m)$ is a measure of the magnitude of the causal effect of a final brief "blip" of treatment a_m in the interval $(t_m, t_{m+1}]$ on the survival experience of this subset, in the sense that it maps percentiles of the random variable $T_{G=(\bar{a}_m,0)}$ into those of the random variable $T_{G=(\bar{a}_{m-1},0)}$. We assume that the random variables, $T_{G=(\bar{a}_m,0)}$ and $T_{G=(\bar{a}_{m-1},0)}$ conditional on $(\bar{l}_m, \bar{a}_m)$ have a density on (m, ∞) that is continuous almost everywhere. Thus, it follows from its definition that $\gamma(t, \bar{l}_m, \bar{a}_m)$ is well defined and satisfies (a) $\gamma(t, \bar{l}_m, \bar{a}_m) > m$; (b) $\gamma(t, \bar{l}_m, \bar{a}_m) = t$ if $a_m = 0$; (c) $\gamma(t, \bar{l}_m, \bar{a}_m)$ is increasing in t; and (d) the derivative of $\gamma(t, \bar{l}_m, \bar{a}_m)$ with respect to t is continuous.

Note, by definition, conditional on $(\bar{L}_m, \bar{A}_m, T > m)$, the random variable $\gamma(T_{G=(\bar{A}_m,0)}, \bar{L}_m, \bar{A}_m)$ has the same distribution as $T_{G=(\bar{A}_{m-1},0)}$. If, conditional on $(\bar{L}_m, \bar{A}_m, T > m)$, these two random variables are equal with probability one, we say there is *local rank preservation*. Local rank preservation is a strong, untestable assumption that would rarely be expected to hold.

For $t \le T$, define $H_{\text{int}(t)}(t) \equiv \mathbf{h}_{\text{int}(t)}(t, \bar{L}(t), \bar{A}(t))$ to be $\gamma(t, \bar{L}_{\text{int}(t)}, \bar{A}_{\text{int}(t)})$ and, for $0 \le m < \text{int}(t)$, define $H_m(t) \equiv \mathbf{h}_m(t, \bar{L}(t), \bar{A}(t))$ to be $\gamma(H_{m+1}(t), \bar{L}_m, \bar{A}_m)$. Define $H(t) \equiv \mathbf{h}(t, \bar{L}(t), \bar{A}(t))$ to be $H_0(t)$. Let $H \equiv H(T)$ and $H_m \equiv H_m(T)$. H is a deterministic function of $(H_m, \bar{L}_{m-1}, \bar{A}_{m-1})$. Note, if we have local rank preservation, $H_m = T_{G=(\bar{A}_{m-1},0)}$ for $T > m$, H is $T_{G=(0)}$ and, therefore,

$$\text{pr}[H_m > t \,|\, \bar{L}_m, \bar{A}_m, T > m] = \text{pr}[T_{G=(\bar{A}_{m-1},0)} > t \,|\, \bar{L}_m, \bar{A}_m, T > m] \quad (A1.5)$$

In fact, in Appendix 3 we prove that, even without local rank preservation,

Theorem A1.1. The consistency assumption 1 implies (A1.5). In particular, $\text{pr}[H > t] = \text{pr}[T_{G=(0)} > t]$ and $\text{pr}[H > t \,|\, R] = \text{pr}[T_{G=(0)} > t \,|\, R]$.

As an immediate consequence, we have

Corollary A1.1. If (A1.1) and CA1 hold, then

$$H_i \amalg R_i \,|\, L_{0,i}^* \quad (A1.6a)$$

and

$$H_i \amalg R_i \qquad\qquad (A1.6b)$$

Corollary A1.2. If the blip null hypothesis

$$\gamma(t, \bar{l}_m, \bar{a}_m) = t \qquad \text{for all } \bar{l}_m, \bar{a}_m \qquad\qquad (A1.7)$$

(A1.1) and CA1 hold, then $H_i = T_i$ and the intention-to-treat null hypotheses (A1.3) hold [but the G-null hypothesis (A1.4) may not hold].

Remark A1.2. Note that the sharp null hypothesis (A1.2) implies the blip null hypothesis (A1.7).

Theorem A1.1 implies that if $\gamma(t, \bar{l}_m, \bar{a}_m)$ were known, we could identify $\text{pr}[T_{G=(0)} > t]$. Unfortunately, it is trivial to construct examples to show that the restrictions (A1.6) implied by (A1.1) do not suffice to identify $\gamma(t, \bar{l}_m, \bar{a}_m)$, yet (A1.6) is the sole restriction placed on $\gamma(t, \bar{l}_m, \bar{a}_m)$ by (A1.1). If we assume the function $\gamma(t, \bar{l}_m, \bar{a}_m)$ is known up to a finite vector of unknown parameters, it often becomes identifiable.

Definition. The population follows a structural nested failure time model (SNFTM) or blip model $\gamma^*(t, \bar{l}_m, \bar{a}_m, \psi)$ with respect to L if (1) $\gamma(t, \bar{l}_m, \bar{a}_m)$ $= \gamma^*(t, \bar{l}_m, \bar{a}_m, \psi_0)$ where $\gamma^*(\cdot, \cdot, \cdot, \cdot)$ is a known function; (2) ψ_0 is a finite vector of unknown parameters to be estimated taking values in R^v; (3) for each value of $\psi \epsilon R^v$, $\gamma^*(t, \bar{l}_m, \bar{a}_m, \psi)$ satisfies the conditions (a)–(d) that were satisfied by $\gamma(t, \bar{l}_m, \bar{a}_m)$ described in the paragraph in which the blip function is defined; (4) $\partial\gamma^*(t, \bar{l}_m, \bar{a}_m, \psi)/\partial\psi'$ and $\partial^2\gamma^*(t, \bar{l}_m, \bar{a}_m, \psi)/\partial\psi'\partial t$ are continuous for all ψ and almost all $t\epsilon(m, \infty)$; and (5) $\gamma^*(t, \bar{l}_m, \bar{a}_m, \psi) = t$ if $\psi = 0$.

Let $H(t, \psi) \equiv \mathbf{h}(t, \bar{L}(t), \bar{A}(t), \psi)$ be defined like $H(t) \equiv \mathbf{h}(t, \bar{L}(t), \bar{A}(t))$ except with $\gamma^*(t, \bar{l}_m, \bar{a}_m, \psi)$ replacing $\gamma(t, \bar{l}_m, \bar{a}_m)$. Define $H(\psi) \equiv H(T, \psi)$ so that $H(\psi_0) = H$. Given an SNFTM w.r.t. L, $h(\cdot, \cdot, \cdot, \cdot)$ is a fixed almost everywhere smooth function, satisfying (1) monotonicity: $h(t, \bar{L}_i(t)\bar{A}_i(t), \psi)$ $> h(u, \bar{L}_i(u), \bar{A}_i(u), \psi)$ if $t > u$; (2) identity: $h(t, \bar{L}_i(t), \bar{A}_i(t), \psi) = t$ if $\bar{A}_i(t)$ is identically zero on $(0, t)$; and (3) $h(t, \bar{L}_i(t), \bar{A}_i(t), 0) = t$.

Example. Suppose

$$\gamma^*(t, \bar{l}_m, \bar{a}_m, \psi_0) = (t - m)\exp(\psi_{0,1}a_m + \psi_{0,2}a_m l_m + \psi_{0,3}a_m r) + m$$

$$\text{if } t < m + 1$$

$$\gamma^*(t, \bar{l}_m, \bar{a}_m, \psi_0) = t + \exp(\psi_{0,1}a_m + \psi_{0,2}a_m l_m + \psi_{0,3}a_m r) - 1$$

$$\text{if } t \geq m + 1 \quad (A1.8)$$

where $\psi_0' = (\psi_{0,1}, \psi_{0,2}, \psi_{0,3})$ and, for concreteness, suppose l_m is the ordinal covariate "number of PCP episodes prior to m." Given $(\bar{a}, \bar{l})$ defined on $(0, \infty)$, write

$$x = \int_0^t \exp\{\psi_{0,1}a(u) + \psi_{0,2}a(u)l(u) + \psi_{0,3}a(u)r\} du \quad (A1.9)$$

Then, under (A1.8), $\mathbf{h}(t, \bar{l}(t), \bar{a}(t))$ equals x.

Note that if subjects with history $(\bar{l}_m, \bar{a}_m)$ on a particular treatment arm, say $r = 1$, are not comparable to subjects with the same history on another treatment arm, say $r = 0$, then $\gamma(t, \bar{l}_m, \bar{a}_m)$ would, as in our example, depend on treatment arm r. *Until Appendix 4, we shall assume all subjects failed by the end of the study so that there is no censoring.*

Corollary A1.3. Given (A1.1), CA1, and a correctly specified SNFTM $\gamma^*(t, \bar{l}_m, \bar{a}_m, \psi)$, then (a)

$$H_i(\psi_0) \amalg R_i \mid L_{0,i}^* \quad (A1.10)$$

is the sole restriction on the joint distribution of the observables $\{T_i, \bar{L}_i(T_i), \bar{A}_i(T_i)\}$ other than (A1.1b); (b)

$$\text{pr}[H(\psi_0) > t] = \text{pr}[T_{G=(0)} > t]$$

(c) $\psi_0 = 0$ implies the ITT null hypothesis (A1.3) but not the G-null hypothesis; (d) ψ_0 is identified if

$$H_i(\psi) \,\, \cancel{\amalg} \,\, R_i \mid L_{0,i}^* \qquad \text{for } \psi \neq \psi_0 \quad (A1.11)$$

(e) there will exist, under regularity conditions, a solution $\tilde{\psi}^\dagger(q)$ to $0 = \sum_{i=1}^n q(R_i, H_i(\psi), L_{0,i}^*) - \int q(r, H_i(\psi), L_{0,i}^*) dF(r)$ that is asymptotically normal and unbiased for ψ_0 where $q(\cdot, \cdot, \cdot)$ is a fixed function chosen by the investigator. The asymptotic variance of $\tilde{\psi}^\dagger(q_{opt}^\dagger)$ attains the semiparametric variance bound for the semiparametric model defined by (A1.10), where $q_{opt}^\dagger(R_i, H_i(\psi_0), L_{0,i}^*) = E[S_{\psi,i} \mid R_i, H_i(\psi_0), L_{0,i}^*]$, where $S_{\psi,i} = S_{\psi,i}(\psi_0)$ and

$S_{\psi,i}(\psi_0)$ is the score for ψ under restriction (A1.10) calculated as follows. Noting the map from $\{T_i, \bar{L}_i(T_i), \bar{A}_i(T_i)\}$ to $\{H_i(\psi_0), \bar{L}_i(T_i), \bar{A}(T_i)\}$ is one to one with strictly positive Jacobian determinant $\partial H_i(\psi_0)/\partial T_i$, we have

$$f_{\{T,\bar{L}(T),\bar{A}(T)\}}\{T_i, \bar{L}_i(T_i), \bar{A}_i(T_i)\}$$

$$= \left\{\frac{\partial H_i(\psi_0)}{\partial T_i}\right\} f_{\{H(\psi_0),\bar{L}(T),\bar{A}(T)\}}\{H_i(\psi_0), \bar{L}_i(T_i), \bar{A}_i(T_i)\}$$

By a decomposition into a product of conditional probabilities, the right-hand side of the previous equation can be written

$$\left[\frac{\partial H_i(\psi_0)}{\partial T_i}\right] f\{H_i(\psi_0)\} f\{L_{0,i}^* | H_i(\psi_0)\} f(R_i)$$

$$\times \prod_{m=0}^{m=\text{int}(T_i)} f\{A_{m,i} | \bar{L}_{m,i}, \bar{A}_{m-1,i}, H_i(\psi_0), T_i > m\}$$

$$\times \prod_{m=1}^{\text{int}(T_i)} f\{L_{m,i} | \bar{L}_{m-1,i}, \bar{A}_{m-1,i}, H_i(\psi_0), T_i > m\} \quad \text{(A1.12)}$$

We have used the fact that, by Theorem A1.1, (A1.1) implies $f[R_i | L_{0,i}^*, H_i(\psi_0)] = f(R_i)$. Finally, we obtain $S_{\psi,i}(\psi_0)$ by differentiating the logarithm of (A.12) w.r.t. ψ_0. [This corollary is relevant to Method 2 in the text. The optimal Robins–Tsiatis rank estimator is, in the absence of censoring, the most efficient estimator of $\psi_0 = (\beta_r^*, \beta_p^*)$ that ignores data on the pretreatment variables L_0^* under the sole restrictions (A1.10) and (A1.1) (Robins and Tsiatis, 1991). However, this optimal rank estimator will be less efficient than $\tilde{\psi}^\dagger(q_{\text{opt}}^\dagger)$ when data on L_0^* is available.]

A1.3. Identification and Estimation of $\text{pr}[T_G > t]$

Although the assumption of an SNFTM w.r.t. L will serve to identify $\text{pr}[T_{G=(0)} < t]$ from the data $(T_i, \bar{L}_i(T_i), \bar{A}_i(T_i))$ when (A1.11) is true, nonetheless, $\text{pr}[T_G < t]$ will not be identifiable for any other treatment regimes without further assumptions. Three such identifying assumptions are given in Theorem A1.2 below. First some definitions are needed.

Definition. For any $\bar{l}_m$, $\bar{a}_m$ and $G^* \in \mathbf{G}$ such that $G^*(\bar{l}_{m-1}) = \bar{a}_{m-1}$, define the function $y(t, \bar{l}_m, \bar{a}_m, G^*)$ by

$$\mathrm{pr}[\,T_{G^*} > y(t, \bar{l}_\mathrm{m}, \bar{a}_\mathrm{m}, G^*)|\bar{l}_\mathrm{m}, \bar{a}_\mathrm{m}, T > m\,]$$

$$= \mathrm{pr}[\,T_{G=(\bar{a}_{\mathrm{m}-1,0})} > t|\bar{l}_\mathrm{m}, \bar{a}_\mathrm{m}, T > m\,] \quad (\mathrm{A1.13})$$

We shall call $y(t, \bar{l}_\mathrm{m}, \bar{a}_\mathrm{m}, G^*)$ the treatment effect transformation function w.r.t. L. It transforms percentiles of the survival curve that would have been observed if subjects with history $(\bar{l}_\mathrm{m}, \bar{a}_\mathrm{m})$ had received *no* further treatment subsequent to time m into percentiles of the survival curve that would have been observed if the same subjects had followed regime G^* subsequent to m.

Definition. We say there is no current treatment interaction w.r.t. L if

$$y(t, \bar{l}_\mathrm{m}, \bar{a}_\mathrm{m}, G^*) \text{ does not depend on } a_\mathrm{m} \text{ for all } G^* \text{ and } m \quad (\mathrm{A1.14})$$

That is, if conditional on $(\bar{l}_\mathrm{m}, \bar{a}_{\mathrm{m}-1})$, the treatment effect transformation function is the same for subsets of the population differing in their observed treatment a_m at m^+.

Definition. A regime G is nondynamic if, for all m, $\bar{l}_\mathrm{m}^{(1)}$, $\bar{l}_\mathrm{m}^{(2)}$, we have $G[\bar{l}_\mathrm{m}^{(1)}] = G[\bar{l}_\mathrm{m}^{(2)}]$. The nondynamic regimes are precisely the regimes $G = (\bar{a})$ defined previously.

Definition. We say there is no current treatment interaction w.r.t. L for non-dynamic regimes if $y(t, \bar{l}_\mathrm{m}, \bar{a}_\mathrm{m}, G^*)$ does not depend on a_m for all nondynamic regimes G^*.

Definition. We have no confounding by unmeasured confounders for survival given L if for all $G \in \mathbf{G}$

$$T_G \amalg A_\mathrm{m}|\bar{L}_\mathrm{m}, G(\bar{L}_{\mathrm{m}-1}), T > m \quad (\mathrm{A1.15})$$

Definition. We have no confounding by unmeasured confounders for survival given (L, H) if for all $G \in \mathbf{G}$

$$T_G \amalg A_\mathrm{m}|\bar{L}_\mathrm{m}, H, G(\bar{L}_{\mathrm{m}-1}), T > m \quad (\mathrm{A1.16})$$

Define the function $\rho(x, \bar{l}_\mathrm{m}, \bar{a}_\mathrm{m})$ recursively for all $\bar{l}_\mathrm{m}, \bar{a}_\mathrm{m}$ and $x\epsilon(0, \infty)$ as follows. $\rho(x, \bar{l}_0, \bar{a}_0) = \gamma^{-1}(x, \bar{l}_0, \bar{a}_0)$ where $\gamma^{-1}(u, \bar{l}_k, \bar{a}_k) \equiv t$ if $\gamma(t, \bar{l}_k, \bar{a}_k) = u$. For $1 \le k \le m$, $\rho(x, \bar{l}_k, \bar{a}_k) = \gamma^{-1}(\rho(x, \bar{l}_{k-1}, \bar{a}_{k-1}), \bar{l}_k, \bar{a}_k)$ if $\rho(x, \bar{l}_{k-1}, \bar{a}_{k-1}) \ge k$; and $\rho(x, \bar{l}_k, \bar{a}_k) = \rho(x, \bar{l}_{k-1}, \bar{a}_{k-1})$ otherwise. We call $\rho(x, \bar{l}_k, \bar{a}_k)$ the recursive blip-up function. Given $(\bar{l}, \bar{a})$, let $\rho(x, \bar{l}, \bar{a}) = \lim_{m\to\infty} \rho(x, \bar{l}_\mathrm{m}, \bar{a}_\mathrm{m})$ if the limit exists and $\rho(x, \bar{l}, \bar{a}) = \infty$, otherwise. In Appendix 3, we prove

Theorem A1.2. If $\gamma(t, \bar{l}_m, \bar{a}_m)$ is identified, CA1 holds, and if (a) there is no current treatment interaction w.r.t. L, (b) Eq. (A1.15) or (c) Eq. (A1.16) holds, then (i) $\mathrm{pr}[T_G > t \mid R = r]$ and $\mathrm{pr}[T_G > t \mid R = r, l_0^*]$ are identified and (ii) the blip-null hypothesis implies the G-null hypothesis. Further, CA1 and (A1.15) imply $\gamma(t, \bar{l}_m, \bar{a}_m)$ is identified. In particular, if (A1.15) or (A1.16) hold, then

$$\mathrm{pr}[T_G > t \mid R = r, l_0^*]$$

$$= \int\!\!\int \cdots \int \left\{ \mathrm{pr}[T > t \mid T > \mathrm{int}(t), \bar{l}_{\mathrm{int}(t)}, G(\bar{l}_{\mathrm{int}(t)}), h] \right.$$

$$\times \prod_{m=1}^{m=\mathrm{int}(t)} \mathrm{pr}[T > m \mid T > m - 1, \bar{l}_{m-1}, G(\bar{l}_{m-1}), h]$$

$$\left. \times \prod_{m=1}^{m=\mathrm{int}(t)} dF[l_m \mid h, T > m, \bar{l}_{m-1}, G(\bar{l}_{m-1})] \right\}$$

$$\times dF_H[h \mid r, l_0^*] \quad \text{(A1.17)}$$

where (i) $\mathrm{pr}[T > t \mid T > m - 1, \bar{l}_{m-1}, G(\bar{l}_{m-1}), h]$, $t \leq m$, is 1, 0, or undefined as $\rho[h, \bar{l}_{m-1}, G(\bar{l}_{m-1})]$ exceeds t, lies in $(m - 1, t]$, or is less than or equal to $m - 1$; (ii) $f[l_m \mid T > m, \bar{l}_{m-1}, G(\bar{l}_{m-1}), h]$ is undefined if $\rho[h, \bar{l}_{m-1}, G(\bar{l}_{m-1})] < m$; and (iii) we assign the value 0 to undefined quantities in (A1.17). Further, if (A1.15) or (A1.16) hold, the following Monte–Carlo algorithm produces independent realizations $t_{v,\text{``G''}}$ of a random variable $T_{v,\text{``G''}}$ whose distribution is that of T_G given $R = r$.

Given a regime G,

Step 1: Set $v = 1$
Step 2: Draw h_v from $f_H(h \mid r)$
Step 3: Draw $l_{0,v}^*$ from $f[l_0^* \mid h_v, r]$
Step 4: Set $m = 1$
Step 5: If $\rho[h_v, \bar{l}_{m-1,v}, G(\bar{l}_{m-1,v})] \leq m$, set $t_{v,\text{``G''}} = \rho[h_v, \bar{l}_{m-1,v}, G(\bar{l}_{m-1,v})]$, increment v by 1 and return to Step 2. If $\rho[h_v, \bar{l}_{m-1,v}, G(\bar{l}_{m-1,v})] > m$, draw $l_{m,v}$ from $f[l_m \mid \bar{l}_{m-1,v}, G(\bar{l}_{m-1,v}), h_v, T > m]$, increment m by 1 and return to Step 5.

Remark A1.3. Suppose we allow the $A(t)$ and $L(t)$ processes to jump at any time t. Consider continuous time feasible treatment regimes G characterized by functions $G(t, \bar{L}(t))$ taking values in the set of possible $a(t)$ values. It then follows from the proofs of the fundamental identities in Robins and Rotnitzky

(1992, Section 3h), that, under conditions (a) and (b) below, we have the identity $\mathrm{pr}[T_G > t \mid R, L_0^*] = E[\tau_G(t)/K_G(t) \mid L_0^*, R]$, where (i) $\tau_G(t) = I(X(G) \geq t)$, where $X(G)$ is the minimum of T and the first time U^* at which $G\{\bar{L}(u)\} \neq \bar{A}(u)$, where $G\{\bar{L}(t)\} = \{G(u, \bar{L}(u)); 0 \leq u < t\}$; and (ii) $K_G(t) \equiv \exp[-\int_0^t \lambda_{X(G),1}(u \mid \bar{L}(u))du]$, where $\lambda_{X(G),1}(u \mid \cdot)$ is the cause-specific hazard of $X(G)$ corresponding to $\sigma_G = 1$ given $\cdot$ with $\sigma_G = I\{X(G) \neq T\}$. Here, conditions (a) and (b) are (a) $\lambda_{X(G),1}(u \mid \bar{L}(u), T_G) = \lambda_{X(G),1}(u \mid \bar{L}(u))$ and (b) $K_G(t) > c > 0$ w.p.1. If $A(t)$ and $L(t)$ can only jump at discrete times m^+ and m, respectively, the above identity remains true except now conditon (a) becomes equation (A1.15), and

$$K_G(t) \equiv \prod_{m=0}^{\mathrm{int}(t)} f[A_m = G(m, \bar{L}_m) \mid \bar{L}_m, T > m, G(\bar{L}_{m-1})]$$

Theorem A1.3. (a) If, for all $\bar{a}$ histories, neither $\gamma(t, \bar{l}_m, \bar{a}_m)$ nor $y(t, \bar{l}_m, \bar{a}_m, G^* = (\bar{a}))$ depend on $\bar{l}_m$ except through r, then $\gamma(t, \bar{l}_m, \bar{a}_m) = \gamma(t, r, \bar{a}_m)$, $y(t, \bar{l}_m, \bar{a}_m, G^* = (\bar{a})) = y(t, r, \bar{a}_m, G^* = (\bar{a}))$, and $\rho(h, \bar{l}, \bar{a}) = \rho(h, r, \bar{a})$ where $\gamma(t, \bar{l}_m, \bar{a}_m)$, $y(t, r, \bar{a}_m, G^* = (\bar{a}))$, and $\rho(h, r, \bar{a})$ are as defined previously except with r replacing $\bar{l}_m$.

(b) If we have no current treatment interaction w.r.t. r, i. e., by definition, $y(t, r, \bar{a}_m, G^* = (\bar{a}))$ does not depend on a_m, then $\mathrm{pr}[T_{G=(\bar{a})} > t \mid R = r] = \mathrm{pr}[\rho(H, r, \bar{a}) > t \mid R = r]$.

Proof. Theorem (A1.3(a)) is an easy calculation. (A1.3(b)) follows from Theorem A1.1 and the proof of Theorem A3.1 in Appendix 3.

Remark A1.4. Hence, if we have a correctly specified SNFTM for $\gamma(t, r, \bar{a}_m)$, we can identify $\mathrm{pr}[T_{G=(\bar{a})} > t \mid R = r]$ without data on any posttreatment covariate $L^*(t)$ provided we can assume no current treatment interaction w.r.t. r. Unfortunately, this latter assumption will be false if there is a time-dependent covariate L_m^* (e. g., red blood count at m) that is (1) a predictor of future treatment and (2) there exists a treatment covariate interaction. [For example, (1) AZT treatment is contraindicated in patients with low red blood counts and (2) AZT is harmful in subjects with very low red blood counts but beneficial in subjects with normal red counts.]

The following proposition provides the logical relationships between the three identifying restrictions of Theorem A1.2. The proofs are omitted or are only sketched.

Proposition A1.1. (a) Equation (A1.15) implies no current treatment interaction w.r.t. L but the converse is not true; (b) (A1.15) neither implies nor is implied by (A1.16); (c) by Theorem A1.1, (A1.15) implies

$$H \amalg A_{\mathrm{m}} \mid \bar{L}_{\mathrm{m}}, \bar{A}_{\mathrm{m}}, T > m \qquad (A1.18)$$

(d) (A1.18) plus (A1.16) imply (A1.15); (e) if $\gamma(t, \bar{l}_{\mathrm{m}}, \bar{a}_{\mathrm{m}})$ does not depend on $\bar{l}_{\mathrm{m}}$ except through r and (A1.16) holds, then there will be no current treatment interaction w.r.t. L for nondynamic regimes, although if (A1.15) is false, there will be current treatment interaction w.r.t. L for dynamic regimes; (f) it follows from Theorem A1.3 that if there is no current treatment interaction w.r.t. L for nondynamic regimes and $\gamma(t, \bar{l}_{\mathrm{m}}, \bar{a}_{\mathrm{m}})$ depends on $\bar{l}_{\mathrm{m}}$ only through r, then (i) $\mathrm{pr}[T_{G=(\bar{a})} > t \mid r] = \mathrm{pr}[\rho(H, r, \bar{a}) > t \mid r]$ and (ii) if R was assigned at random so (A1.1) holds, neither $\gamma(t, r, \bar{a}_{\mathrm{m}})$ nor $\rho(H, r, \bar{a})$ will depend on r; and, finally, (g) if $\gamma(t, \bar{l}_{\mathrm{m}}, \bar{a}_{\mathrm{m}})$ depends on $\bar{l}_{\mathrm{m}}$ and (A1.15) is false, then, in general, even for nondynamic regimes G, (i) it is not possible both for there to be no current interaction w.r.t. L and for (A1.16) to be true, and (ii) if there is no current treatment interaction w.r.t. L, the right-hand side of (A1.17) does not equal $\mathrm{pr}[T_{G} > t \mid R, l_{0}^{*}]$.

The following example gives an explicit demonstration of point g above.

Example. Suppose $l_{0} = r$. Further, a_{0}, a_{1}, and l_{1} are each dichotomous (0, 1) variables, and, conditional on $R = r$, $\mathrm{pr}[A_{1} = 0] = 0$, and $\mathrm{pr}[A_{0} = 1] = \pi$ where we have suppressed the conditioning event $R = r$ throughout this example. Suppose there exists a constant c, $c > 2$, such that, conditional on $R = r$, (1) $\mathrm{pr}[H < 2] = 0$, (2) $\mathrm{pr}[H < c \mid A_{0} = 0] = 1$, (3) $\mathrm{pr}[H < c \mid A_{0} = 1] = 1/2$, (4) $H \amalg A_{0} \mid H < c$, (5) $0 = \mathrm{pr}[L_{1} = 1 \mid H, A_{0} = 1, H < c] = 1 - \mathrm{pr}[L_{1} = 1 \mid H, A_{0} = 1, H > c]$, (6) $\gamma^{-1}(u, \bar{l}_{0}, \bar{a}_{0}) = u$, (7) $\gamma^{-1}(u, \bar{l}_{1}, \bar{a}_{1}) = u$ if $l_{1} = 0$ and $1 \leq \gamma^{-1}(u, \bar{l}_{1}, \bar{a}_{1}) < 2$ if $l_{1} = 1$. Then, given $R = r$, with $t = 2$ the right-hand side of (A1.17) equals $\pi \mathrm{pr}[T > 2 \mid A_{0} = 1] + (1 - \pi)$ for $G = (a_{0} = 1, a_{1} = 1, 0)$ so

$$\mathrm{pr}[T_{G=(a_{0}=1, a_{1}=1, 0)} > 2] = \pi \mathrm{pr}[T > 2 \mid A_{0} = 1] + (1 - \pi)$$

if (A1.16) holds. On the other hand, it is easy to calculate that, given r, (1)–(7) above imply $\mathrm{pr}[T_{G=(a_{0}=1, a_{1}=1, 0)} > 2] = \pi \mathrm{pr}[T > 2 \mid A_{0} = 1]$ under the assumption of no current treatment interaction w.r.t. L. [Note (1)–(7) imply (A1.18) is false so (A1.15) must be false.]

We next turn our attention to the substantive plausibility of the identifying restrictions. (A1.15) will be true if all risk factors for (i. e., predictors of) T_{G} that are used by patients and physicians to determine their treatment dosage at m^{+} are recorded in $\bar{L}_{\mathrm{m}}, \bar{A}_{\mathrm{m}-1}$. Thus, an investigator could try to ensure that (A1.15) was justifiable by trying to measure all such risk factors.

We next consider what beliefs an investigator would need to hold to accept (A1.16) but not (A1.15) as true.

Definition. We have no unmeasured confounding for survival given "L and current risk" if, for all $G \in \mathbf{G}$,

$$\bar{A}_m \amalg T_G | \bar{L}_m, T_{G=(\bar{A}_{m-1},0)}, G(\bar{L}_{m-1}), T > m \qquad (A1.19)$$

We would believe (A1.19) held, but (A1.15) did not if, using standard epidemiologic parlance, we thought $T_{G=(\bar{A}_{m-1},0)}$ effectively controlled residual confounding by those unmeasured risk factors for T_G not contained in $(\bar{L}_m, \bar{A}_{m-1})$.

Lemma A1.1. If we have local rank preservation and (A1.19) holds, then (A1.16) holds [since local rank preservation implies that $H_m = T_{G=(\bar{A}_{m-1},0)}$, and H is a deterministic function of $(H_m, \bar{L}_m, \bar{A}_{m-1})$].

In standard epidemiologic parlance, the assumption of local rank preservation is the assumption that all modifiers of the effect of a single blip of exposure a_m at m^+ are contained in $(\bar{L}_m, \bar{A}_{m-1})$. It is my opinion that (A1.15) might often adequately approximate the beliefs of an investigator. Occasionally, an investigator might accept that (A1.16) was approximately true as a consequence of (A1.19) and local rank preservation, even if (A1.15) was not accepted. It is hard to imagine settings in which the assumption of no current treatment interaction w.r.t. L would adequately represent an investigator's beliefs, when (A1.15) did not.

A1.4. Efficiency Considerations

We have seen in Corollary A1.3 that given (A1.1), CA1, (A1.11), and a correctly specified SNFTM, $\tilde{\psi}^\dagger(q^\dagger_{opt})$ is semiparametric efficient for ψ_0. If we impose the added restriction (A1.16) to identify $\mathrm{pr}[T_G > t | R]$, $G \in \mathbf{G}$, $\tilde{\psi}^\dagger(q^\dagger_{opt})$ is no longer semiparametric efficient [unless $\gamma^*(t, \bar{l}_m, \bar{a}_m, \psi)$ depends only on l_0^* and $\bar{a}_m$]. To see why, note (i) (A1.1) implies $\mathrm{pr}[T_G > t | l_0 \equiv (r, l_0^{*\prime})']$ does not depend on r; (ii) (A1.1) plus (A1.16) imply [although (A1.10) plus (A1.16) do not imply] that $\mathrm{pr}[T_G > t | l_0]$ is given by the right-hand side of (A1.17); and (iii) points (i) and (ii) constitute all additional restrictions on the joint distribution of the observables beyond (A1.10) and (A1.1b) obtained by imposing (A1.16).

Similarly the imposition either of the assumption of no current treatment interaction w.r.t. L or of (A1.15) implies $\tilde{\psi}^\dagger(q^\dagger_{opt})$ is no longer efficient.

Furthermore, imposition of (A1.15) implies more restrictions on the distribution of the observables than does imposing (A1.16). Specifically, by Robins (1989b) and Theorem A1.1, (A1.15) plus CA1 imply that $\gamma(t, \bar{l}_m, \bar{a}_m)$ and $\mathrm{pr}[T_G > t | r, l_0^*]$ are identified and that (A1.18) holds [without imposing either the assumption (A1.1) of randomization or the assumption of a correctly specified SNFTM].

(A1.15), CA1, plus a correctly specified SNFTM $\gamma^*(t, \bar{l}_m, \bar{a}_m, \psi)$ imply

$$A_m \amalg H(\psi_0) | \bar{L}_m, \bar{A}_m, T > m \qquad \text{(A1.20)}$$

Robins (1989b) and Robins *et al.* (1992) propose a class of G-estimators $\tilde{\psi}(q)$ that are consistent for ψ_0 under (A1.20) and drive an estimator $\tilde{\psi}(q_{opt})$ that is semiparametric efficient under the sole restriction (A1.20). Specifically, $\tilde{\psi}(q)$ solves

$$0 = S_\theta(\tilde{\alpha}, 0, \psi) \equiv \sum_{i=1}^{n} \sum_{m=0}^{\text{int}(T_i)} Q_{m,i}\{A_{m,i}, H_i(\psi)\}$$

$$- \int Q_{m,i}\{a_m, H_i(\psi)\} f(a_m | \bar{L}_{m,i}, \bar{A}_{m-1,i}; \tilde{\alpha}) d\mu(a_m) \qquad \text{(A1.21)}$$

where $\tilde{\alpha}$ is the partial maximum likelihood estimator of the parameter α_0 in a correctly specified model for the density $f[a_m | \bar{L}_m, \bar{A}_{m-1}, T > m]$ with respect to a measure μ and $Q_{m,i}\{A_{m,i}, H_i(\psi)\} \equiv q(A_{m,i}, H_i(\psi), \bar{A}_{m-1,i}, \bar{L}_{m,i}) \epsilon R^v$ where $q(\cdot, \cdot, \cdot, \cdot)$ is a fixed function.

Under the restrictions (A1.15) and (A1.6a), an inverse variance weighted average of $\tilde{\psi}(q_{opt})$ and $\tilde{\psi}^\dagger(q_{opt}^\dagger)$ will be semiparametric efficient where $q_{opt}(A_m, H(\psi_0), \bar{A}_{m-1}, \bar{L}_m) = E[S_\psi | \bar{L}_m, \bar{A}_m, H(\psi_0), T > m]$ and S_ψ and $q_{opt}^\dagger$ are as defined above. [Note $S_\psi \equiv S_\psi(\psi_0)$ can now also be obtained by removing $H(\psi_0)$ from the terms $f(A_m | \bar{L}_m, \bar{A}_{m-1}, H(\psi_0), T > m)$ in (A1.12), and then differentiating the logarithm of (A1.12) w.r.t. ψ_0.] In contrast, this inverse variance weighted average will not be efficient under (A1.1) and (A1.15) since (A1.1) and (A1.15) imply [but (A1.15) and (A1.6a) do not imply] the additional restriction that the right-hand side of (A1.17) does not depend on r [except when $\gamma^*(t, \bar{l}_m, \bar{a}_m, \psi)$ only depends on l_0^* and $\bar{a}_m$]. This is relevant to efficient estimation under Method 3 in the text.

Instrumental Variables

Suppose next that $A_m = (A_m^{(1)}, A_m^{(2)})'$ is two-dimensional and that one is willing to assume

$$A_m^{(1)} \amalg T_G | \bar{L}_m, G(\bar{L}_{m-1}), T > m \qquad \text{(A1.22)}$$

is true but that (A1.15) is not.

$A_m^{(1)}$ would be called an instrument for $A_m^{(2)}$. Then $\tilde{\psi}^{(1)}(q^{(1)})$ solving (A1.21) with $A_{m,i}$ and a_m replaced by $A_{m,i}^{(1)}$ and $a_m^{(1)}$ (but $\bar{A}_{m-1,i}$ unchanged) would be asymptotically normal and unbiased for ψ_0. Further, under (A1.1), (A1.22), and CA1, the inverse variance weighted average of $\tilde{\psi}^\dagger(q_{opt}^\dagger)$ and $\tilde{\psi}^{(1)}(q_{opt}^{(1)})$ will be semiparametric efficient where $q_{opt}^{(1)}(A_m^{(1)}, H(\psi_0), \bar{A}_{m-1}, \bar{L}_m) = E[S_\psi \mid A_m^{(1)}, \bar{L}_m, \bar{A}_{m-1}, H(\psi_0), T > m]$ and S_ψ and $q_{opt}^\dagger$ are as defined previously. [Note that $S_\psi(\psi_0)$ can now also be obtained by replacing the term $f[A_m \mid \bar{L}_m, \bar{A}_{m-1}, H(\psi_0), T > m]$ in (A1.12) with $f[A_m^{(1)} \mid \bar{L}_m, \bar{A}_{m-1}, T > m] \times f[A_m^{(2)} \mid A_m^{(1)}, \bar{L}_m, \bar{A}_{m-1}, H(\psi_0), T > m]$, and then differentiating the natural log of (A1.12) w.r.t. ψ_0.] [If (A1.15) is not true, even given (A1.1), (A1.22), CA1, and a correctly specified SNFTM $\gamma^*(t, \bar{l}_m, \bar{a}_m, \psi)$, $\text{pr}[T_G > t \mid r, l_0^*]$ is not identified for regimes other than $G = (0)$, unless we assume either (A1.16) or no current treatment interaction w.r.t. L.]

A1.5. Implications of No Unmeasured Confounders for L^*-History and Death

We shall next assume there exists $\bar{L}_{i,G}^*(T_{i,G})$ representing the L^*-history that would be observed if subject i had followed regime G. (Remember that L^*-history is L-history ignoring treatment arm.) Furthermore, we make the following consistency assumption.

CA2. If $T_i > m$ and $G(\bar{L}_{m-1,i}^*) = \bar{A}_{m-1,i}$, then $\bar{L}_{m,i,G}^* = \bar{L}_{m,i}^*$.

We assume physical randomization of R in the trial implies

$$\{T_G, \bar{L}_G^*(T_G); G \in \mathbf{G}\} \amalg R \qquad (A1.23)$$

which generalizes (A.1).

Definition. There exists no unmeasured confounders jointly for survival and L^*-history given L if, for all $G \in \mathbf{G}$, and all m

$$\{T_G, \bar{L}_G^*(T_G)\} \amalg A_m \mid \bar{L}_m, G(\bar{L}_{m-1}), T > m \qquad (A1.24)$$

Note (A1.24) implies (A1.15). *Furthermore, in Appendix 2, we argue that it would essentially never make substantive sense to believe that (A1.15) were true but (A1.24) false!*

We now show that when (A1.23) and (A1.24) hold, the sufficient statistics for ψ_0 and for $\text{pr}(T_G > t)$ do not depend on the data through R_i so that R_i could be completely ignored in the analysis without loss of efficiency and it is irrelevant that the data arose from a randomized trial. This result is based on the following two lemmas.

Lemma A1.2. If (A1.23), (A1.24), and CA1 and CA2 hold, then

$$\text{pr}[L_\text{m} | \bar{L}^*_{\text{m}-1}, T > m, G(\bar{L}^*_{\text{m}-1}), R]$$

$$= \text{pr}[L_\text{m} | \bar{L}^*_{\text{m}-1}, T > m, G(\bar{L}^*_{\text{m}-1})] \quad (\text{A1.25})$$

and, for $t \leq m$,

$$\text{pr}[T > t | \bar{L}^*_{\text{m}-1}, T > m - 1, G(\bar{L}^*_{\text{m}-1}), R]$$

$$= \text{pr}[T > t | \bar{L}^*_{\text{m}-1}, T > m - 1, G(\bar{L}^*_{\text{m}-1})] \quad (\text{A1.26})$$

Lemma A1.3. If (A1.24), CA1 and CA2, (A1.25) and (A1.26) are known to hold, then

a. $(T_\text{G}, \bar{L}^*_\text{G}(T_\text{G})) \amalg A_\text{m} | \bar{L}^*_\text{m}, G(\bar{L}^*_{\text{m}-1}), T > m$ (A1.27)

b. $\gamma(t, \bar{l}_\text{m}, \bar{a}_\text{m})$, $\rho(x, \bar{l}_\text{m}, \bar{a}_\text{m})$, $h(t, \bar{l}(t), \bar{a}(t))$, and $y(t, \bar{l}_\text{m}, \bar{a}_\text{m}, G^*)$ do not depend on r; thus, $H(\psi)$ and $\partial H(\psi)/\partial T$ do not depend on r

c. $H \amalg R | \bar{A}_\text{m}, \bar{L}^*_\text{m}, T > m$

d. The likelihood function (A1.12) can be written

$$\left[\frac{\partial H_\text{i}(\psi_0)}{\partial T_\text{i}} \right] f\{H_\text{i}(\psi_0)\}$$

$$\times \prod_{m=0}^{m=\text{int}(T_\text{i})} f\{L^*_{\text{m,i}} | \bar{L}^*_{\text{m}-1,\text{i}}, \bar{A}_{\text{m}-1,\text{i}}, H_\text{i}(\psi_0), T_\text{i} > m\}$$

$$\times \prod_{m=0}^{m=\text{int}(T_\text{i})} f(A_{\text{m,i}} | \bar{L}^*_{\text{m,i}}, \bar{A}_{\text{m}-1,\text{i}}, T_\text{i} > m) f[R_\text{i} | \bar{A}_{\text{int}(T_\text{i}),\text{i}}, \bar{L}^*_{\text{int}(T_\text{i}),\text{i}}] \quad (\text{A1.28})$$

e. A semiparametric efficient estimator $\tilde{\psi}^*(q^*_\text{opt})$ of ψ_0 does not depend on the data through R, where $\tilde{\psi}^*(q)$ is defined like $\tilde{\psi}(q)$ except with $\bar{L}^*_\text{m}$ replacing $\bar{L}_\text{m}$ and $q^*_\text{opt}(A_\text{m}, H(\psi_0), \bar{A}_{\text{m}-1}, \bar{L}^*_\text{m})$ is the conditional expectation of S_ψ [which now equals the derivative of the logarithm of (A1.28) w.r.t. ψ_0] given $\{\bar{A}_\text{m}, \bar{L}^*_\text{m}, H(\psi_0)\}$

f. The Monte–Carlo algorithm of Theorem 2 produces draws from $\text{pr}(T_\text{G} > t) = \text{pr}(T_\text{G} > t | r)$ when all references to "r" are deleted

Remark A1.3. Even part (f) is false if (A1.15) and (A1.23) hold, but (A1.24) does not.

Proof of Lemma A1.2. Given (A1.24) and CA1 and CA2, the left-hand sides of (A1.25) and (A1.26) equal $\mathrm{pr}[L_{m,G} | \bar{L}^*_{m-1,G}, T_G > m, R]$ and $\mathrm{pr}[T_G > t | \bar{L}^*_{m-1,G}, T_G > m - 1, R]$, $t < m$, respectively, by Theorem 4.1 of Robins (1986). But, by (A1.23), neither of these conditional probabilities depends on R, proving the lemma.

Proof of Lemma A1.3. Parts (a)–(c) follow directly from Theorem 7 of Robins *et al.* (1992) if R is identified with $\bar{L}^{(2)}_m$ and $\bar{L}^*_m$ is identified with $\bar{L}^{(1)}_m$. Robins *et al.* (1992) did not prove part (b) of their Theorem 7 on which parts (b) and (c) of this lemma depend. Therefore, we give the proof of part (b) of Theorem 7 of Robins *et al.* (1992) in Lemma A3.1 of Appendix 3. The proof of part (d) proceeds as follows. (A2.30) of Robins *et al.* (1992) implies that their (A2.5) can be written

$$\{\partial H(\psi_0)/\partial T\} f[H(\psi_0)] \{ \prod_{m=0}^{\mathrm{int}(T_i)} f[L_m^{(1)} | \bar{L}_{m-1}^{(1)}, \bar{A}_{m-1}, H(\psi_0), T$$

$$> m] f[A_m | \bar{L}_m, \bar{A}_{m-1}, T > m] \} f[\bar{L}^{(2)}_{\mathrm{int}(T)} | \bar{L}^{(1)}_{\mathrm{int}(T)}, \bar{A}_{\mathrm{int}(T)}, H(\psi_0)]$$

But by (A2.31) of Robins *et al.* (1992), $f[\bar{L}^{(2)}_{\mathrm{int}(T)} | \bar{L}^{(1)}_{\mathrm{int}(T)}, \bar{A}_{\mathrm{int}(T)}, H(\psi_0)]$ does not depend on $H(\psi_0)$. Part (e) follows from (d) and the proof of semiparametric efficiency in Robins (1993b) [part (e) remains true if the marginal law of R is known. In this case, a proof uses part (c) of Corollary A3.1 to rewrite the likelihood (A1.12).]. Part (f) follows from part (a) and Theorem 3 in Robins *et al.* (1992).

APPENDIX 2: PLAUSIBLE VERSUS MATHEMATICAL ASSUMPTIONS

In this appendix we argue that in the context of an AIDS study, it is not plausible to assume (A1.15) is true when (A1.24) is false. In the context of a study of the effect of a workplace exposure on occupational mortality, Robins (1987b) presented a plausible scenario under which it would make substantive sense to believe the assumption (A1.15) of no unmeasured confounders for survival given L was true for the regime $G = (0)$ but the assumption (A1.24) of no unmeasured confounders jointly for survival and L^*-history given L was false. He was unable to provide a scenario in which (A1.15) was true but (A1.24) was false for any other regime. Here we translate Robins's scenario into our AIDS context and show, in this context, it is no longer substantively plausible to assume that (A1.15) is true but (A1.24) is false, even for a regime $G = (0)$. We shall use the results and the notation collected in Robins (1986, 1987a,b, 1989a,b, 1992). Figure 2a is a causal tree graph representing the expected data from a simplified hypothetical version of trial 002 in which L_m^* is a dichotomous (0, 1) variable representing the absence and presence of anemia (low red blood cell count), respectively, $A_0^{(1)}$ represents the AZT treatment arm to which a subject was randomized, and $(A_0^{(2)}, A_1^{(2)})$ represents prophylaxis treatment at time 0 and 1. We assume that $L_0^* = 0$ for all subjects, follow-up ends at time 2, and all deaths occur just prior to time 2. Further, we assume that (A1.24) holds. In the occupational study context, $L_1 = 1$ represents a subject "off work" (i. e., unemployed), $L_1 = 0$ represents a subject "at work," $(A_0^{(2)}, A_1^{(2)})$ represents exposure to a workplace chemical, and $A_0^{(1)}$ represents a genetic sensitivity to eye irritants. Figure 2a captures the scenario described by Robins (1987b). We represent the eight nondynamic treatment regimes in Fig. 2a as $G^{(a)} = [(a_0^{(1)}, a_0^{(2)}), a_1^{(2)}]$ where the superscript "a" refers to Fig. 2a and for example $G^{(a)} = [(1, 0), 1]$ is the regime in which a subject is randomized to the high-dose arm at time 0, takes no prophylaxis at time 0 but takes prophylaxis at time 1. Using the G-computation algorithm described by Robins (1986, 1987a,b, 1989a,b), we see that the G-null hypothesis holds for Fig. 2a and $\mathrm{pr}[T_{G^{(a)}} > 2] = 0.75$ for all $G^{(a)}$. As a consequence, we say that neither AZT treatment arm nor prophylaxis has a direct, indirect, or overall effect on survival. In contrast,

$$5/6 = \mathrm{pr}[L_{1,G^{(a)}=[(1,a_0^{(2)}),a_1^{(2)}]} = 1] \neq \mathrm{pr}[L_{1,G^{(a)}=[(0,a_0^{(2)}),a_1^{(2)}]} = 1] = 1/6 \quad (A2.1)$$

But,

$$\mathrm{pr}[L_{1,G^{(a)}=[(0,0),a_1^{(2)}]} = 1] = \mathrm{pr}[L_{1,G^{(a)}=[(0,1),a_1^{(2)}]} = 1] = 1/6 \quad (A2.2)$$

and

$$\mathrm{pr}[L_{1,G^{(a)}=[(1,0),a_1^{(2)}]} = 1] = \mathrm{pr}[L_{1,G^{(a)}=[(1,1),a_1^{(2)}]} = 1] = 5/6 \quad (A2.3)$$

by the G-computation algorithm. (A2.1) implies that AZT protocol $A_0^{(1)}$ has a direct effect on L_1 controlling for prophylaxis. (A2.2) and (A2.3) imply prophylaxis has no direct effect on L_1 controlling for AZT protocol. For later reference, we note it follows from (A2.2) and (A2.3) that

$$\mathrm{pr}[L_{1,G^{(a)}=[(A_0^{(1)},0),a_1^{(2)}]} = 1] = \mathrm{pr}[L_{1,G^{(a)}=[(A_0^{(1)},1),a_1^{(2)}]} = 1] \quad (A2.4)$$

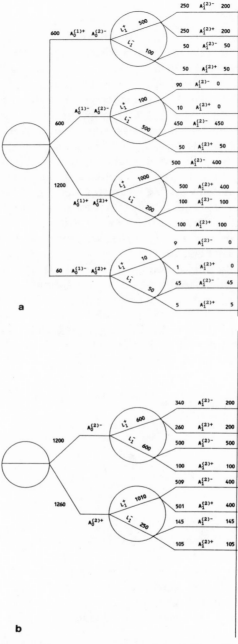

Figure 2. $A_0^{(1)+}$ ($A_0^{(1)-}$), assigned to high (low) AZT protocol; $A_m^{(2)+}$ ($A_m^{(2)-}$), taking (not taking) prophylaxis therapy at time m; L_1^+ (L_1^-), presence (absence) of anemia at time 1; whole numbers, numbers of subjects with a given history at a given time.

where, e. g., $\text{pr}[L_{1,G^{(a)}=[(A_0^{(1)},0),a_1^{(2)}]} = 1] = [5/6]\text{pr}[A_0^{(1)} = 1] + (1/6)$
$\text{pr}[A_0^{(1)} = 0]$ since $A_0^{(1)}$ is random.
Similarly,

$$\text{pr}\{T_{G^{(a)}=[(A_0^{(1)},a_0^{(2)}),a_1^{(2)}]} > 2\} = 3/4 \tag{A2.5}$$

Figure 2b represents the expected data when data on AZT protocol $A_0^{(1)}$ are missing and thus have been collapsed over. The outcomes under the four nondynamic regimes of Fig. 2b, i. e., $T_{G^{(b)}} = [a_0^{(2)}, a_1^{(2)}]$ are defined in terms of the outcomes under regimes $G^{(a)}$ as follows. $T_{G^{(b)}=[a_0^{(2)},a_1^{(2)}]}$ $= T_{G^{(a)}=[(A_0^{(1)},a_0^{(2)}),a_1^{(2)}]}$ and $L_{1,G^{(b)}=[a_0^{(2)},a_1^{(2)}]} = L_{1,G^{(a)}=[(A_0^{(1)},a_0^{(2)}),a_1^{(2)}]}$. Thus, by (A2.4),

$$\text{pr}\{L_{1,G^{(b)}=[1,a_1^{(2)}]}\} = \text{pr}\{L_{1,G^{(b)}=[0,a_1^{(2)}]}\} \tag{A2.6}$$

But, since

$$1/2 = \text{pr}[L_1 = 1 \mid A_0^{(2)} = 0] \neq \text{pr}[L_1 = 1 \mid A_0^{(2)} = 1] = 1010/1260 \tag{A2.7}$$

it follows that $L_{1,G^{(b)}} \amalg A_0^{(2)}$ so (A1.24) is false for Fig. 2b [since (A2.6) plus (A1.24) implies (A2.7) would be an equality]. (A1.24) is false for Fig. 2b because the (unrecorded) causal risk factor $A_0^{(1)}$ for L_1 is correlated with $A_0^{(2)}$.

In this setting, Robins (1987b) claimed that if (i) Fig. 2a satisfied (A1.24) and (ii) the unmeasured factor $A_0^{(1)}$ was not a direct causal risk factor for death controlling for $\bar{A}_1^{(2)}$, (A1.15) might hold on Fig. 2b for the regime $G^{(b)}$ = [0, 0]. But, if (A1.15) were true, by the G-computation algorithm formula, $3/4 = \text{pr}[T_{G^{(b)}=[(0,0)]} > 2]$ would have to equal $\text{pr}[L_1 = 1 \mid A_0^{(2)} = 0]\,\text{pr}[T > 2 \mid \bar{A}_1^{(2)} = (0, 0), L_1 = 1] + \text{pr}[L_1 = 0 \mid A_0^{(2)} = 0]\,\text{pr}[T > 2 \mid \bar{A}_1^{(2)} = (0, 0), L_1 = 0] = (1/2)(200/340) + (1/2)(500/500) = 27/34$. But it does not. We now discuss why not. One can show that, when (A1.24) is true for Fig. 2a, then with $G^{(b)}$ set equal to $G^{(b)} = [0, 0]$, $T_{G^{(b)}} \amalg A_m^{(2)} \mid G^{(b)}(\bar{L}_{m-1}), \bar{L}_m$, for $m = 0, 1$, is true for Fig. 2b $except$ at $L_1 = 1$. [It is true at $L_1 = 0$ because on Fig. 2a $T \amalg A_0^{(1)} \mid A_0^{(2)}, L_1 = 0$. However, $T \amalg A_0^{(1)} \mid A_0^{(2)}, L_1 = 1$.]

Thus, if $\text{pr}[A_1^{(2)} = 1 \mid L_1 = 1, A_0^{(2)}] = 0$, (A1.15) would hold for Fig. 2b and we would indeed obtain the correct result $3/4$ by using the above G-computation algorithm formula. Robins (1987b) assumed, in his plausible scenario, that $\text{pr}[A_1^{(2)} = 1 \mid L_1 = 1, A_0^{(2)}] = 0$ since $L_1 = 1$ represented subjects "off work" and $A_1^{(2)}$ denoted exposure to a workplace chemical. In fact, if $1 \neq \text{pr}[A_1^{(2)} = 1 \mid L_1, A_0^{(2)}] \neq 0$, then if, as in Fig. 2a, (i) $L_1 \amalg A_0^{(1)} \mid A_0^{(2)}$, (ii) $L_1 \amalg T \mid A_0^{(1)}, \bar{A}_1^{(2)}$, and (iii) $A_1^{(2)} \amalg A_0^{(1)} \mid L_1, A_0^{(2)}$, then when (A1.24) holds for Fig. 2a, it is not possible for (A1.15) to hold for Fig. 2b since it cannot be the case that for $G^{(b)}$ equal to $G^{(b)} = [0, 0]$, $T_{G^{(b)}} \amalg A_1^{(2)} | A_0^{(2)} = 0$, $L_1 = 1$ and $T_{G^{(b)}} \amalg A_1^{(2)} | A_0^{(2)} = 0$, $L_1 = 0$ are both true. Given (A1.24), (i) states that AZT protocol $A_0^{(1)}$ is a direct causal risk factor for anemia L_1 controlling for prophylaxis $\bar{A}_1^{(2)}$; (ii) states that that anemia is an independent prognostic factor for death controlling for AZT and prophylaxis history; and (iii) states that given a subject's prophylaxis treatment at time 0 and anemia status at time 1, the probability a physician chooses to provide prophylaxis therapy at time 1 depends on a subject's AZT protocol $A_0^{(1)}$. (i)–(iii) would all be expected to be substantively true in an actual AIDS study.

APPENDIX 3: PROOFS OF SOME THEOREMS

Proof of Theorem A1.1. Given $(\bar{L}_m, \bar{A}_m)$, define $t = \gamma(u, \bar{L}_m, \bar{A}_m)$ and let G refer to the regime $G = (\bar{A}_m, 0)$. Then, by definition,

$$\mathrm{pr}[T_G > u | \bar{L}_m, \bar{A}_m] = \mathrm{pr}[T_{G=(\bar{A}_{m-1},0)} > t | \bar{L}_m, \bar{A}_m] \qquad (A3.1)$$

Case A3.1. Suppose $m + 1 \geq u > m$. Then

$$\mathrm{pr}[T_G > u | \bar{L}_m, \bar{A}_m] = \mathrm{pr}[T > u | \bar{L}_m, \bar{A}_m] = \mathrm{pr}[H_m > t | \bar{L}_m, \bar{A}_m] \qquad (A3.2)$$

where the first equality is from CA1 and the second from $T > u \Leftrightarrow H_m(T, \bar{L}(T), \bar{A}(T)) > H_m(u, \bar{L}(u), \bar{A}(u)) \equiv t$ by the monotonicity of H_m. (A3.1) and (A3.2) prove Theorem A1.1 in Case A3.1.

Case A3.2. $u > m + 1$. Proof by induction. Assume the theorem is true with $m + 1$ replacing m. We now show it is true for m. $\mathrm{pr}[T_G > u | \bar{L}_m \bar{A}_m]$ equals

$$\mathrm{pr}[T > m + 1 | \bar{L}_m, \bar{A}_m] \int \mathrm{pr}[T_G > u | l_{m+1}, a_{m+1}, \bar{L}_m, \bar{A}_m]$$
$$\times dF[a_{m+1}, l_{m+1} | \bar{L}_m, \bar{A}_m, T > m + 1] \qquad (A3.3)$$

By the induction assumption, $\mathrm{pr}[T_G > u | l_{m+1}, a_{m+1}, \bar{L}_m, \bar{A}_m] = \mathrm{pr}[H_{m+1} > u | \bar{L}_m, \bar{A}_m, a_{m+1}, l_{m+1}]$. Hence, (A3.3) equals $\mathrm{pr}[H_{m+1} > u | \bar{L}_m, \bar{A}_m]$ since, by the definition of H_{m+1}, given $\bar{L}_m, \bar{A}_m$, and $u > m + 1$, then $H_{m+1} > u \Rightarrow T > m + 1$. But, by definition, $H_{m+1} > u$ if and only if $H_m > t$, proving the theorem.

Proof of Theorem A1.2. When (A1.16) holds, (A1.17) is a restatement of Theorem (A.1) in Robins (1989a) or Theorem 1 in Robins *et al.* (1992) with H simply an additional pretreatment variable. When (A1.15) holds, the identifiability of $\gamma(t, \bar{l}_m, \bar{a}_m)$ and (A1.17) is proved in the appendix of Robins *et al.* (1993b) and in Robins (1989a). When supposition (a) of Theorem A1.2 holds, Theorem A1.2 is a corollary of the following theorem.

Theorem A3.1. If there is no current treatment interaction with respect to L and the function $\gamma(t, \bar{l}_m, \bar{a}_m)$ is identified, then, for any $G^* \in \mathbf{G}$ and $m \geq 0$,

$$\text{pr}[T_{G^*} > t \,|\, \bar{L}_m, G^*(\bar{L}_m)] \qquad (A3.4)$$

and

$$\text{pr}[T_{G^*} > t \,|\, \bar{L}_m, G^*(\bar{L}_{m-1})] \qquad (A3.5)$$

are identified.

Proof. First we show that under the suppositions of the theorem, if we assume (A3.4) is identified, then (A3.5) is identified. Now (A3.4) equals

$$\text{pr}\{ T_{G=[G^*(\bar{L}_{m-1}),0]} < y^{-1}[u, \bar{L}_m, G^*(\bar{L}_{m-1}), G^*] \,|\, \bar{L}_m, G^*(\bar{L}_m)\} \quad (A3.6)$$

since, by the assumption of no current treatment interaction w.r.t. L, we can write $G^*(\bar{L}_{m-1})$ rather than $G^*(\bar{L}_m)$ in $y^{-1}[u, \bar{L}_m, G^*(\bar{L}_{m-1}), G^*]$ where $y^{-1}(t, \bar{l}_m, \bar{a}_m, G^*)$ is the inverse of $y(t, \bar{l}_m, \bar{a}_m, G^*)$ with respect to its first argument. Therefore, since (a) (A3.4) is identified by assumption and (b) by Theorem A1.1, the law of $T_{G=[G^*(\bar{L}_{m-1}),0]}$ conditional on $[\bar{L}_m, G^*(\bar{L}_m)]$ is identified if $\gamma(t, \bar{l}_m, \bar{a}_m)$ is identified, it follows that $y^{-1}[u, \bar{L}_m, G^*(\bar{L}_{m-1}), G^*]$ is itself identified. But, the assumption of no current treatment interaction w.r.t. L implies $\text{pr}[T_{G^*} < u \,|\, \bar{L}_m, G^*(\bar{L}_{m-1}), A_m]$ equals

$$\text{pr}\{ T_{G=[G^*(\bar{L}_{m-1}),0]} < y^{-1}[u, \bar{L}_m, G^*(\bar{L}_{m-1}), G^*] \,|\, \bar{L}_m,$$
$$G^*(\bar{L}_{m-1}), A_m\} \quad (A3.7)$$

Therefore, by Theorem A1.1 and the fact that $\gamma(t, \bar{l}_m, \bar{a}_m)$ is identified, it follows that $\text{pr}[T_{G^*} < u \,|\, \bar{L}_m, G^*(\bar{L}_{m-1}), A_m]$ is identified. It follows that (A3.5) is identified.

We now prove that (A3.4) is identified.

Case A3.2. $u \leq m + 1.$ (A3.4) equals

$$\text{pr}[T_{G=[G^*(\bar{L}_{m-1}),0]} < u \,|\, \bar{L}_m, G^*(\bar{L}_m)] \tag{A3.8}$$

by CA1. By the definition of the function γ^{-1}, (A3.8) equals

$$\text{pr}\{\gamma^{-1}[T_{G=[G^*(\bar{L}_{m-1}),0]}, \bar{L}_m, G^*(\bar{L}_m)] < u \,|\, \bar{L}_m, G^*(\bar{L}_m)\} \tag{A3.9}$$

But (A3.9) is identified by Theorem A1.1 and the fact that, by supposition, $\gamma(t, \bar{l}_m, \bar{a}_m)$ is identified.

Case A3.3. $u > m + 1.$ We proceed by induction. Specifically, we assume the theorem is true with $m + 1$ replacing m and show it is true for m. Now $\text{pr}[T_{G^*} > u \,|\, \bar{L}_m, G^*(\bar{L}_m)]$ equals

$$\text{pr}[T_{G^*} > u \,|\, \bar{L}_m, G^*(\bar{L}_m),$$
$$T > m + 1]\text{pr}[T_{G^*} > m + 1 \,|\, \bar{L}_m, G^*(\bar{L}_m)] \tag{A3.10}$$

where we have used the fact that for subjects with history $[\bar{L}_m, G^*(\bar{L}_m)]$, it follows from CA1 that $T > m + 1 \Leftrightarrow T_{G^*} > m + 1$.

Since, by Case A3.2 above, the right-hand term in (A3.10) is identified, it follows that (A3.4) is identified if the left-hand term in (A3.10) is identified. The left-hand term of (A3.10) equals

$$\int \text{pr}[T_{G^*} > u \,|\, \bar{L}_m, G^*(\bar{L}_m), L_{m+1}] dF[L_{m+1} \,|\, \bar{L}_m, G^*(\bar{L}_m),$$
$$T > m + 1] \tag{A3.11}$$

From the induction assumption that the theorem holds with $m + 1$ replacing m, expression (A3.11) is identified which completes the proof.

Proof of Part (b) of Theorem 7 of Robins *et al.* (1992)

Lemma A3.1. Under (A2.15), (A2.29a), and (A2.29b) of Robins *et al.* (1992) and the consistency assumptions, $\text{pr}[H_k > t \,|\, T > k, \bar{L}_k, \bar{A}_k] = \text{pr}[H_k > t \,|\, \bar{L}_k^{(1)}, \bar{A}_k, T > k].$

Proof. For G equal to $G = (\bar{A}_{k-1}, 0)$,

$$\text{pr}[H_k > t \mid T > k, \bar{L}_k, \bar{A}_k] = \text{pr}[T_G > t \mid T > k, \bar{L}_k, \bar{A}_k] \quad (A3.12)$$

by Theorem 2 of Robins *et al.* (1992). But by Theorem 1 of Robins *et al.* (1992), the right-hand side of (A3.12) equals

$$\iint \text{pr}[T > t \mid T > \text{int}(t), \bar{l}_{\text{int}(t)}, G(\bar{l}_{\text{int}(t)})]$$

$$\times \prod_{m=k+1}^{\text{int}(t)} \{\text{pr}[T > m \mid T > m - 1, \bar{l}_{m-1}, G(\bar{l}_{m-1})]$$

$$\times dF[l_m^{(1)} \mid T > m, \bar{l}_{m-1}, G(\bar{l}_{m-1})]\}$$

$$\times \prod_{m=k+1}^{\text{int}(t)} dF[l_m^{(2)} \mid T > m, \bar{l}_{m-1}, l_m^{(1)}, G(\bar{l}_{m-1})] \quad (A3.13)$$

By (A2.29a) and (A2.29b) of Robins *et al.* (1992), (A3.13) equals

$$\int \text{pr}[T > t \mid T > \text{int}(t), \bar{l}_{\text{int}(t)}^{(1)}, G(\bar{l}_{\text{int}(t)}^{(1)})] \prod_{m=k+1}^{\text{int}(t)} \{\text{pr}[T > m \mid T > m - 1,$$

$$\bar{l}_{m-1}^{(1)}, G(\bar{l}_{m-1}^{(1)})] dF[l_m^{(1)} \mid T > m, \bar{l}_{m-1}^{(1)}, G(\bar{l}_{m-1}^{(1)})]\}$$

$$\times \int \prod_{m=k+1}^{\text{int}(t)} dF[l_m^{(2)} \mid T > m, \bar{l}_{m-1}, l_m^{(1)}, G(\bar{l}_{m-1})].$$

But $\int \prod_{m=k+1}^{\text{int}(t)} dF[l_m^{(2)} \mid T > m, \bar{l}_{m-1}, l_m^{(1)}, G(\bar{l}_{m-1})]$ equals one. Hence, $\text{pr}[H_k > t \mid T > k, \bar{L}_k, \bar{A}_k]$ does not depend on $\bar{L}_k^{(2)}$, proving the lemma.

Thus, we have shown $H_k \amalg \bar{L}_k^{(2)} \mid T > k, \bar{L}_k^{(1)}, \bar{A}_k$ and, thus, by choosing $k = \text{int}(T)$, we see that $\gamma(t, \bar{l}_m, \bar{a}_m)$ does not depend on $\bar{l}_m^{(2)}$. Finally, to show that this implies (A2.31) of Robins *et al.* (1992), we note that H is a deterministic function of $H_k, \bar{L}_k^{(1)}, \bar{A}_k$ when (A2.29a) and (A2.29b) hold since $\gamma(t, \bar{l}_m, \bar{a}_m)$ does not depend on $\bar{l}_m^{(2)}$. This completes the proof.

Corollary A3.1. The suppositions of Lemma A3.1 also imply that (a) $H \amalg L_m^{(2)} \mid \bar{L}_m^{(1)}, \bar{L}_{m-1}^{(2)}, \bar{A}_{m-1}$; (b) $L_m^{(1)} \amalg \bar{L}_{m-1}^{(2)} \mid \bar{L}_{m-1}^{(1)}, \bar{A}_{m-1}, H$; and

(c) $f(L_m \mid \bar{L}_{m-1}, \bar{A}_{m-1}, T > m, H)$

$\qquad = f(L_m^{(2)} \mid \bar{L}_{m-1}, L_m^{(1)}, \bar{A}_{m-1}, T > m) f(L_m^{(1)} \mid T > m, \bar{L}_{m-1}^{(1)}, \bar{A}_{m-1}, H).$

Proof. Part (a) follows from Lemma A3.1 and the fact that by Theorem 2 of Robins *et al.* (1992), their (A2.15) implies their (A2.20). Part (b) follows from Bayes Theorem by part (a) and Eqs. (A2.29) and (A2.20) of Robins *et al.* (1992). Part (c) is an immediate consequence of parts (a) and (b).

APPENDIX 4: CENSORING

A4.1. Known Potential Censoring Time

In this section, we shall consider the following restricted type of censoring. We suppose that in our trial, follow-up ends on a particular calendar date and staggered entry is allowed. Let C record the known potential censoring time defined as the difference between the end of follow-up date and the date a subject was enrolled in the trial. We now observe for $i = (1, \ldots, n)$

$$V_i = \{ C_i, X_i^* = \min(T_i, C_i), \bar{L}_i(X_i^*), \bar{A}_i(X_i^*), \Delta_i^*$$

$$= I(T_i < C_i) \} \qquad\qquad\qquad\qquad (A4.1)$$

rather than

$$\{ T_i, \bar{L}_i(T_i), \bar{A}_i(T_i) \} \qquad\qquad\qquad\qquad (A4.2)$$

where, again, $L_0 = (R, L_0^*)$ and L_0^* are the pretreatment variables. Since C is the known potential end of follow-up time, we can and do include it in L_0^* and write $L_0^* = (L_0^{**}, C)$. Further, $H(\psi)$ is the "residual" on the ψ-time scale of Appendix 1. The notation in this section is consistent with that of Appendix 1. We make no effort here to keep the notation consistent with that in the main body of the chapter.

Let model (aj) be a semiparametric model for $\psi_0, j = 0, 1, 2, 3$, characterized by (i) the data (A4.1), (ii) the restriction (A1.10), and (iii) a model (j) for $f(Z_1 \mid Z_2)$ with $R \equiv Z_1$ and $L_0^* \equiv Z_2$, defined as follows. Given random variables (Z_1, Z_2), we consider four models, indexed by j, for $f(Z_1 \mid Z_2)$. Model (1) is a correctly specified parametric model $f(Z_1 \mid Z_2; \eta)$ with η finite dimensional with true value η_0; model (2) assumes Z_1 and Z_2 are independent; model (3) places no restrictions on the law of Z_1 given Z_2 and thus is completely nonparametric; model (0) assumes $f(Z_1 \mid Z_2)$ is completely known.

Note that in a completely randomized trial in which R was assigned at random, we would expect that all four models could be correctly specified by the data analyst, since $f(R|L_0^*)$ is a known function of R alone. However, in an observational study, we might wish to only entertain the completely nonparametric model (3) if we were uncertain about how R was assigned. [In order to allow our results to applied observational studies, we shall no longer assume that R is necessarily discrete or that (A1.1) necessarily holds.]

We shall need the following notation. Letting j, $j = (0, 1, 2, 3)$, index the model and given any function $g(Z_1, Z_2)$, define $\tilde{E}^{(j)}[g(Z_1, Z_2)|Z_2] = \int g(z_1, Z_2)\tilde{f}^{(j)}(z_1|Z_2)dz_1$ where $\tilde{f}^{(j)}(Z_1|Z_2)$ (i) is $f(Z_1|Z_2; \hat{\eta})$ with $\hat{\eta}$ the MLE of η_0 under model (1), (ii) places mass $1/n$ at each of the n observed values of Z_1 under model (2), so $\tilde{E}^{(j)}[g(Z_1, Z_2)|Z_2] = n^{-1} \sum_{i=1}^{n} g(Z_{1i}, Z_2)$, (iii) is a completely nonparametric estimate, e. g., a multivariate kernel estimate, of $f(Z_1|Z_2)$, under model (3), and (iv) is $f(Z_1|Z_2)$ under model (0) so $\tilde{E}^{(0)}$ is a true expectation. We now have

Theorem A4.1. Under the semiparametric model (aj) for ψ_0, for each choice of functions $\theta = \theta(u, l_0^*)$, $b = b(u, r, l_0^*)$, $b^* = b^*(u, r, l_0^*)$, and each collection of sets, $\mathbf{K}(R, L_0^*)$ indexed by R, L_0^* of $[\bar{l}(C), \bar{a}(C)]$ histories satisfying

$$1 = \text{pr}\{[\bar{L}(C), \bar{A}(C)] \in \mathbf{K}(R, L_0^*)| R, L_0^*, T > C\} \qquad \text{(A4.3)}$$

subject to regularity conditions, there will exist an asymptotically normal and unbiased estimator $\tilde{\psi}^{(j)} = \tilde{\psi}^{(j)}(b, \theta, b^*, \mathbf{K})$ of ψ_0 solving $n^{1/2}\tilde{E}[\tilde{D}^{(j)}(\psi)] = o_p(1)$, where

$$\tilde{E}(Z) \equiv n^{-1} \sum_{i=1}^{n} Z_i, \; \tilde{D}^{(j)}(\psi) = \tilde{D}^{(j)}(\psi, b, \theta, b^*, \mathbf{K})$$

$$= \int_0^{\infty} \{dN_{H(\psi)}(u) - \theta(u, L_0^*)I[\nu(\psi) > u]du\}B^*(u)\{B(u)$$

$$- \tilde{\mathcal{L}}^{(j)}(u, \psi, b, b^* \mid L_0^*)\},$$

$$N_{H(\psi)}(u) = I[H(\psi) \leq u, \Delta(\psi) = 1], \; \Delta(\psi) = I[H(\psi) \leq \mu(\psi)],$$

$$\mu(\psi) = \mu(\psi, R, L_0^*, \mathbf{K}) = \inf\{h[C, \bar{l}(C), \bar{a}(C); \psi];$$

$$[\bar{l}(C), \bar{a}(C)] \in \mathbf{K}(R, L_0^*)\},$$

$$\nu(\psi) = \nu(\psi, R, L_0^*, \mathbf{K}) = \min\{\mu(\psi), H(\psi)\}, B(u) = b(u, R, L_0^*),$$

$$B^*(u) = b^*(u, R, L_0^*), \tilde{\mathcal{L}}^{(j)}(u, \psi, b, b^*| L_0^*)$$

$$= \tilde{E}^{(j)}\{B(u)B^*(u)I[\mu(\psi) > u]| L_0^*\}/\tilde{E}^{(j)}\{B^*(u)I[\mu(\psi) > u]| L_0^*\}$$

Further,

$$n^{1/2}(\tilde{\psi}^{(j)} - \psi_0) = n^{1/2}\tilde{E}[\kappa^{-1}U_{\mathrm{f}}^{(j)}] + o_{\mathrm{p}}(1) \qquad (A4.4)$$

$U_{\mathrm{f}}^{(j)} \equiv D - D_{\mathrm{adj}}^{(j)}$, $D \equiv \tilde{D}^{(0)}(\psi_0)$, $D_{\mathrm{adj}}^{(0)} \equiv 0$, $D_{\mathrm{adj}}^{(1)} \equiv \mathrm{ls}(D, S_\eta)$, $\mathrm{ls}(A, B) \equiv E[AB']\{E[BB']\}^{-1}B$, $S_\eta \equiv \partial \ln f(R|L_0^*; \eta_0)/\partial \eta$; $D_{\mathrm{adj}}^{(2)} \equiv E[D|R]$; $D_{\mathrm{adj}}^{(3)} \equiv E[D|R, L_0^*]$, and $\kappa \equiv -\partial E[D^{(0)}(\psi_0)]/\partial \psi' = E[DS_\psi^{\mathrm{cen}'}]$, $S_\psi^{\mathrm{cen}} = E[S_\psi | V]$, V is given by (A4.1), and S_ψ is the score for ψ in a model characterized by the sole restriction (A1.10) in the absence of censoring [i. e., based on data (A4.2)]. [S_ψ is the derivative of the logarithm of (A1.12) w.r.t. ψ_0.] In addition, $\mathrm{Var}^{\mathrm{A}}[n^{1/2}(\tilde{\psi}^{(j)} - \psi_0)] = \kappa^{-1}\,\mathrm{Var}[U_{\mathrm{f}}^{(j)}](\kappa^{-1})'$.

Sketch of Proof. One can calculate that (A1.10) implies $E[D] = 0$. Next one shows that $n^{1/2}\tilde{E}[\tilde{D}^{(j)}(\psi_0)] = n^{1/2}\tilde{E}[U_{\mathrm{f}}^{(j)}] + o_{\mathrm{p}}(1)$ by arguments similar to those in the proof of Theorem A.2 in Appendix 3 of Robins and Rotnitzky (1992) and/or by using Theorem 4.3 in Newey (1990). Under regularity conditions, $\tilde{\psi}^{(j)}$ will be regular so that $\kappa = [U_{\mathrm{f}}^{(j)}S_\psi^{\mathrm{cen}'}]$ by Theorem 2.2 of Newey (1990). That $\kappa = E[DS_\psi^{\mathrm{cen}'}]$ follows from $E[D_{\mathrm{adj}}^{(j)}S_\psi^{\mathrm{cen}'}] = 0$ since $D_{\mathrm{adj}}^{(j)}$ is a function of (R, L_0^*) and $E[S_\psi^{\mathrm{cen}}|R, L_0^*] = 0$ by ancillarity of R, L_0^* for ψ.

Remark A4.1. The use of b^* in $\tilde{\mathcal{L}}^{(j)}$ is nonstandard. Its usefulness will become clear later.

Optimal Estimation

Let $\mathbf{K}_{\mathrm{op}} = \mathbf{K}_{\mathrm{op}}(R, L_0^*)$ be the smallest set satisfying (A4.3) with associated $\mu_{\mathrm{op}}(\psi)$, $\nu_{\mathrm{op}}(\psi)$, $\Delta_{\mathrm{op}}(\psi)$. Let $b_{\mathrm{op}}^*(u, R, L_0^*)$ be the constant 1. $\theta_{\mathrm{op}}(u, L_0^*) \equiv \lambda_{\mathrm{H}}(u|L_0^*)$, $b_{\mathrm{op}}(u, R, L_0^*) \equiv q_{\mathrm{op}}(u, R, L_0^*) - E[q_{\mathrm{op}}(H, R, L_0^*)|H > u, R, L_0^*]$ where $q_{\mathrm{op}}(u, R, L_0^*) = E[S_\psi | H = u, R, L_0^*]$.

Remark A4.2. $D_{\mathrm{adj}}^{(j)} = 0$ if $\theta = \theta_{\mathrm{op}}$.

Define $\tilde{D}_{\mathrm{op}}^{(j)}(\psi) = \tilde{D}^{(j)}(\psi, b_{\mathrm{op}}, \theta_{\mathrm{op}}, b_{\mathrm{op}}^*, \mathbf{K}_{\mathrm{op}})$ and let $\tilde{\psi}_{\mathrm{op}}^{(j)}$ solve $n^{1/2}\tilde{E}[\tilde{D}_{\mathrm{op}}^{(j)}(\psi)] = o_{\mathrm{p}}(1)$. Set $D_{\mathrm{op}} = \tilde{D}_{\mathrm{op}}^{(0)}(\psi_0)$. Then we have

Theorem A4.2. (a) $\mathrm{Var}^{\mathrm{A}}[n^{1/2}(\tilde{\psi}_{\mathrm{op}}^{(j)} - \psi_0)] = \{E[D_{\mathrm{op}}D_{\mathrm{op}}']\}^{-1}$ does not depend on j and is less than or equal to $\mathrm{Var}^{\mathrm{A}}[n^{1/2}(\tilde{\psi}^{(j)}) - \psi_0]$. Furthermore, $D_{\mathrm{op,adj}}^{(j)} = 0$ for all j and $\kappa(b, \theta, b^*, \mathbf{K}) = E[D(b, \theta, b^*, \mathbf{K})D_{\mathrm{op}}']$. (b) D_{op} is the efficient score for ψ_0 in all four models (aj) and $E[D_{\mathrm{op}}D_{\mathrm{op}}']$ is the semiparametric information bound (SIB), if

$$\text{pr}[\gamma = \mu_{\text{op}}|R, L_0^*, H, H > \mu_{\text{op}}] > c > 0 \qquad (A4.5)$$

for some constant c w.p.1, where $\gamma \equiv h(C, \bar{L}(C), \bar{A}(C), \psi_0)$ if $\Delta^* = 0$ and $\gamma \equiv \infty$ if $\Delta^* = 1$. [Here and throughout we use the convention that we drop the ψ argument for functions evaluated at ψ_0, e. g., we write $\mu(\psi_0)$ as μ.]

Definition. We say that $h(t, \bar{l}(t), \bar{a}(t), \psi)$ is standard if it does not depend on any posttreatment variable $l^*(t), t > 0$.

Definition. We shall say there is complete compliance if for $u < T$, $\bar{A}(u)$ is a deterministic function of R and L_0^*. We then have the following obvious corollary.

Corollary A4.1. If $h(t, \bar{l}(t), \bar{a}(t), \psi)$ is standard and there is complete compliance, then (A4.5) holds and D_{op} is the efficient score under each model (aj). [We do not know as yet the form of the efficient score when (A4.5) is false.] (A4.5) may be true even if the supposition of the corollary is false, especially if $[\bar{L}(C), \bar{A}(C)]$ is, for fixed C, a discrete random variable w.p.1.

Remark A4.3. If L_0^* consists only of C, model (a3) is called the (nonlinear) limited information model with known potential censoring time (Newey, 1990). Typically, one would obtain the limited information model by taking the pretreatment variables L_0^{**} other than C that are initially included in L_0^* and incorporating them in A_0 (i. e., in "exposure" at time zero), so that the residual $h(T, \bar{L}(T), \bar{A}(T), \psi) = H(\psi)$ would now also model the variation in failure times as a function of the pretreatment covariates L_0^{**}. For example, if L_0^{**} consisted (only) of "age" at entry, we might add a term $\psi_{0,4}$ "age" to the right-hand side of (A1.9) in defining $h(t, \bar{l}(t), \bar{a}(t), \psi)$ and "age" would no longer need be included in L_0^*.

Sketch of Proof of Theorem A4.2a

We note that for fixed θ, b, b^*, $\mathbf{K}(R, L_0^*)$, the asymptotic variance of $\tilde{\psi}^{(3)}$ is less than or equal to that of any other $\tilde{\psi}^{(j)}$ since $\text{Var}[U_f^{(3)}] = \text{Var}\{D - E[D|L_0^*, R]\} \leq \text{Var}\{D - g(L_0^*, R)\}$ for any $g(\cdot, \cdot)$. Next, as in Lemma (3.4) of Robins and Rotnitzky (1992), one can use integration by parts to show that $U_f^{(3)} = \int_0^\infty dM_H(u)\{G(u) - E[G(u)|\nu > u, L_0^*]\}$ for some $G(u) = g(u, R, L_0^*)$ depending on b, b^*, θ where $M_H(u) = N_H(u) - \int_0^u \lambda_H[x|L_0^*]I[\nu > x]dx$ is a martingale adapted to the filtration $\mathbf{F}(u,$

$L_0^*) = \sigma[L_0^*, R, \{N_H(x), I(\nu \geq x); x \leq u\}]$.

Let $M_{H,op}(u)$, $F_{op}(u, L_0^*)$, $N_{H,op}(u)$ be based on $\mathbf{K}_{op}$ and ν_{op}. Then $U_f^{(3)} = \int_0^\infty dM_{H,op}(u)I(\nu > u)\{G(u) - E[G(u)|\nu > u, L_0^*]\}$. $U_f^{(3)}$ is thus also a martingale adapted to $F_{op}(u, L_0^*)$ since $I(\nu > u)$ is $F_{op}(u, L_0^*)$-predictable. In the next paragraph, we use this latter representation of $U_f^{(3)}$ to show that $\kappa = E[U_f^{(3)}D_{op}']$. Therefore, $\text{Var}^A[n^{1/2}(\check\psi^{(3)} - \psi_0)]$ $= [E\{U_f^{(3)}D_{op}'\}]^{-1}\text{Var}[U_f^{(3)}]\{E[D_{op}U_f^{(3)\prime}]\}^{-1}$ which, by Cauchy-Schwartz, is minimized at $U_f^{(3)} = D_{op}$, proving Theorem A4.2a.

To show $\kappa = E[U_f^{(3)}D_{op}']$, note that, with $\Delta_{op} = I[H < \mu_{op}]$, κ $= E[U_f^{(3)}S_\psi^{cen\prime}] = E\{U_f^{(3)}E[S_\psi^{cen\prime}|\nu_{op}, \Delta_{op}, R, L_0^*]\} = E[U_f^{(3)}\{D_{op}'$ $+ \int_0^\infty dM_{H,op}(u)E[B_{op}'(u)|\nu_{op} > u, L_0^*]\}] = E[U_f^{(3)}D_{op}']$ since, by standard martingale arguments, for any $h(u, L_0^*)$, $E[U_f^{(3)}\{\int_0^\infty dM_{H,op}(u)h(u, L_0^*)\}]$ $= E[\int_0^\infty h(u, L_0^*)\lambda_H(u|L_0^*)E[I(\nu_{op} > u)I(\nu > u)\{G(u) - E[G(u)|\nu > u, L_0^*]\}|L_0^*]] = 0$ [because $I(\nu_{op} > u)I(\nu > u) = I(\nu > u)$].

Sketch of Proof of Theorem A4.2b

First consider model ($a0$). By standard arguments for missing data problems as in Bickel *et al.* (1993), Newey (1990), or Robins and Rotnitzky (1992), the nuisance tangent space under model ($a0$) is $\Lambda = $ closure $\{P$ $= \Delta^*(P^{(1)} + P^{(2)}) + (1 - \Delta^*)E[P^{(1)} + P^{(2)}|J(\gamma), H > \gamma]; |\text{Var}(P^{(1)})|$ $< \infty, P^{(1)} = p^{(1)}(H, L_0^*) \in R^v; E[P^{(1)}|L_0^*] = 0, P^{(2)} = P^{(2)}(J(H), H, L_0)$ $\in R^v, E[P^{(2)}|H, L_0] = 0, |\text{Var}(P^{(2)})| < \infty\}$ where the closure is taken with respect to the Hilbert space of random variables with finite variance with the inner product of A and B given by $E(AB)$. Here $L_0 = (R, L_0^*)$ and $J(u) = [\bar L\{\rho(u, \bar L_{int(T)}, \bar A_{int(T)}, \psi_0)\}, \bar A\{\rho(u, \bar L_{int(T)}, \bar A_{int(T)}, \psi_0)\}]$ (with ρ as defined in Appendix 1) is covariate and treatment history up to u on the ψ_0-residual time scale. Let $\Lambda^\perp$ be the orthogonal complement of Λ.

We now show that, given any random variable $G^* = g^*(V) \equiv I(H \leq \gamma)g_1^*\{H, J(H)\} + I(H > \gamma)g_2^*[\gamma, J(\gamma)]$, when (A4.5) is true,

$$\amalg[g^*(V)|\Lambda^\perp] = d(G^*)$$

$$\equiv \int_{-\infty}^\infty dM_{H,op}(u)\{B(u) - E[B(u)|\nu_{op} > u, L_0^*]\}$$

$$\text{(A4.5a)}$$

where $\amalg$ is the Hilbert space projection operator, $B(u) = q(u, R, L_0^*) - E[q(H, R, L_0^*)|H > u, R, L_0^*]$, $q(u, R, L_0^*) = E[G|H = u, R, L_0^*]$, $G = g[H, J(H)]$, and $g[u, J(u)] \equiv I(u < \gamma)g_1^*[u, J(u)] + I(u \geq \gamma)[g_2^*(\gamma, J(\gamma))]$. If $g^*(V) = E(S_\psi|V) \equiv S_\psi^{cen}$, one can calculate $d(G^*)$ $= D_{op}$ and $B(u)$ is $B_{op}(u)$.

It is not difficult to show $d(G^*)$ is in $\Lambda^\perp$. So to prove (A4.5a), it remains to show that $G^* - d(G^*) \in \Lambda$. Now let $h(u, L_0^*) = E[B(u)|\nu_{op} > u, L_0^*]$. Define $\mathring{P}^{(1)} = h(H, L_0^*) - \int_0^H \lambda_H(u|L_0^*)h(u, L_0^*)du$. Define $\mathring{P}^{(2)} = I(H < \mu_{op})\{G - E(G|H, R, L_0^*)\} + I(H > \mu_{op})I(\gamma \neq \mu_{op})\{G - E[G|H > \mu_{op}, L_0] + E[\mathring{P}^{(1)}|H > \mu_{op}, L_0^*] - \mathring{P}^{(1)}\} + I(H > \mu_{op})I(\gamma = \mu_{op})\{-E[\mathring{P}^{(2)}|H, L_0, \gamma \neq \mu_{op}]\text{pr}[\gamma \neq \mu_{op}|H, L_0]/\text{pr}[\gamma = \mu_{op}|H, L_0]\}$. $E[\mathring{P}^{(1)}|L_0^*] = 0$ by results in Ritov and Wellner (1988). By construction, $E[\mathring{P}^{(2)}|H, L_0] = 0$. $\mathring{P}^{(2)}$ has finite variance since (A4.5) is true. Some tedious calculation then shows that $\mathring{P} = \Delta^*(\mathring{P}^{(1)} + \mathring{P}^{(2)}) + (1 - \Delta^*)E[\mathring{P}^{(1)} + \mathring{P}^{(2)}|J(\gamma), H > \gamma]$ equals $G^* - d(G^*)$.

The efficient score under any of the models $(a1)-(a3)$ is the same as that under model $(a0)$ since the nuisance tangent space under any of $(a1)-(a3)$ simply adds to Λ functions of (R, L_0^*) and the score w.r.t. ψ remains S_ψ^{cen}. But $E[S_\psi^{cen}|R, L_0^*] = 0$, so the projection of S_ψ^{cen} on the nuisance tangent space remains D_{op} when (A4.5) is true.

M-Estimator Representation

We now provide conditions under which the "martingale-like" score function $\tilde{D}^{(j)}$ can be represented as an "M-estimator like" score function.

Define $\mu^{min}(\psi) = \mu^{min}(\psi, L_0^*, \mathbf{K}) = \inf_R \{\mu(\psi, R, L_0^*, \mathbf{K})\}$; $\nu^{min}(\psi) = \min(H(\psi), \mu^{min}(\psi))$; and $\Delta^{min}(\psi) = I[H(\psi) < \mu^{min}(\psi)]$. Let $q[R, \nu^{min}(\psi), \Delta^{min}(\psi), L_0^*] \equiv Q(\psi) = \int_0^\infty I[\mu^{min} > u]\{dN_{H(\psi)}(u) - \theta(u, l_0^*)I[\nu(\psi) > u]du\}B^*(u)B(u)$.

Corollary A4.2. If $b^*(u, R, L_0^*)$ does not depend on R, and (a) $\mu(\psi, R, L_0^*, \mathbf{K})$ does not depend on R, (b) R is dichotomous, or (c) for each C, $[\bar{A}(C), \bar{L}(C)]$ takes on at most two values w.p.1, then, under model (aj), $\tilde{D}^{(j)}(\psi) = Q(\psi) - \int q(r, \nu^{min}(\psi), \Delta^{min}(\psi), L_0^*)\tilde{f}^{(j)}(r|L_0^*)dr$, and $D = Q - E[Q|L_0^*, \nu^{min}, \Delta^{min}]$, $U_f^{(2)} = D - E[Q|R] + E(Q)$; $U_f^{(3)} = D - E[Q|L_0^*, R] + E(Q|L_0^*)$.

Corollary A4.3. If (a) μ_{op} does not depend on R, (b) R is dichotomous, or (c) for each $C, [\bar{A}(C), \bar{L}(C)]$ is dichotomous w.p.1, then D_{op} under model $(aj), j = (0, 1, 2, 3)$, is $Q_{op} - E[Q_{op}|L_0^*, \nu_{op}^{min}, \Delta_{op}^{min}]$ where $Q_{op} = E[S_\psi|R, L_0^*, \nu_{op}^{min}, \Delta_{op}^{min}]$.

Proofs. Under supposition (a), the corollaries are a consequence of the identity

$$\tilde{\mathcal{L}}^{(j)}(u, \psi, b, b^*|L_0^*) = \tilde{E}^{(j)}[B(u)|L_0^*] \qquad (A4.6)$$

for all u. Under supposition (b) or (c) for times u, $u > \mu^{\min}(\psi)$, $B(u)$ $= \hat{\mathcal{L}}^{(j)}(u, \psi, b, b^* \mid L_0^*)$. Further, for times $u < \mu^{\min}(\psi)$, (A4.6) holds [since then $I[\mu(\psi) > u] = 1$ w.p.l].

Remark A4.4. If $\psi_0 = 0$, then $\mu_{\mathrm{op}} = C$ and thus does not depend on R. For $\psi_0 \neq 0$, μ_{op} may or may not depend on R.

Rank Estimators

Now suppose $L_0^* = C = c_{\max}$ is a fixed nonrandom constant so that there is no staggered entry. Then models $(a0)$–$(a3)$ are the same model (a). We can then estimate ψ_0 under model (a) using a generalized weighted rank estimator $\tilde{\psi}^{(r)}$ with the superscript "(r)" signifying "rank." Specifically, define $\tilde{D}^{(r)}(\psi) = \tilde{D}^{(r)}(\psi, b, b^*, \mathbf{K}) = \int_0^\infty dN_{H(\psi)}(u)B^*(u)[B(u) - \hat{\mathcal{L}}^{(r)}(u, \psi, b, b^*)]$ where $\hat{\mathcal{L}}^{(r)}(u, \psi, b, b^*) = \tilde{E}\{B(u)B^*(u)I[\nu(\psi) > u]\}/\tilde{E}\{B^*(u) I[\nu(\psi) > u]\}$. We have the important identity $\tilde{E}[\tilde{D}^{(r)}(\psi)] = \tilde{E}[\tilde{U}_f^{(r)}(\psi)]$, where $\tilde{U}_f^{(r)}(\psi) = \int_0^\infty \{dN_{H(\psi)}(u) - \lambda_{H(\psi)}[u]I[\nu(\psi) > u]du\}B^*(u)[B(u) - \hat{\mathcal{L}}^{(r)}(u, \psi, b, b^*)]$. We can then prove:

Lemma A4.1. If $L_0^* = C = c_{\max}$, then under model (a), subject to regularity conditions, $n^{1/2}\tilde{E}[\tilde{U}_f^{(r)}(\psi_0)] = n^{1/2}\tilde{E}[U_f^{(r)}] + o_p(1)$ where $U_f^{(r)} = U_f^{(r)}(\psi_0)$ replaces $\tilde{E}$ by the true expectation E in the definition of $\tilde{U}_f^{(r)}(\psi_0)$. Also $U_f^{(r)}$ $= D(b, \theta_{\mathrm{op}}, b^*, \mathbf{K})$. Further, there exists a solution $\tilde{\psi}^{(r)}$ to $n^{1/2}\tilde{E}[\tilde{D}^{(r)}(\psi)]$ $= o_p(1)$ such that $n^{1/2}(\tilde{\psi}^{(r)} - \psi_0) = n^{1/2}\tilde{E}[\{\kappa^{(r)}\}^{-1}U_f^{(r)}] + o_p(1)$ where $\kappa^{(r)}$ $= \kappa(b, \theta_{\mathrm{op}}, b^*, \mathbf{K})$ so that $\tilde{\psi}^{(r)}(b_{\mathrm{op}}, b_{\mathrm{op}}^*, \mathbf{K}_{\mathrm{op}})$ will be asymptotically equivalent to $\tilde{\psi}_{\mathrm{op}}^{(j)}$. The estimator $\tilde{\psi}^{(r)}$ was originally proposed by Fu-Chang Hu.

A consistent estimator of $\mathrm{Var}[U_f^{(r)}]$ is $\hat{\mathrm{Var}}\{U_f^{(r)}(\psi)\} \equiv \tilde{E}[\tilde{\Omega}(\psi)]$, with $\tilde{\Omega}(\psi) = \int_0^\infty dN_{H(\psi)}(u)B^*(u)[B(u) - \hat{\mathcal{L}}^{(r)}(u, \psi, b, b^*)]\{B^*(u)[B(u) - \hat{\mathcal{L}}^{(r)}(u, \psi, b, b^*)]\}'$ evaluated at $\tilde{\psi}^{(r)}$. $\kappa^{(r)}$ is estimated by taking numerical derivatives of $\tilde{E}[\tilde{D}^{(r)}(\psi)]$ with step size $O(n^{-1/2})$.

Proof of Lemma A4.1. Since $\tilde{E}[\tilde{U}_f^{(r)}(\psi_0)]$ is a martingale adapted to the filtration that records the information in each of the n-subject-specific filtrations $\mathbf{F}(u, L_0^*)$, Lemma A4.1 follows immediately from results in Tsiatis (1990) and Robins and Tsiatis (1991).

Standard Independent Censoring

In analyzing censored survival data, it is commonly assumed (but not often checked) that

$$C \amalg H(\psi_0) \mid R, L_0^{**} \qquad\qquad (A4.7a)$$

That is, censoring is independent of baseline failure time $H(\psi_0)$ given treatment arm R and other pretreatment variables L_0^{**}. Now given (A1.10), (A4.7a) is implied by

$$C \amalg H(\psi_0) \mid L_0^{**} \qquad\qquad (A4.7b)$$

Hence, let semiparametric models $(bj), j = (0, 1, 2, 3)$, be characterized by (A4.7b), the data (A4.1), restriction (A1.10), and a model j for $f(Z_1 \mid Z_2)$ with $Z_1 = (R, C)$, $Z_2 = L_0^{**}$ [where $L_0^* \equiv (C, L_0^{**})$]. We then have

Theorem A4.3. Under semiparametric model (bj), subject to regularity conditions, there will exist a solution $\tilde{\psi}^{(bj)}$ to $n^{1/2} \tilde{E}[\tilde{D}^{(bj)}(\psi)] = o_p(1)$ such that $n^{1/2}(\tilde{\psi}^{(bj)} - \psi_0) = n^{1/2} \tilde{E}[\{\kappa^{(b)}\}^{-1} U_f^{(bj)}] + o_p(1)$ where $\tilde{D}^{(bj)}(\psi)$, $D^{(b)}$, $\kappa^{(b)}$ are defined just like their counterparts above except $\tilde{\mathcal{L}}^{(j)}(u, \psi, b, b^* \mid L_0^{**})$ replaces $\tilde{\mathcal{L}}^{(j)}(u, \psi, b, b^* \mid L_0^*)$, and $\tilde{E}^{(j)}$ used in defining $\tilde{\mathcal{L}}^{(j)}(u, \psi, b, b^* \mid L_0^{**})$ is based on $Z_1 = (R, C)$ and $Z_2 = L_0^{**}$. Further, $U_f^{(bj)} = D^{(b)} - D_{adj}^{(bj)}$ with $D_{adj}^{(b0)} = 0$, $D_{adj}^{(b1)} = \mathbf{ls}(D^{(b)}, S_\eta^{(b)})$, $S_\eta^{(b)} = \partial \ln f(R, C \mid L_0^{**}, \eta_0)/\partial \eta$, $D_{adj}^{(b2)} = E[D^{(b)} \mid R, C]$, $D_{adj}^{(b3)} = E[D^{(b)} \mid R, L_0^*]$.
Set $D_{op}^{(b)} = \tilde{D}_{op}^{(b0)}(\psi_0)$, $\tilde{D}_{op}^{(b)}(\psi) = \tilde{D}^{(bj)}(\psi, b_{op}, \theta_{op}, b_{op}^*, \mathbf{K}_{op})$. Then we have

Theorem A4.4. $\mathrm{Var}^A[n^{1/2}(\tilde{\psi}_{op}^{(bj)} - \psi_0)] = \{E[D_{op}^{(b)} D_{op}^{(b)\prime}]\}^{-1}$ does not depend on j and is less than or equal to $\mathrm{Var}^A[n^{1/2}(\tilde{\psi}^{(bj)} - \psi_0)]$. Further, $D_{op}^{(b)}$ is the efficient score for ψ_0 in all four models (bj) if (A4.5) holds.

The proofs of Theorems A4.3 and A4.4 are similar to their counterparts for models (aj) and will not be given except to note that $h(u, L_0^*)$ in the proof of Theorem A4.2b is now replaced by $h(u, L_0^{**}) \equiv E[B(u) \mid \nu_{op} > u, L_0^{**}]$, since $P^{(1)}$ will now represent functions of (H, L_0^{**}) with mean 0 given L_0^{**}.

It is of interest to determine the conditions under which prior knowledge that (A4.7) is true provides additional information about ψ_0 in the sense that $\mathrm{Var}[D_{op}^{(b)}] > \mathrm{Var}[D_{op}^{(a)}]$ where we have added the superscript "(a)" to previously defined quantities related to model (a).

To do so, note $D_{op}^{(a)}$ and $D_{op}^{(b)}$ can be written $D_{op}^{(a)} = \int_0^\infty dM_{H,op}(u)\{B_{op}(u) - E[B_{op}(u) \mid \mu_{op} > u, C, L_0^{**}]\}$ and $D_{op}^{(b)} = \int_0^\infty dM_{H,op}(u)\{B_{op}(u) - E[B_{op}(u) \mid \mu_{op} > u, L_0^{**}]\}$ which are martingales adapted to $\mathbf{F}_{op}(u, L_0^*)$ under model $(b3)$.

It follows that $\mathrm{Var}[D_{op}^{(a)}] = \mathrm{Var}[D_{op}^{(b)}]$ if and only if $E[B_{op}(u) \mid \mu_{op} > u, C, L_0^{**}]$ does not depend on C. Given (A4.7b) is true, sufficient and essentially necessary (joint) conditions for this are

i. $\mu_{op}(\psi_0, R, C, L_0^{**})$ does not depend on R,
ii. $b_{op}(u, R, C, L_0^{**})$ does not depend on C, and
iii. $R \amalg C | L_0^{**}$

As discussed above, (i) will always be true at $\psi_0 = 0$ and sometimes at all values of ψ_0 [note that (i) cannot be replaced by the condition that R is dichotomous]. (iii) will be true in a completely randomized trial since (C, L_0^{**}) are pretreatment variables. With $\bar{L}^{**}(t)$ defined to be $\bar{L}(t)$ less C, (ii) will be true if either

iv.a $h(t, \bar{l}(t), \bar{a}(t), \psi)$ does not depend on C and

$$(\bar{L}^{**}(T), \bar{A}(T)) \amalg C | R, H(\psi_0), L_0^{**} \qquad (A4.8a)$$

or

iv.b our SNFTM is fully "standard" and

$$\bar{A}(T) \amalg C | R, H(\psi_0), L_0^{**} \qquad (A4.8b)$$

where we say that our SNFTM is fully standard if $h(t, \bar{l}(t), \bar{a}(t), \psi)$ does not depend on C or on any posttreatment variables $l^*(t)$, $t > 0$. Note complete compliance implies (A4.8b). However, (iv.b) implies that (i) is false if $\psi_0 \neq 0$.

To see why (iv.a) and (iv.b) imply (ii), note (iv.a) and/or (iv.b) guarantee first S_ψ is not a function of C and second that $E[S_\psi | H(\psi_0) = u, L_0^{**}, R, C] \equiv q_{op}(u, R, L_0^{**})$ does not depend on C. Finally, (A4.7a) implies that $E[q_{op}(H, R, L_0^{**}) | H > u, R, L_0^{**}, C]$ and thus, by definition, $b_{op}(u, R, L_0^*)$ does not depend on C.

Remark A4.5. If $L_0^* = C$, then, under model (b), we can estimate ψ_0 using the generalized rank estimator $\tilde{\psi}^{(r)}$ defined in Lemma A4.1 even if C is random. This follows from

Lemma A4.2. If $L_0^* = C$, then, under model (b), and subject to regularity conditions, $n^{1/2}(\tilde{\psi}^{(r)} - \psi_0) = n^{1/2}\tilde{E}[\{\kappa^{(r)}\}^{-1}U_f^{(r)}]$ where, now, $\kappa^{(r)} = \kappa^{(b)}(b, \theta_{op}, b^*, \mathbf{K})$, $U_f^{(r)} = D^{(b)}(b, \theta_{op}, b^*, \mathbf{K})$. In particular, $\tilde{\psi}^{(r)}(b_{op}, b_{op}^*, \mathbf{K})$ is optimal.

Note to compute $\tilde{\psi}^{(r)}$, we, in general, require data on C even for subjects who failed prior to C, since, even if $T < C$, $\Delta(\psi)$ may equal 0 if $\psi \neq 0$. Thus, data on C are necessary to compute $\Delta(\psi)$. However, data on C for subjects with $T < C$ are not necessary for (a) testing the null hypothesis $\psi_0 = 0$ or (b) for calculating $\tilde{\psi}^{(r)}$ if our SNFTM is fully standard and there is complete compliance since, then, $T < C \Leftrightarrow \Delta(\psi) = 1$.

Comparisons with the Robins–Tsiatis (1991) Rank Estimators

Since (A4.7b) would not be expected to hold if there were secular changes in baseline risk over time, yet R will be independent of C in a randomized trial, it is of interest to determine whether one can construct generalized rank estimators for ψ_0 that are guaranteed to be asymptotically normal and unbiased under model $(a2)$ when $L_0^* = C$. Robins and Tsiatis (1991) show this is possible and propose a specific class of rank estimators $\tilde{\psi}^{RT}$ with influence functions $E[D^{RT} S_\psi^{cen'}]^{-1} D^{RT}$. $D^{RT} \equiv D^{RT}(g^{(0)}, g^{(1)}, \mathbf{K})$ [depending on functions $g^{(k)}(u, R)$, $k = 0, 1$, chosen by the data analyst] is $\sum_{k=0}^{1} \int_0^\infty dM_{\nu\min}^{(k)}(u)\{g^{(k)}(u, R) - E[g^{(k)}(u, R)]\}$ where $M_{\nu\min}^{(k)}(u) = N_{\nu\min}^{(k)}(u) - \int_0^u \lambda_{\nu\min}^{(k)}(x)I[\nu^{\min} > x]dx$, $N_{\nu\min}^{(k)}(u) = I[\nu^{\min} \leq u, \Delta^{\min} = k]$ and $\lambda_{\nu\min}^{(k)}(u)I[\nu^{\min} > u]$ is the intensity process (i. e., cause-specific hazard) corresponding to $N_{\nu\min}^{(k)}(u)$ w.r.t. the filtration $\mathbf{F}(u) = \sigma[R, \{N_{\nu\min}^{(k)}(x), I[\nu^{\min} \geq x]; x \leq u\}]$. [Note C is not included in the filtration $\mathbf{F}(u)$.]

Sufficient conditions for the asymptotic variance of $\tilde{\psi}^{RT}$ to equal $\{\mathrm{Var}[D_{op}^{(a)}]\}^{-1}$ are that (1) $\mathbf{K} = \mathbf{K}_{op}$ so $\nu^{\min} = \nu_{op}^{\min}$; (2) (A4.7) holds so $\lambda_{\nu\min}^{(1)}(u) = \lambda_H(u)$; (3) $b_{op}(u, R, C)$ does not depend on C; (4) supposition (a), (b), or (c) of Corollary A4.3 holds; and (5) $g^{(1)}(u, R) = b_{op}(u, R)$ and $g^{(0)}(u, R) = 0$. When (1)–(5) hold, $D^{RT} = D_{op}^{(a)}$. We believe but have not proved that unless (1)–(5) hold, $\tilde{\psi}_{op}^{(aj)}$ will have strictly smaller variance than $\tilde{\psi}^{RT}$.

Remark A4.6. If $\mu(\psi, R, C)$ does not depend on R, $\tilde{\psi}^{(r)}(b, b^*, \mathbf{K})$ equals $\tilde{\psi}^{RT}(g^{(0)}, g^{(1)}, \mathbf{K})$ if (i) the function b^* is the constant 1, (ii) $b(u, r, c) = g^{(1)}(u, r)$, and (iii) $g^{(0)}(u, r) = 0$. In fact, under model $(a2)$, $\tilde{\psi}^{(r)}(b, b^*, \mathbf{K})$ will be asymptotically normal and unbiased for ψ_0 even if (A4.7b) is false and $L_0^* = C$ is nonconstant, provided $\mu(\psi, R, C)$ does not depend on R and the functions b^* and b do not depend on C.

A.4.2. Adjustment for Censoring by Competing Risks

Let Q represent time to a censoring (or competing risk) event other than C. For example, Q might be time to initiation of prophylaxis, and $A(u)$ might be actual AZT treatment and $L(u)$ does not contain $I(Q = u)$. Let T^* be the possibly counterfactual variable recording time to failure in the absence of censoring by Q (i. e., if prophylaxis were never initiated), so $T^* = T$ if $T < Q$. Redefine $H(\psi) = h(T^*, \bar{L}(T^*), \bar{A}(T^*), \psi)$. For notational convenience write $[\bar{L}(u), \bar{A}(u)]$ as $\overline{LA}(u)$.

If we discard data on $L(u), A(u)$, and T subsequent to Q, the observable data are now

$$\{ C_i, X_i = \min(Q_i, T_i, C), \overline{LA}(X_i), \tau_i$$

$$= I[X_i \neq Q_i], \Delta_i^* \tau_i \}, i = 1, \ldots, n \quad (A4.9)$$

We shall assume the cause-specific hazard for censoring satisfies

$$\lambda_Q(u \mid \overline{LA}(u), H(\psi_0)) = \lambda_Q(u \mid \overline{LA}(u)) \quad (A4.10)$$

where $\lambda_Q(u \mid \cdot) = \lim_{h \to 0} h^{-1} \operatorname{pr}[u \leq X < u + h, \tau = 0 \mid X \geq u, \cdot]$. Define $K(t) \equiv \exp\{-\int_0^t \lambda_Q[u \mid \overline{LA}(u)] du\}$. We suppose we have a correctly specified stratified time-dependent Cox model

$$\lambda_Q[u \mid \overline{LA}_i(u)] = \lambda_{S_i^*}(u) \exp[\alpha_0' W_i(u)] \quad (A4.11)$$

where α_0 is a parameter vector, $W_i(u)$ is a vector of functions $w(\overline{LA}_i(u))$ of $\overline{LA}_i(u)$, $S_i^* \equiv S_i^*(u)$ is a time-dependent discrete stratification variable that is a function of $\overline{LA}_i(u)$, and the $\lambda_{S_i^*}(u)$ are unspecified stratum specific baseline hazard functions. Let $\hat{\alpha}$ be the Cox maximum partial likelihood estimator of α_0. To obtain $\hat{\alpha}$ one can use standard time-dependent Cox proportional hazards model software by regarding the subjects with $X_i = Q_i$ as the "failures." Let

$$\hat{\lambda}_{S_j^*}(X_j) = (1 - \tau_j)[\sum_{i=1}^n e^{\hat{\alpha}' \cdot W_i(X_j)} Y_i(X_j) I[S_i^*(X_j) = S_j^*(X_j)]]^{-1} \quad (A4.12)$$

where $Y_i(u) = I[X_i \geq u]$ records "at-risk" status at u. $\hat{\lambda}_{S_j^*}(X_j)$ is the Cox baseline hazard estimator for censoring at X_j in stratum S_j^*. Finally,

$$\hat{K}_i(u) \equiv \prod_{\{j; X_j \leq u, \tau_j = 0\}} [1 - \hat{\lambda}_{S_j^*}(X_j) e^{\hat{\alpha}' \cdot W_i(X_j)}]^{I[S_i^*(X_j) = S_j^*(X_j)]} \quad (A4.13)$$

We will sometimes write $\hat{K}_i \equiv \hat{K}_i(X_i)$ as $\hat{K}_i^w$ to stress its dependence on $W_i(u)$. $\hat{K}_i$ is an $n^{1/2}$-consistent estimator of $K_i(X_i)$.

Define, for any random N, $\hat{E}\{N\} \equiv n^{-1}\Sigma_i(\tau_i/\hat{K}_i)N_i$. Also define $\hat{D}^{(r)}(\psi)$ like $\tilde{D}^{(r)}(\psi)$ except with $\hat{\mathcal{L}}^{(r)}$ replacing $\tilde{\mathcal{L}}^{(r)}$, where $\hat{\mathcal{L}}^{(r)}$ is defined like $\tilde{\mathcal{L}}^{(r)}$ but with $\hat{E}$ replacing $\tilde{E}$. Define $\hat{U}_f^{(r)}(\psi)$ analogously in terms of $\tilde{U}_f^{(r)}(\psi)$. Let $\hat{\psi}^{(aj)}$ solve $n^{1/2}\hat{E}[\tilde{D}_{(4)}^{(aj)}] = o_p(1)$ and similarly for $\hat{\psi}^{(bj)}$. Let $\hat{\psi}^{(r)}$ solve $n^{1/2}$ $\hat{E}[\hat{D}^{(r)}(\psi)] = o_p(1)$. The following theorem is true for models (aj) and (bj) [given the data $(A4.9)$] when appropriate superscripts (aj) or (bj) are added. That is, $\hat{\psi}$ and $\tilde{D}$ will refer to $\hat{\psi}^{(aj)}$ and $\tilde{D}^{(aj)}$ under model (aj). First define $N_Q(x) = I[X \leq x, \tau = 0]$, $Y(u) = I[X \geq u]$, $M_Q(x) \equiv N_Q(x)$ $- \int_0^x \lambda_Q[u|\overline{LA}(u)]Y(u)du$. $M_Q(x)$ is, by $(A4.10)$, a subject-specific martingale with respect to the filtration $\mathbf{F}^Q(u)$ that records $[C, H(\psi_0),$ $\overline{LA}\{\min(T, u)\}, \{N_Q(x), Y(x); 0 \leq x \leq u\}]$. For a random $H(u)$, define $\Phi^Q(H, u, s) \equiv H(u) - \mathcal{L}^Q(H, u, s)$ with $\mathcal{L}^Q(H, u, s)$ $\equiv E\{H(u)Y(u)e^{\alpha_0'W(u)}I[S^*(u)=s(u)]\}/E\{Y(u)e^{\alpha_0'W(u)}I[S^*(u)=s(u)]\}$. Set $\Gamma(H) \equiv \int_0^\infty dM_Q(u)\Phi^Q(H, u, S^*)$.

Theorem A4.5. Subject to regularity conditions, under models (aj) or (bj), if $(A4.10)$ and $(A4.11)$ hold, and if $K(X) > \sigma > 0$ for some σ w.p.1

$$n^{1/2}\hat{E}[\tilde{D}(\psi_0)] = n^{-1/2}\Sigma_i U_i + o_p(1)$$

$$n^{1/2}(\hat{\psi} - \psi_0) = n^{-1/2}\Sigma_i\kappa^{-1}U_i + o_p(1) \qquad (A4.14)$$

$n^{1/2}\hat{E}[\tilde{D}(\psi_0)]$ and $n^{1/2}(\hat{\psi} - \psi_0)$ are asymptotically normal with mean 0 and asymptotic variances $\text{Var}(U) = \text{Var}(U_f) + \text{Var}(U_{\text{mis}}) - \text{Var}(U_{\text{rec}})$ and $\kappa^{-1}\text{Var}(U)\kappa^{-1'}$; $U = U_f - U_{\text{mis}} + U_{\text{rec}}$; $U_{\text{mis}} = \Gamma(H_{\text{mis}})$, with $H_{\text{mis}}(u) = D/K(u)$; and $U_{\text{rec}} = \mathbf{ls}(U_{\text{mis}}, U_w)$, where $U_w = \Gamma(W)$ with W the function $W(u)$. Further, $\text{Var}[U_{\text{rec}}] = E[U_{\text{mis}}U_w']\{E[U_wU_w']\}^{-1}E[U_wU_{\text{mis}}']$ and $E[U_{\text{mis}}U_{\text{rec}}'] = E[U_{\text{rec}}U_{\text{rec}}']$ where $E[\Gamma(H_1)\Gamma(H_2)'] = E[\int_0^\infty dN_Q(u)$ $\times \{\mathcal{L}^Q(H_1H_2', u, S^*) - \mathcal{L}^Q(H_1, u, S^*)\mathcal{L}^Q(H_2, u, S^*)'\}]$ when $H_1(u)$, $H_2(u)$ are $\mathbf{F}^Q(u)$ predictable. Note $E[U_fU_{\text{mis}}'] = E[U_fU_{\text{rec}}'] = 0$ since U_f is $\mathbf{F}^Q(0)$-predictable. The noncentrality parameter of the test based on $n^{1/2}$ $\hat{E}[\tilde{D}(\psi)]$ is $\{\kappa^{-1}\text{Var}(U)\kappa^{-1'}\}^{-1}$.

The proof is like that of Theorem 3.4 in Robins and Rotnitzky (1992).

Remark A4.7. If $(A4.5)$ holds, it follows from $(A4.5a)$ in the proof of Theorem A4.2b of this chapter and from Theorems 3.5, 4.1, 4.3, and 4.4 of Robins and Rotnitzky (1992) that, for some function b, $\hat{\psi}(b, \theta_{\text{op}}, b_{\text{op}}^*, \mathbf{K}_{\text{op}})$ is semiparametric efficient under the suppositions of Theorem A4.5. The optimal b is the solution to an integral equation that does not exist in closed form. The bound is unchanged if the data in $(A4.1)$ are available in addition to the data $(A4.9)$. Further, we have

Corollary A4.4. Theorem A4.5 is true with $\hat{\psi}$ defined to be $\hat{\psi}^{(r)}$ with $\hat{D}^{(r)}(\psi_0)$ replacing $\tilde{D}(\psi_0)$ and with $H_{\text{mis}} = U_f^{(r)}/K(u)$ if either (i) model (a) holds and $L_0^* = c_{\text{max}}$ or (ii) model (b) holds and $L_0^* = C$. This also follows from the proof to Theorem 3.4 in Robins and Rotnitzky (1992).

It follows from the decomposition of $\text{Var}(U)$ that $\hat{\text{Var}}\{U(\hat{\psi})\}$ can be based on consistent estimators of $\text{Var}(U_f)$ and $E[\Gamma(H_1)\Gamma(H_2)']$ for $H_1(u)$, $H_2(u) \in \{H_{\text{mis}}(u), W(u)\}$. Turning first to the rank estimators, a consistent estimator $\hat{\text{Var}}\{U_f^{(r)}(\hat{\psi})\}$ of $\text{Var}(U_f^{(r)})$ is $\hat{\text{Var}}[U_f^{(r)}(\hat{\psi})] \equiv \hat{E}\{\hat{\Omega}(\hat{\psi})\}$ where $\hat{\Omega}(\psi)$ is defined like $\tilde{\Omega}(\psi)$ with $\hat{\mathcal{L}}$ replacing $\tilde{\mathcal{L}}$. $E[\Gamma(H_1)\Gamma(H_2)']$ can be consistently estimated by $\tilde{E}[\int_0^\infty dN_Q(u)\{\hat{\mathcal{L}}^Q(\hat{H}_1\hat{H}_2', u, S^*) - \hat{\mathcal{L}}^Q(\hat{H}_1, u, S^*)\hat{\mathcal{L}}^Q(\hat{H}_2, u, S^*)'\}$ where $\hat{H}_1(u)$ and $\hat{H}_2(u)$ are consistent for $H_1(u)$ and $H_2(u)$; $\hat{\mathcal{L}}^Q(H, u, s) = Z(H, u, s)/Z(1, u, s)$ with $\mathbf{1}(u) = 1$, and $Z(H, u, s) = \sum_{i=1}^n \{\tau_i \hat{K}_i(u)/\hat{K}_i(X_i)\}Y_i(u)H_i(u)e^{\hat{\alpha}'w_i(u)}I[S_i(u) = s(u)]$. Thus, it only remains to provide a consistent estimator for $\hat{H}_{\text{mis}}(u, \hat{\psi})$ for $H_{\text{mis}}(u)$ as follows. $\hat{H}_{\text{mis}}(u, \hat{\psi}) \equiv \{\hat{K}(u)\}^{-1}\hat{U}_f^{(r)}(\psi)$ where $\hat{U}_f^{(r)}$ is $\hat{U}_f^{(r)}(\psi)$ with $\lambda_{H(\psi)}(u)$ replaced by $\hat{\lambda}_{H(\psi)}(u) = \hat{E}[dN_{H(\psi)}(u)]/\hat{E}[I(\nu(\psi) > u)]$.

Turning now to the nonrank estimators $\hat{\psi}$, i. e., $\hat{\psi}^{(aj)}$ and $\hat{\psi}^{(bj)}$, $\hat{\text{Var}}\{U_f(\hat{\psi})\} = \hat{E}[\hat{U}_f(\hat{\psi})\hat{U}_f(\hat{\psi})']$ where $\hat{U}_f(\hat{\psi}) = \tilde{D}(\hat{\psi}) - \hat{D}_{\text{adj}}(\hat{\psi})$, $\hat{D}_{\text{adj}}^{(1)}(\hat{\psi}) = \hat{I}s[\tilde{D}^{(1)}(\hat{\psi}), S_\eta(\hat{\eta})]$, $\hat{I}s(A, B) = \hat{E}(AB')\{\hat{E}[BB']\}^{-1}B$, a consistent but inefficient estimator $\hat{D}_{\text{adj}}^{(2)}(\hat{\psi})$ of $D_{\text{adj}}^{(2)}$ is obtained by the predicted value from a nonparametric regression of $\tau\tilde{D}^{(2)}/\hat{K}$ on R in model (a2) and on (R, C) in model (b2); similarly, $\hat{D}_{\text{adj}}^{(3)}(\hat{\psi})$ is the predicted value from a nonparametric regression of $\tau\tilde{D}^{(3)}/\hat{K}$ on (R, L_0^*) in both models (a3) and (b3). [However, $\tilde{D}^{(3)}$ still depends on the model (a) versus (b).] More efficient estimators of $D_{\text{adj}}^{(2)}$ and $D_{\text{adj}}^{(3)}$ can be obtained as in Section 3j of Robins and Rotnitzky (1992) although only consistency is necessary for variance estimation. Estimates of $\text{Var}(U_{\text{mis}})$ and $\text{Var}(U_{\text{rec}})$ are as described for the rank estimators except $\hat{H}_{\text{mis}}(u) = \tilde{D}^{(j)}/\hat{K}(u)$.

Robins and Rotnitzky (1992) consider the interpretation of the components of the variance decomposition $\text{Var}(U) = \text{Var}(U_f) + \text{Var}(U_{\text{mis}}) - \text{Var}(U_{\text{rec}})$. An alternative variance decomposition with its own interesting interpretation follows from the identities $U_f + U_{\text{mis}} = \tau U_f/K(X) + U_{\text{rec}}^*$ and $E[\{\tau U_f/K(X)\}U_{\text{rec}}^{s*'}] = -\text{Var}(U_{\text{rec}}^*)$ leading to $\text{Var}(U) = \text{Var}\{\tau U_f/K(X)\} - \text{Var}(U_{\text{rec}}^*) - \text{Var}(U_{\text{rec}})$. Here, $U_{\text{rec}}^* = \int_0^\infty dM_Q(u)\mathcal{L}^Q(H_{\text{mis}}, u, S^*)$. Now $\kappa^{-1}\text{Var}\{\tau U_f/K(X)\}\kappa^{-1'}$ is the asymptotic variance of $\hat{\psi}$ or $\hat{\psi}^{(r)}$ if we had used $K(X)$ instead of $\hat{K}(X)$. $\kappa^{-1}[\text{Var}\{\tau U_f/K(X)\} - \text{Var}(U_{\text{rec}}^*)]\kappa^{-1'}$ is the asymptotic variance of $\hat{\psi}$ or $\hat{\psi}^{(r)}$ if $\hat{K}(X)$ is calculated with α_0 replacing $\hat{\alpha}$ in (A4.12) and (A4.13). Hence, $\kappa^{-1}\text{Var}(U_{\text{rec}}^*)\kappa^{-1'}$ is the savings in variance attributable to estimating the hazards $\lambda_{s^*}(u)$. $\kappa^{-1}\text{Var}(U_{\text{rec}})\kappa^{-1'}$ is the additional savings attributable to estimating α_0 by $\hat{\alpha}$.

An alternative estimator of $\text{Var}(U)$ is obtained by (i) estimating $\text{Var}\{\tau U_f/K(X)\}$ by $\tilde{E}\{\tau[\hat{U}_f/\hat{K}(X)]^{[2]}\}$ where $\hat{U}_f$ denotes $\hat{U}_f(\hat{\psi})$ or $\hat{U}_f^{(r)}(\hat{\psi})$ for nonrank and rank estimators, respectively, and $A^{[2]} \equiv AA'$; (ii) estimating $\mathrm{Var}(U_{\mathrm{rec}}^*)$ by $\tilde{E}[\int_0^\infty dN_Q(u)\{\hat{\mathcal{L}}^Q(\hat{H}_{\mathrm{mis}}, u, S^*)\}^{[2]}]$; and (iii) estimating $\mathrm{Var}(U_{\mathrm{rec}})$ as above.

The results of this subsection and Sections A4.3–A4.5 depend critically on results in Robins and Rotnitzky (1992). A clear understanding of Robins and Rotnitzky (1992) requires the correction of several typographical errors. (See the listing of corrections to the above article at the end of this chapter.)

A4.3. An Improvement on the Usual Rank Estimator

Suppose our SNFTM is fully standard with complete compliance and $L_0^* = C$. Then we can define $\rho(u, R, \psi)$ such that $\rho(u, R, \psi) = t$ if and only if $h(t, \bar{L}(t), \bar{A}(t), \psi) = u$.

Suppose

$$\lambda_Q[u \mid \overline{LA}(u)] = \lambda_Q(u \mid R) \qquad (A4.15)$$

so $K(u) \equiv k(u, R)$ is a function only of R. Let $\hat{K}_i^0$ be $\hat{K}_i^w$ with $\hat{\alpha} \equiv 0$ in (A4.12) and (A4.13) and with $S_i^*(u) = R_i$, R_i discrete. $\hat{K}_i^0$ is the *treatment-arm-specific* Kaplan–Meier estimator of $K_i(u)$ evaluated at $u = X_i$.

Let $\hat{\psi}^0$ and $\hat{\psi}^w$ represent the estimator of $\hat{\psi}$ when $\hat{E}$ is based on $\hat{E}^0$ and $\hat{E}^w$, respectively, where $\hat{E}^0$ uses $\{\hat{K}_i^0\}^{-1}$ and $\hat{E}^w$ uses $\{\hat{K}_i^w\}^{-1}$. [In the Cox model for censoring used in computing $\hat{K}_i^w$, $S_i^*(u)$ is chosen so that R_i is a function of $S_i^*(u)$.]

If (A4.15) holds, then, under the suppositions of Theorem A4.5, $\hat{\psi}^0$ and $\hat{\psi}^w$ are both asymptotically normal and unbiased but asymptotic variance of $\hat{\psi}^w$ is less than or equal to that of $\hat{\psi}^0$.

Suppose further that $L_0^* = C = c_{\max}$ and model (a) is true. Then $\hat{\psi}^{0,(r)}$ is asymptotically normal and unbiased but with asymptotic variance greater than $\hat{\psi}^{w,(r)}$. Further, by Appendix 3 of Robins and Rotnitzky (1992), $\hat{\psi}^{0,(r)}(b, b^*, \mathbf{K})$ has, under regularity conditions, the same limiting distribution as $\hat{\psi}^{0,(r)}(b, \hat{b}, \mathbf{K})$ where $\hat{b}$ converges to b^* in probability. Now set $\hat{b}(u, R) = \hat{K}^0\{\rho(u, R, \psi), R\}$ and let $b^*(u, R)$ be its limit. Then $\hat{\psi}^{0,(r)}(b, \hat{b}, \mathbf{K})$ is precisely $\tilde{\psi}^{(r)}(b, b_{\mathrm{op}}^*, \mathbf{K})$ provided (i) we replace C by $\min(Q, c_{\max})$ in computing $\tilde{\psi}^{(r)}(b, b_{\mathrm{op}}^*, \mathbf{K})$ and (ii) if, in any arm R, the largest value of X_i has $\tau_i = 0$, we set that subject's τ_i to one in computing $\hat{\psi}^{0,(r)}(b, \hat{b}, \mathbf{K})$.

Thus, under (A4.15), $\hat{\psi}^{w,(r)}(b, \hat{b}, \mathbf{K})$ is more efficient than $\tilde{\psi}^{(r)}(b, b_{\mathrm{op}}^*, \mathbf{K})$. It is for this improvement that we introduced the function b^* initially. Similar remarks hold under model (b) if $L_0^* = C$ except in computing $\tilde{\psi}^{(r)}(b, b_{\mathrm{op}}^*, \mathbf{K})$ we replace C by $\min(Q, C)$. These remarks justify the results in Section 3.5 of the text. As in Robins and Rotnitzky (1992), a small modification in the notation allows us to obtain analogous results for the Cox proportional hazards model. As a consequence, we obtain an estimator of the proportional hazards β that will always be more efficient than the Cox partial likelihood estimator under an independent censoring assumption.

A4.4. Adjustment for Dependent Censoring and Recovery of Information with Independent Censoring

Throughout this section, we shall assume that the only form of censoring is by end of follow-up so $T^* = T$ and $h(t, \bar{l}(t), \bar{a}(t), \psi)$ does not depend on the potential censoring time C. (A4.7a) plus the condition (iv.a), Eq. (A4.8a), imply

$$C \amalg \{H(\psi_0), \bar{L}^{**}(T), \bar{A}(T)\} \mid R, L_0^{**} \qquad (A4.16a)$$

(A4.16a) implies

$$\lambda_C[u \mid \bar{L}^{**}(T), \bar{A}(T), R, H(\psi_0)] = \lambda_C[u \mid \bar{L}^{**}(u), \bar{A}(u), R] \quad (A4.16b)$$

(A4.16b) implies

$$\lambda_C[u \mid \bar{L}^{**}(u), \bar{A}(u), R, H(\psi_0)] = \lambda_C[u \mid \bar{L}^{**}(u), \bar{A}(u), R] \quad (A4.16c)$$

Note (A4.7a) can be written

$$\lambda_C[u \mid R, L_0^{**}, H(\psi_0)] = \lambda_C[u \mid R, L_0^{**}] \qquad (A4.16d)$$

Further, (A4.16d) is implied by (A4.16a). Also, given (A4.16c), (A4.16d) is implied by the identifiable restriction

$$\lambda_C[u \mid \bar{L}^{**}(u), \bar{A}(u), R] = \lambda_C[u \mid R, L_0^{**}] \qquad (A4.17)$$

Often, from a substantive point of view, one would not believe (A4.7a) held unless one believed (A4.16c) were true. But, given (A4.16c), we can test whether (A4.7a) holds by testing whether (A4.17) holds.

Suppose that we assume

$$H(\psi_0) \amalg R \mid L_0^{**} \qquad (A4.18)$$

(A4.7a) plus (A4.18) imply $H(\psi_0) \amalg (R, C) \mid L_0^{**}$ which, in turn, implies (A1.10) and (A4.7b).

Let the semiparametric model (cj) for $\psi_0, j = 0, 1, 2, 3$, be characterized by the data (A4.1), restrictions (A4.16c) and (A4.18), and a model j for $f(Z_1 | Z_2)$ with $Z_1 = R$, and $Z_2 = L_0^{**}$. We then have by a straightforward examination of the likelihood functions that

Theorem A4.6. The semiparametric efficiency bound for ψ_0 in model (cj) does not depend on j and is the same as that in the more restrictive models that impose one or more of the restrictions (A4.17) [so (A4.7a), (A4.7b), and (A1.10) hold], (A4.16b), and (A4.16a).

Remark A4.8. It follows that when both model $(c3)$ and (A4.17) are given *a priori* so that model $(b3)$ holds [since (A4.7b) and (A1.10) hold], the SIB for model $(c3)$ is greater than or equal to that for model $(b3)$ since model $(c3)$ and (A4.17) imply model $(b3)$.

To estimate ψ_0 under model (cj), recode censoring time by end of follow-up as Q, recode c_{max} as C, and then use the methods of Section A4.2 to estimate ψ_0.

Remark A4.9. Also note that in a semiparametric model characterized by (i) (A1.10) and (ii) $C \amalg R \mid L_0^{**}$, the SIB of that model is equal to that of model $(a3)$ and, furthermore, (A4.18) holds. Thus, if we are willing to impose the additional restriction (iii) (A4.16c), model $(c3)$ will hold, the SIB of the model characterized by (i), (ii), and (iii) equals that of model $(c3)$ and is greater than or equal to that of model $(a3)$.

A4.5. Estimation under Observational Study Assumptions in the Presence of Censoring

In this section we suppose (A1.23) and (A1.24) are true and the available data are given by (A4.1). If data (A4.2) were available, by Lemma A1.3, the model would be defined by the likelihood function (A1.28).

Now define θ_m, b_m, b_m^*, $\mathbf{K}_m$, μ_m, ν_m, B_m, B_m^*, $\check{\mathcal{L}}_m^{(j)}$, $\tilde{E}_m^{(j)}$, $U_{f,m}^{(j)}$, D_m, $\check{D}_m^{(j)}$, $D_{adj,m}^{(j)}$, κ_m as in Theorem A4.1 but with (i) $(\bar{L}_m^*, \bar{A}_{m-1})$ replacing L_0^* and (ii) A_m replacing R. The parameter vectors η_m, $m = 1, 2, \cdots$, in the parametric models for $f[A_m | \bar{L}_m^*, \bar{A}_{m-1}]$ are assumed variation independent.

For any variable N_m, let $N = \sum_{m=0}^{int(X^*)} N_m$, so, for example, $\check{D}^{(j)}$ is now $\sum_{m=0}^{int(X^*)} \check{D}_m^{(j)}$. Then, under a semiparametric model characterized by (A1.23), (A1.24), and models indexed by j_m for $f[A_m | \bar{L}_m^*, \bar{A}_{m-1}]$, $\check{\psi}^{(j)}$ solving $n^{1/2} \tilde{E}[\check{D}^{(j)}(\psi)] = o_p(1)$ will be asymptotically normal with mean 0 and asymptotic variance $\kappa^{-1} \operatorname{Var}[U_f^{(j)}](\kappa^{-1})'$, where $\kappa = E[DS_\psi^{cen'}]$.

This result follows from the proof of Theorem A4.1 and the nested martingale structure with increasing m. The optimal estimator $\tilde{\psi}_{op}^{(j)}$ is based on using $b_{op,m}^*$, $\mathbf{K}_{op,m}$, $b_{op,m}$, $\theta_{op,m}$ defined as above with R and L_0^* replaced by A_m and $(\bar{L}_m^*, \bar{A}_{m-1})$, respectively. $\tilde{\psi}_{op}^{(j)}$ is an improvement (in terms of efficiency) on the estimator $\tilde{\psi}^c(q_{opt}^{mod})$ of Section (A2.8) of Robins *et al.* (1992). Further, in the presence of censoring by competing risks satisfying (A4.10) and (A4.11), Theorem A4.5 remains true with $H_{mis}(w) \equiv \sum_{m=0}^{int(X)} D_m I(w > m)/K(w)$. This is relevant to the results stated in Section A2.11 of Robins *et al.* (1992).

Corrections for Robins and Rotnitzky (1992)

Page	Line	Uncorrected	Corrected
302	Eq. (3.3b)	$I[S_i^* = S_j^*][1 - \hat{\lambda}_{S_j^*}(X_j)e^{\hat{\alpha}' \cdot W_i(X_j)}]$	$[1 - \hat{\lambda}_{S_j^*}(X_j)e^{\hat{\alpha}' \cdot W_i(X_j)}]^{I[S_i^* = S_j^*]}$
311	Third to last	$\lambda_0(u)I\{X^* \geq u\}$	$\lambda_0(u)e^{\beta_0 Z}I\{X^* \geq u\}$
311	Second to last	$\lambda_0(u)I(X^* \geq u)$	$\lambda_0(u)e^{\beta_0 Z}I(X^* \geq u)$
313	Eq. (3.10a)	$\lambda_Q(x)$	$\lambda_Q(x\|\bar{L}(x), Z)$
313	Eq. (3.10b)	$\lambda_Q(x)$	$\lambda_Q(x\|\bar{L}(x), Z)$
317	Second paragraph line 12	$\|A\|$	$\|A\|^2$
318	Following Eq. (4.4)	Π	π
320	Second	$\mathbf{m}(D) = \bar{\pi}_m$	$\mathbf{m}(D) = \bar{\pi}_M$
327	Eq. (A.5)	$\Pi[S_\beta^{(F)}\|\Lambda^{(F),\perp}]$	$\Pi[S_\beta^{(F)}\|\Lambda_0^{(F)}]$

ACKNOWLEDGMENT. We are indebted to Dr. Margaret Fischl for making the data from ACTG Trial 002 available and to James Wiley for making data from the San Francisco Men's Health Study available. This work was in part supported by NIH grants K04-ES00180, 5-P30-ES00002, RO1-AI32475, and R01-ES03405 from NIEHS. Ron Kessler, Sander Greenland, and Fu Chang Hu provided valuable suggestions.

REFERENCES

Bickel, P., Klassen, C., Ritov, Y., and Wellner, J. (1993). Efficient and adaptive inferences in semiparametric models (to be published).

Cox, D. R. (1972). Regression models and life tables (with discussion). *J. R. Stat. Soc. Ser B* **34**:187–220.

Cox, D. R., and Oakes, D. (1984). *Analysis of survival data.* London: Chapman & Hall.

Fischl, M., *et al.* (1990). Randomized controlled trial of a reduced daily dose of zidovudine in patients with the acquired immunodeficiency syndrome. *N. Engl. J. Med.* **323**:1009–1019.

Greenland, S., and Robins, J. M. (1986). Identifiability, exchangeability and confounding. *Int. J. Epidemiol.* **15**:413–419.

Heckman, J. J., and Robb, R. (1985). Alternative methods for evaluating the impact of interventions. In J. J. Heckman and B. Singer (eds.), *Longitudinal analysis of labor market data*. London: Cambridge University Press, pp. 156–246.

Holland, P. (1986). Statistics and causal inference. *J. Am. Stat. Assoc.* **81**:945–961.

Kalbfleisch, J. D., and Prentice, R. L. (1980). *The statistical analysis of failure time data*. New York: Wiley.

Lagakos, S., Lim, L., and Robins, J. M. (1990). Adjusting for early treatment termination in comparative clinical trials. *Stat. Med.* **9**:1417–1424.

Lang, W., Anderson, R. A., Perkins, H., Grant, R. M., Lyman, D., Winkelstein, W., Royce, R., and Levy, J. A. (1987). Clinical, immunologic and serologic findings in men at risk for acquired immunodeficiency syndrome. The San Francisco Men's Health Study. *J. Am. Med. Assoc.* **257**:326–330.

Louis, T. A. (1981). Nonparametric analysis of an accelerated failure time model. *Biometrika* **68**:381–390.

Mark, S. D., and Robins, J. M. (1993a). Estimating the causal effect of smoking cessation in the presence of confounding factors using a rank preserving structural failure time model. *Stat. Med.* (in press).

Mark, S., and Robins, J. (1993b). A method for the analysis of randomized trials with compliance information: An application to the multiple risk factor intervention trial. *Controlled Clinical Trials* **14**:79–97.

Newey, W. K. (1990). Semiparametric efficiency bounds. *J. Appl. Econom.* **5**:99–135.

Ritov, Y., and Wellner, J. A. (1988). Censoring, martingales, and the Cox model. *Contemp. Math. Stat. Inf. Stoch. Process.* **80**:191–220.

Robins, J. M. (1986). A new approach to causal inference in mortality studies with sustained exposure periods—Application to control of the healthy worker survivor effect. *Math. Model.* **7**:1393–1512.

Robins, J. M. (1987a). A graphical approach to the identification and estimation of causal parameters in mortality studies with sustained exposure periods. *J. Chronic Dis.* Suppl. 2, **40**: 139s–161s.

Robins, J. M. (1987b). Addendum to "A new approach to causal inference in mortality studies with sustained exposure periods—Application to control of the healthy worker survivor effect." *Comput. Math. Appl.* **14**:923–945.

Robins, J. M. (1989a). The control of confounding by intermediate variables. *Stat. Med.* **8**:679–701.

Robins, J. M. (1989b). The analysis of randomized and non-randomized AIDS treatment trials using a new approach to causal inference in longitudinal studies. In L. Sechrest, H. Freeman, and A. Mulley (eds.), *Health Service research methodology: A focus on AIDS*. NCHSR, U.S. Public Health Service, pp. 113–159.

Robins, J. (1992). Estimation of the time-dependent accelerated failure time model in the presence of confounding factors. *Biometrika* **79**:321–334.

Robins, J. M. (1993a). Correcting for non-compliance in randomized trials using structural nested mean models. *Commun. Stat.* (in press).

Robins, J. M. (1993b). Estimating the causal effect of a time-varying treatment on survival using a new class of failure time models. *Commun. Stat.* (in press).

Robins, J. M., and Greenland, S. (1992). Identifiability and exchangeability for direct and indirect effects. *Epidemiology* **3**:143–155.

Robins, J. M., and Rotnitzky, A. (1992). Recovery of information and adjustment for dependent censoring using surrogate markers. In N. Jewell, K. Dietz, and V. Farewell (eds.), *AIDS epidemiology—Methodological issues.* Boston: Birkhäuser, pp. 297–331.

Robins, J. M., and Tsiatis, A. (1991). Correcting for non-compliance in randomized trials using rank-preserving structural failure time models. *Commun. Stat.* **20**:2609–2631.

Robins, J., and Tsiatis, A. A. (1992). Semiparametric estimation of an accelerated failure time model with time-dependent covariates. *Biometrika* **79**:311–319.

Robins, J. M., and Tsiatis, A. A. (1993). Correcting for non-compliance in randomized clinical trials using the strong version of the accelerated failure time model. *Stat. Med.* (provisionally accepted).

Robins, J. M., Blevins, D., Ritter, G., and Wulfsohn, M. (1992). G-estimation of the effect of prophylaxis therapy for pneumocystis carinii pneumonia on the survival of AIDS patients. *Epidemiology* **3**:319–336.

Rubin, D. B. (1978). Bayesian inference for causal effects: The role of randomization. *Ann. Stat.* **6**:34–58.

Tsiatis, A. A. (1990). Estimating regression parameters using linear rank tests for censored data. *Ann. Stat.* **18**:354–372.

Wei, L. J., Ying, Z., and Lin, D. Y. (1990). Linear regression analysis of censored survival data based on rank tests. *Biometrika* **77**:845–852.

Winkelstein, W., Jr., Lyman, D., and Padian, N., Grant, R., Samuel, M., Wiley, J. A., Anderson, R. E., Lang, W., Riggs, J., and Levy, J. A. (1987). Sexual practices and risk of infection by the human immunodeficiency virus. The San Francisco Men's Health Study. *J. Am. Med. Assoc.* **257**:321–325.

Zeger, S. L., and Liang, K.-Y. (1986). Longitudinal data analysis for discrete and continuous outcomes. *Biometrics* **42**:121–130.

10

The Design and Analysis of Partner Studies of HIV Transmission

NICHOLAS P. JEWELL and
STEPHEN C. SHIBOSKI

1. INTRODUCTION

Common goals in epidemiologic studies of infectious diseases include identification of the infectious agent, description of the modes of transmission,
and characterization of factors that influence the probability of transmission
from infected to uninfected individuals. In the case of AIDS, the agent has
been identified as the human immunodeficiency virus (HIV), and transmission
is known to occur through a variety of contact mechanisms including unprotected sexual intercourse, transfusion of infected blood products, and sharing
of needles in intravenous drug use. Relatively little is known about the probability of HIV transmission associated with the various modes of contact, or
the role that other cofactors play in promoting or suppressing transmission.
Here, transmission probability refers to the probability that the virus is transmitted to a susceptible individual following exposure consisting of a series of
potentially infectious contacts. The infectivity of HIV for a given route of
transmission is defined to be the per contact probability of infection. Knowledge of infectivity and its relationship to other factors is important in understanding the dynamics of the AIDS epidemic and in suggesting appropriate
measures to control its spread.

NICHOLAS P. JEWELL • Program in Biostatistics and Department of Statistics, University of
California, Berkeley, California 94720.   *STEPHEN C. SHIBOSKI* • Department of Epidemiology and Biostatistics, University of California, San Francisco, California 94143-0560.

Methodological Issues in AIDS Behavioral Research, edited by David G. Ostrow and Ronald C.
Kessler. Plenum Press, New York, 1993.

The primary source of empirical data about infectivity comes from sexual partners of infected individuals. Partner studies consist of a series of such partnerships, usually heterosexual and monogamous, each composed of an initially infected "index case" and a partner who may or may not be infected by the time of data collection. However, because the infection times of both partners may be unknown and the history of contacts uncertain, any quantitative characterization of infectivity is extremely difficult. Thus, most statistical analyses of partner study data involve the simplifying assumption that infectivity is a constant common to all partnerships.

The major objectives of this chapter are to describe and discuss the design and analysis of partner studies, providing a general statistical framework for investigations of infectivity and risk factors for HIV transmission. The development here is largely based on three papers: Jewell and Shiboski (1990), Kim and Lagakos (1990), and Shiboski and Jewell (1992).

Section 2 introduces some simple models for transmission of an infectious disease, motivates the use of partner studies of transmission, and reviews basic concepts and previous work on HIV transmission. Section 3 defines the basic data structures obtained from partner studies, and outlines basic study designs and data collection issues, while Section 4 presents models for transmission probabilities and describes their relationship to data collected in partner studies. In Section 5, techniques for estimation and inference are reviewed, and in Section 6 these are applied to data from two partner studies for illustration. Section 7 presents conclusions and briefly reviews topics of interest that are not addressed in the chapter.

2. BACKGROUND

2.1. The Use of Models in Studying Infectious Disease Transmission

2.1.1. The Transmission Process

Transmission of an infectious disease takes place when a susceptible individual is exposed to the disease agent through contact with an infected individual or *infective,* and the exposure is sufficient to induce infection. Following infection, newly infected individuals usually undergo a latent stage during which the infection develops, after which they become infectious themselves. Once infectious, the degree of infectiousness may vary considerably depending on the natural history of the disease and factors in the infected host such as immune function. In many diseases the infectious period may last indefinitely (i. e., until the host is removed from the population of infectives, or becomes immune), while for diseases that are eliminated from the host (i. e., no immunity is conferred), the host again becomes susceptible. Thus, the probability that the disease is transmitted to a susceptible following an exposure consisting of a series of identical contacts with the same infective depends on a number of factors including

1. the nature of the contacts (i. e., type, number, and frequency)
2. factors influencing the susceptibility of the potential host
3. factors influencing the infectiousness of the infective
4. the timing of the contacts relative to the infective's time of infection

2.1.2. Infectivity and Transmission Probability

The *infectivity* of a disease—the probability of transmission associated with a single exposure to an infective—is often used as a measure of the "force of infection" acting on a susceptible individual, analogous to the role of the hazard function in measuring current mortality risk in survival analysis. Similarly, the *transmission probability* is related to the survival function, being defined as the cumulative probability of transmission given a fixed length of exposure or contact. Infectivity is defined on a time scale relative to the time of infection of an infective, and because transmission to a susceptible can only occur during the infectious period, the infectivity is by definition zero outside of this period. In addition to indicating the degree of infectiousness of the infective, the infectivity also reflects susceptibility of the susceptible; separation of these two influences is impossible unless specific assumptions are made about their relative influence. Because the infectivity may be different for different types of exposures, any investigation of its properties must specify clearly what constitutes a single exposure. For sexually transmitted diseases this may be a single act of intercourse, while for an airborne agent it may consist of a set period of time spent in the proximity of an infective. The correspondences with survival analytic quantities and specific examples of possible expressions for infectivities and transmission probabilities will be worked out in detail below.

2.1.3. Modeling Transmission

Unlike diseases with completely unknown etiologies, the agents of infectious diseases are often known and the mechanisms of transmission somewhat understood. Thus, even a greatly oversimplified mathematical description of transmission can capture essential elements of the transmission process and provide useful insights into factors influencing the spread of an infectious disease. For this reason, epidemiologists often rely on simple models of transmission to assist in understanding the relative importance of factors influencing exposure, infectiousness, and susceptibility. The remainder of this section will be concerned with a particular model, both to gain a historical perspective on the use of such models, and to motivate applications to HIV transmission.

2.1.4. The Chain Binomial Model of Infectious Disease Transmission

The earliest transmission models were constructed to represent the spread of a disease through a closed group or household of susceptibles initiated by one or multiple infectives, and are called *chain binomial models* (Dietz and Schenzle, 1985; Becker, 1989). Although very simple in nature, these models illustrate many features of transmission and form the starting point for derivations of many more complex models. The development below follows Becker (1989) and Dietz and Schenzle (1985).

The aspect of transmission modeled by the chain model is the probability distribution of new cases arising in a given generation of the epidemic, where each generation consists of newly infected individuals arising from contact with infectives of the previous generation, the first generation consisting of the initial infective(s). An epidemic chain can be written symbolically as $i_1 \rightarrow i_2 \rightarrow \ldots \rightarrow i_r$, where i_t denotes the number of new cases arising in generation t, and no new cases occur after the rth generation. Let N_t be a random variable representing the number of susceptibles remaining at generation t, I_t the number of infectives resulting from new infections in generation $t - 1$, and $P(i)$ the probability that a given susceptible is infected by at least one of the $I_t = i$ infectives.

Then, the probability of observing y new infectives at the end of the succeeding time interval is given by

$$\mathrm{pr}(I_{t+1} = y \,|\, N_t = n, I_t = i) = \binom{n}{y} P(i)^y (1 - P(i))^{(n-y)}, \qquad y = 0, \ldots, n \quad (1)$$

There are many assumptions regarding transmission implicit in (1). In particular, the probability $P(i)$ depends only on the number of infectives to which a susceptible is exposed, and any dependence on the degree of infectiousness of the infectives (e. g., infectivity) or the degree of exposure (e. g., number of contacts or length of exposure) to the infectives is suppressed. Also, the binomial form implicitly assumes that contacts with infectives are made independently, and that encounters between a susceptible and any of the infectives are equally likely.

Two assumptions are commonly made regarding the form of $P(i)$ in (1). These are intended to distinguish between infectious diseases that require close contact for transmission to occur (e. g., sexual transmission) and those where no such contact is necessary (e. g., airborne agents). The first is the Reed–Frost assumption, which states that

$$(1 - P(i)) = (1 - P)^i$$

where $P = P(1)$. Therefore, the probability that a susceptible exposed through independent contacts to i infectives escapes infection is the same as the probability of escaping infection following i contacts with a single infective. This assumption is attributed to W. H. Frost and L. J. Reed, and was developed around 1928, although formal publication did not occur until 1976 (Frost, 1976). While this assumption may hold approximately for diseases such as the common cold, which are readily transmitted in close contacts, the assumption that a single constant P suffices to describe exposure, infectiousness, and susceptibility for all susceptible–infective contacts is certainly an oversimplification.

The second fundamental assumption is the *Greenwood* assumption after M. Greenwood (Greenwood, 1931):

$$(1 - P(i)) = (1 - P)$$

This assumption is directed at infectious diseases where the number of infectives to which a susceptible is exposed in a given time interval is irrelevant in determining transmission risk. For virulent infectious diseases such as measles, presence of a single infective in a closed household or group may be equivalent to the presence of several in determining transmission risk.

2.1.5. Models for Susceptible–Infective Pairs

From the standpoint of investigating the infectivity as defined above, model (1) is of very limited value since all information about the influence of varying degrees of exposure, infectiousness, and susceptibility is tied up in the constant $P(i)$. In particular, the transmission probability $P(i)$ does not depend directly on the number of contacts between the susceptible and the available infectives, so its relationship to the underlying infectivity is indeterminate. For a more detailed look at how varying exposure, infectiousness, and susceptibility affect transmission, and, in particular, to understand how transmission probabilities depend on the infectivity, more structure needs to be added to the definition of $P(i)$ in (1).

In chain models for transmission within a group, each susceptible can have infectious contacts with multiple infectives, each of whom may be at different stages of infectiousness. Accounting for this in the definition of $P(i)$

would require extensive modifications of the chain model. Consideration of a single susceptible–infective pair with no outside exposure (i. e., a "chain" consisting of a single generation) presents fewer complications because all factors relating to exposure, infectiousness, and susceptibility pertain only to two individuals. This is the primary motivation for partner studies of sexually transmitted diseases such as AIDS, where sexual partnerships consisting of a previously infected infective, often called the index case, and a susceptible partner form naturally occurring pairs that fit this description. Because the sequel will focus on sexual transmission of HIV, the terms *index case* and *partner* will usually be used in place of *infective* and *susceptible.*

For a partnership consisting of an index case and susceptible partner, (1) becomes

$$\mathrm{pr}(I_{t+1} = y \mid N_t = 1, I_t = 1) = P(\cdot)^y(1 - P(\cdot))^{(1-y)} \qquad (y = 0 \text{ or } 1) \quad (2)$$

where $P(\cdot)$ signifies the possible dependence of the transmission probability on additional factors relating to exposure, infectiousness, and susceptibility. As stated, (2) makes no assumptions about the transmission process and only requires that the binary indicator Y of transmission to the partner following an interval of exposure to the index case follows a Bernoulli distribution with parameter $P(\cdot)$. Since the transmission probability in (2) depends only on properties of exposure, infectiousness, and susceptibility for two individuals, deriving specific models for $P(\cdot)$ is feasible, as we will see in Section 4.

2.1.6. The Constant Infectivity Model

To take a simple example of a model for the transmission probability in (2), let K be a random variable representing the number of contacts following infection of the index case, and assume that contacts are made independently, each carrying equal transmission risk λ for the partner. Then

$$P(k) = 1 - (1 - \lambda)^k \tag{3}$$

This is a version of the *constant infectivity model,* with λ representing the infectivity. Comparison of equation (3) with the definition of the Reed–Frost assumption above reveals that the constant infectivity model can be viewed as the analogue of the latter, with multiple exposures to a single infective replacing a single exposure to multiple infectives. This model asserts that transmission depends only on the number of contacts, and not on the length of the period over which the exposure occurred, the placement of the contacts relative to the time of infection of the index case, or other factors related to the infectiousness of the index case and susceptibility of the partner. This may be plausible for certain sexually transmitted diseases.

The analogue of the Greenwood assumption for contact exposure with a single infective yields another variant of the constant infectivity model:

$$P(k) = \lambda \qquad (4)$$

Here, transmission risk is the same regardless of the number of contacts.

2.1.7. Deviations from the Constant Infectivity Model

The assumption of constant infectivity is fundamental to most mathematical and statistical work on disease transmission, and is usually made as a matter of mathematical convenience rather than a reflection of any real properties of transmission. However, it plays a role similar to the Reed–Frost and Greenwood assumptions associated with the classical chain binomial model, in that it provides a parsimonious description of infectivity and provides a useful "null" model against which more complex models may be compared. Following the previous discussion, particular deviations from constant infectivity are expected if infectiousness and/or susceptibility vary systematically or randomly over time within a partnership. Further, even if a constant infectivity seemed reasonable for a given partnership, in applying the model to a series of partnerships, we would not expect that a single infectivity would accurately reflect infectiousness and susceptibility for each of them. Thus, even if the form of the transmission probability [(3) or (4)] is accepted, *random heterogeneity* of infectivity across partnerships may be a source of disagreement between observed data and the assumption of constant infectivity.

Section 4 will present generalizations of the chain binomial model (2) appropriate for examining transmission within a single susceptible–infective pair or partnership. In these models, the infectivity associated with a single infective–susceptible contact will be considered as a parameter and methods for its estimation developed. Techniques for examining deviations of infectivity from a constant will also be presented. The resulting methods will be employed to investigate HIV transmission using data from epidemiologic partner studies.

There is an extensive literature on applications of mathematics and statistics to the study of infectious diseases. Good basic references include Bailey (1975) and Dietz and Schenzle (1985), both of which provide a historical perspective and reviews of mathematical and statistical techniques of epidemic modeling; the recent book by Becker (1989) concentrates on modern statistical methods. Each of these references covers the chain binomial model in detail.

2.2. The Natural History of AIDS

The natural history of AIDS, including properties of the infectivity and the length of the latent and infectious periods, is only partially understood, and continues to be the focus of much research. Infection with HIV can occur through a wide variety of contact mechanisms, all of which involve transfer of bodily fluids containing the virus. Well-known examples include sexual contact, blood transfusion, needle sharing among i.v. drug users, and medical accidents involving transfer of contaminated fluids. Following infection, HIV can be detected only when a sufficient quantity of antibodies is present in the host's bloodstream; this stage is termed *seroconversion* and is thought to occur weeks to months after infection. Although there are frequently flulike symptoms associated with the seroconversion period, the onset of symptoms signaling a more advanced stage of the disease may take many years. The period between infection and development of symptoms signaling onset of the disease is termed the *incubation period,* and for AIDS has been estimated to vary considerably around a median length of approximately 10 years (see, e. g., Bacchetti and Moss, 1989). Figure 1 provides a schematic of the natural history of HIV infection, illustrating the key points in disease transmission and development.

Very little is known about the nature of latent and infectious periods associated with AIDS. However, recent research on viral titer and antigen level in the blood of infected hosts suggests that the potential for transmission of HIV is high close to the time of seroconversion and again in the later symptomatic stages of the disease (Anderson, 1988; Ho *et al.,* 1989; Holmberg *et al.,* 1989). This may imply that the latent period as defined above is short, or nonexistent, and that the infectious period may vary considerably in length and intensity, possibly extending to the final disease stages. There is also limited epidemiologic evidence suggesting that symptomatic individuals may transmit infection more efficiently than asymptomatic individuals (Goedert *et al.,* 1987; European Study Group, 1989).

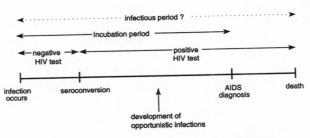

Figure 1. Diagram of the natural history of AIDS.

From the perspective of modeling transmission, AIDS has several features that simplify model formulation: First, the mechanisms of HIV transmission have been fairly well understood since the early 1980s, and epidemiologic studies of the various routes of transmission have been completed or are under way. Second, tests for antibodies to HIV are very reliable, and once infected, an HIV antibody-positive person will almost certainly remain positive (and potentially infective) indefinitely. Finally, as a sexually transmitted disease, exposures can be clearly defined as sexual contacts (e. g., vaginal or anal intercourse with ejaculation).

2.3. Why Is Infectivity Information Important?

Intuitively, it is clear that the level of infectivity must play an important role in influencing the rate of growth of the epidemic and in quantifying the impact of various interventions. This is supported by various kinds of simple deterministic transmission models. These models also indicate that other properties of infectivity are key components of epidemic modeling; e. g., how long is an infective infectious, does the level of infectivity vary according to how long an individual has been infected or the infective's stage of disease? Thus, an understanding of infectivity and its related properties is an important aspect of building more realistic transmission models.

Perhaps of more importance is the need to understand individual characteristics that may influence the probability of transmitting the AIDS virus. Such characteristics may be associated with either the infective or the susceptible partner in a sexual contact and may include descriptions of the nature of contact (e. g., practice of anal sex, use of contraceptives, occurrence of bleeding during intercourse, current or past infection with other sexually transmitted diseases). The relevance of such information to infectivity is of importance not only in epidemic modeling (e. g., can the distribution of such characteristics explain, at least in part, differences in epidemic growth patterns between certain populations?) but also as a guide to intervention and health education efforts designed to reduce and eliminate viral transmission.

Next, the manner in which an individual's infectiousness changes as the disease moves through various stages is not only of interest to modelers but may also be relevant to an understanding of how infectivity may be affected by prophylactic treatment. This issue is critical to any discussion of whether treatments like zidovudine should be systematically offered to asymptomatic individuals, underscoring "the need . . . to assess the degree to which antiviral drug treatment or immunotherapy suppresses infectiousness" (Anderson *et al.*, 1991).

Finally, since "infectiousness" cannot be measured directly (nor "susceptibility"), it would be of value to determine the extent to which serological measurements on an infected individual correlate with the ability to transmit the virus by a specific route. For example, does p24 antigenemia correlate with infectious HIV titers in the blood, and do either or both of these relate to the infectiousness of a sexual contact with the infected individual (Weiss, 1991)? These kinds of questions are, of course, closely related to the relationships, described above, between characteristics of either sexual partner and the likelihood of transmission.

2.4. Previous Literature on Statistical Work on HIV Transmission

Existing quantitative work on HIV transmission can be roughly classified into statistical analyses of data from epidemiologic studies and mathematical models of transmission dynamics. The emphasis of most statistical analyses has been on investigating risk factors for transmission based on data from heterosexual partner studies and prospective studies of HIV infection in homosexual men. Mathematical models have focused on a theoretical understanding of the complex interactions between biological and behavioral factors in controlling the spread of the epidemic. One common interest of both areas of investigation is in estimating the infectivity of HIV.

Grant *et al.* (1987) applied a version of the constant infectivity model (3) to data from a prospective study of San Francisco homosexual men, and produced the first published estimate of per-partner HIV infectivity. Virtually all estimates of infectivity made to date are based on the constant (per-contact) infectivity model. For sexual transmission they range from 0.001 to 0.1 per contact (Holmberg *et al.*, 1989). However, as noted by Kaplan (1990), in most cases the constant model fits the observed data poorly.

A number of papers, including De Gruttola *et al.* (1989), Wiley *et al.* (1989), Jewell and Shiboski (1990), and Kim and Lagakos (1990), have examined the possibility of heterogeneity of infectivity across partnerships as a possible explanation for the poor fit of the constant model to observed data. Jewell and Shiboski (1990) presented techniques for examining the plausibility of the constant infectivity assumption and examined measurement error in exposure data as a further explanation for lack of fit of the constant model. Variation in infectiousness with time following infection and with stage of disease has been incorporated into mathematical models by Blythe and Anderson (1988) and statistical models by Longini *et al.* (1989), Kim and Lagakos (1990), and Shiboski and Jewell (1992). Kaplan (1990) and Shiboski and Jewell (1992) develop a nonparametric estimate of a contact-dependent transmission probability function that makes no assumption about the underlying infectivity.

Jewell (1990) reviews applications of statistics to AIDS research, including material on studying infectivity based on partner study data. Anderson (1989) and Isham (1988) provide overviews of the mathematical modeling approach to studying HIV transmission. The review paper of Fusaro *et al.* (1989) is a comprehensive annotated bibliography of statistical methods in AIDS research, and includes a number of papers on HIV transmission from statistical and mathematical perspectives.

3. PARTNER STUDIES OF HIV TRANSMISSION

3.1. Definition of a Partner Study

As indicated in Section 2, partnerships form natural experimental units for studying transmission of sexually transmitted diseases, and epidemiologic studies of partners of HIV-infected index cases provide valuable information about risk factors for HIV transmission. A partner study consists of a series of partnerships, each composed of an infected index case and an (initially) uninfected partner. Following the infection of the index case, the partner is exposed to infection through a series of contacts with the index case. The *exposure history* of the partnership includes information on variables such as the nature, number, and frequency of contacts, and the length of exposure. Because of the potential differences in efficiency between the various routes of transmission, most partner studies are designed to investigate a particular type of contact in a select type of partnership (e. g., heterosexual transmission in monogamous couples). However, the definition of contacts may vary across studies and includes (1) sexual contacts and (2) sharing of needles in intravenous drug use. In the sequel, contacts are assumed to represent a single route of transmission. It also is assumed that for each partnership, the index case can be identified, and that infection of the partner occurs solely through contact with the index case, and not via other sources of transmission. Partnerships that fail to meet these criteria are usually excluded from the analysis, although studies that relax these restrictions are discussed briefly in Section 7.

3.2. Data Structures for Partner Studies

Since the partnership may have commenced after infection of the index case, define U to be the time since infection of the index case at the point the partnership is initiated. For *long-term partnerships,* in existence at the time of the index case's infection, we set $U \equiv 0$. The partnership is first observed or enrolled after a period of time (of length T time units) following the infection of the index case or the origination of the partnership, whichever occurred later in chronological time. (Thus, at the time of enrollment, the partner has been "exposed" to an infected index case for T time units.) For convenience we denote the chronological time of infection of the index case by t_I and the chronological time of enrollment by t_E. Let K denote the number of contacts during the exposure period. At the end of this period the serostatus of the originally uninfected partner is ascertained. The definitions of variables are illustrated in Fig. 2, and are given as follows for the ith partnership:

$$U_i = \begin{cases} \text{time since infection of index case when partnership was formed} \\ \qquad\qquad\qquad\qquad\qquad\qquad \text{(after index case's infection)} \\ 0 \qquad \text{if partnership was formed prior to infection of index case,} \end{cases}$$

T_i = length of time of exposure,

$\qquad K_i$ = number of contacts with index case during exposure period,

$$Y_i = \begin{cases} 1 \qquad \text{if partner is infected at time of data collection} \\ 0 \qquad \text{if partner remains seronegative at time of data collection.} \end{cases}$$

Another random variable of interest is the rate of contacts between partners, usually assumed constant throughout the exposure. This will be denoted by M_i, or by $M_i(\cdot)$ to indicate time dependence. Frequently, this may be measured as an alternative to K_i. Finally, if $Y = 1$ (i. e., infection has occurred in the partner), the random variable V denotes the chronological time of infection of the partner. Note that, for $Y = 1$, $t_I < V < t_E$, whereas for $Y = 0$, $V > t_E$.

3.3. Study Designs for Partner Studies

We now discuss several designs for data collection from partner studies. For each design considered, we initially assume that a partnership enrolled

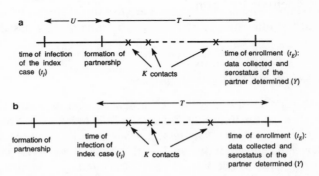

Figure 2. Schematic of data collected in retrospective partner study: partnership formed (a) after and (b) before infection of the index case.

at t_E is randomly selected from all partnerships of a specified nature in the population. For reasons discussed in Section 3.4, this kind of random sampling is not feasible in practice. Furthermore, even when such random sampling is possible, selection forces are still operating that can produce biased samples. For example, partnerships of shorter lengths are likely to be undersampled relative to long-term partnerships. Note that partnerships of short duration may arise naturally, or may result from a short incubation period for either partner. Throughout the following we indicate the impact of this and other forms of selection bias on the statistical approaches outlined. However, in describing differences between the various designs we emphasize the extent to which each of the random variables defined above can be measured, rather than the importance of selection phenomena.

3.3.1. Cross-sectional Designs

In such designs, the time of infection of the index case t_I, is unknown, apart from the knowledge that $t_I < t_E$, the time of partnership enrollment. Thus, neither the time of exposure T nor the number of contacts K during the exposure period can be evaluated although retrospective information may be collected on the history of the rate of contacts between index case and partner, $M(\cdot)$. The partner's serostatus at the time of enrollment, Y, is measured at enrollment.

In the absence of knowledge about the number of contacts during the exposure period, it is clearly not possible to quantify a per-contact infectivity using cross-sectional data. Essentially, only the proportion of partners who are infected at enrollment can be estimated. While this proportion is influenced by the infectivity, it also depends on other factors (including the partnership distribution of the number of exposed contacts) even in the simplest infectivity models. Extreme caution must therefore be used in comparing such transmission proportions across subgroups, since differences may be caused by variation in the contact distributions rather than differences in infectivity. Infectivity patterns across subgroups can only be reliably inferred if one is willing to assume that there is no variation in the contact distribution across the groups in question. This will usually be a heroic assumption since the contact distribution will depend on both the distribution of times of infection of the index case and the pattern of contact rates. Hence, the observation that infectivity varies according to the mode of infection of the index case based on comparison of cross-sectional infection prevalences of partners (see, e. g., Holmes and Kreiss, 1988) could be very misleading since index cases infected by intravenous drug abuse or through homosexual contacts may have been infected at different chronological times during the course of the epidemic and may have differing rates of contacts with their sexual partners.

3.3.2. Retrospective Designs

In these designs, the time of infection of the index case, t_I, is assumed known at least to some level of accuracy. However, this information is collected retrospectively at the time of enrollment. Furthermore, with this date in mind, data on the exposure period and number of contacts during the exposure period can also be collected retrospectively. The partner's serostatus, Y, is measured at enrollment. However, even when $Y = 1$, the exact chronological time of infection of the partner, V, is not observed; only the fact that $t_I < V < t_E$ can be determined in such cases. Nevertheless, because retrospective studies typically contain partnerships with exposure intervals of varying lengths, and a range of reported contact frequencies, they can still provide more information than cross-sectional designs about the dependence of transmission probabilities on exposure, and thus about the infectivity.

3.3.3. Prospective Designs

This design applies only to partnerships that are ongoing at the time of enrollment. Here the time of infection of the index case is unknown, apart from the fact that $t_I < t_E$; also, past history on exposure and the rate and number of contacts is also unknown or unreliable. Furthermore, only partnerships when the partner is uninfected at the time of enrollment [$Y(t_E) = 0$] are retained for follow-up. These partnerships are subsequently routinely monitored with regard to the serostatus of the partner [$Y(t): t > T_E$], in addition to potential longitudinal measurement of key variables including the number and type of contacts, concurrent covariate information on the index case and/ or partner including, perhaps, immunological measurements and the use of therapy for the index case. Thus, in principle, the time of infection of the partner (V) is known should it occur, at least to some level of accuracy, depending on the frequency of monitoring. Also, contact information is available for the period from t_E until infection occurs or follow-up ceases on the partnership (e. g., if the partnership dissolves, or the study is ended, or the partnership is lost to follow-up).

3.3.4. Hybrid Designs

In practice, a partner study may combine characteristics of cross-sectional, retrospective, and prospective designs. For example, in many studies partnerships are recruited without knowledge of the time of index case infection, making the overall design cross-sectional. However, initial interviews frequently provide retrospective data on the number and rate of contacts occurring between partners prior to enrollment. By combining available information on the source of infection for the index cases with data on the rate of new infections in the population, these data can often be adjusted to more accurately reflect exposure, and subsequently analyzed using methods developed for retrospective designs. Retrospective and cross-sectional samples may also form the basis of a prospective study. In such cases, partnerships with uninfected partners on recruitment are subsequently enrolled into a prospective study consisting of regular follow-up visits for counseling, HIV testing, behavioral questionnaires and physical examinations as described below in Section 3.4.

3.4. Data Collection Issues

Partner studies present a number of challenges from the standpoint of data collection, including identification and recruitment of eligible partnerships and determination of accurate exposure information, such as the time of infection of the index case and the frequency and nature of contacts. This section briefly reviews these topics.

3.4.1. Selection of Partners

Partnerships in which one individual can be clearly identified as the index case, and in which there is no other known source of infection risk for the partner are relatively rare. For this reason, partner studies are generally not based on random samples and recruit partnerships using a variety of methods. For retrospective and cross-sectional designs, potentially eligible partnerships are identified either through knowledge of the source of infection of index cases (e. g., transfusion or drug abuse), or by advertising for individuals who are past or current partners of known index cases. Identified partnerships are screened to determine eligibility and enrolled on a volunteer basis. Prospective studies are frequently formed as continuations of retrospective or cross-sectional designs (as discussed above), and eligibility criteria carry the added restriction that partners are uninfected at enrollment.

Because of the nature of recruitment, partner studies do not necessarily yield samples that can be considered random and representative in the statistical sense. In particular, the sampling probability for partnerships with infected partners may differ from that for partnerships with uninfected partners. Statistical techniques for assessing the impact of this bias on estimates are discussed in Section 5.

3.4.2. Measurement of Key Variables

Obtaining accurate exposure history information is a major challenge in conducting partner studies. Perhaps the most difficult variable to measure is the time of infection of the index case; except in rare situations (e. g., infection by transfusion), this time is either completely unknown or can be determined only to lie in a broad interval. Because of its importance in defining the duration of exposure of partner to index, some knowledge of the time of index infection is essential in estimating transmission probabilities and the associated infectivity. When an estimate of the time (or interval) of index infection is available, reported data on duration, frequency, and type of contacts can be adjusted to more accurately reflect exposure. However, because of uncertainty in the estimate, all related exposure data are subject to measurement error, a fact that must be accounted for when the data are analyzed.

Data on other exposure variables such as rate, number, and type of contacts are generally collected using interview techniques in which the partner and/or index case are asked to recall details of their sexual history. In retrospective studies, because of the retrospective nature of data collection, these variables are also particularly subject to measurement error and must be viewed as estimates for the purpose of analysis. There are a number of techniques that can be used to assess and perhaps improve the accuracy of these data, including the comparison of responses between partners.

Other variables that may yield important information about infectiousness and susceptibility include disease status of the index case (as measured by CD4 lymphocyte count, p24 antigen levels, and stage of disease for AIDS cases) and details on sexual practices including mode of intercourse and use of contraception. These variables may be available only at enrollment in retrospective and cross-sectional studies, but can be measured at regular intervals in prospective designs. With regard to measurement of serostatus of the partner at enrollment (Y), antibody tests can be repeated soon after enrollment to ensure that the variable Y accurately reflects the infection status of the partner. Repeated monitoring of Y is, of course, an integral component of a prospective design; however, a major drawback of such studies from the standpoint of studying transmission is that ethical considerations demand that the partners receive counseling to ensure that no transmission occurs. Hence, very few partner infections may be observed in a prospective study so that the resulting data may contain little information about infectivity.

4. TRANSMISSION MODELS FOR PARTNER STUDY DATA

Recalling the discussion of AIDS natural history and HIV transmission in Section 2, a realistic model for sexual transmission of HIV between partners must account for several factors, including temporal and individual variations in infectiousness and susceptibility, degree and duration of exposure, and the influence of behavioral variables such as contraceptive use and sexual practices.

Accordingly, a statistical analysis of transmission based on partner study data should provide a means of evaluating the relative importance of these factors. The next section applies concepts from survival analysis to develop expressions for the probability that the partner will remain infection-free following a series of contacts occurring during an exposure period of specified length. (In the notation of Section 2.1, this probability is $1 - P$, i. e., the complement of the transmission probability.) These expressions form a basis for statistical models for partner study data, which, in addition to providing a general framework in which to view HIV transmission, include the constant infectivity model as a special case, and can thus be used to evaluate the plausibility of the assumption of constant infectivity. The models can also be modified to incorporate covariates for investigations of the impact of additional factors on transmission risk.

4.1. Time-Dependent Transmission Probabilities

As indicated in Section 2.1, the transmission probability is related to a survival function, and the infectivity can be interpreted as a hazard function in a special sense. However, in describing dependence of the transmission probability on the infectivity, both number (or rate) of contacts and length of exposure need to be considered. Knowledge of the length of exposure alone provides incomplete information about the probability of transmission unless contacts are known to have occurred in the exposure interval. Similarly, a time-varying infectivity implies not all contacts will carry the same transmission risk. Thus, inferences about transmission based solely on knowledge of either the number of exposed contacts or length of exposure may be less informative than those made when both factors are considered together.

The infectivity associated with a specific contact will be denoted by λ. Suppose that λ varies according to the time of contact relative to the date of infection of the index case, i. e., $\lambda = \lambda(x)$ where x denotes time since infection of the index case. For now, the form of the function $\lambda(\cdot)$ will not be specified (some specific models will be considered below) and the infectivity function will be assumed to be the same for all partnerships, an assumption that is routinely made for the hazard function in most applications of survival analysis.

4.1.1. Concepts from Survival Analysis

Consider the case of a partnership for which exposure begins at time $U = u$ following infection of the index case. Since, as indicated, infectivity varies with time since infection of the index case (denoted here and below by x), in order to describe the risk of transmission associated with a particular exposure history it is necessary to specify when the contacts occur after time u. For simplicity, assume the contacts after u occur according to a nonhomogeneous Poisson process, $\{K(x)\}_{x \geq u}$, with intensity function $M(\cdot) = \mu(\cdot)$. Let V be a random variable representing the time of infection of the partner measured in the same time units as U. If u and the entire sample path of $\{K(x)\}_{x \geq u}$ are known, then the hazard function associated with V is discrete, with values given by the infectivity function $\lambda(\cdot)$ evaluated at the time points where contacts are made, i. e., for $v \geq u$,

$$h(v \mid u, K(x): x \geq u) \equiv \lim_{\Delta \to 0^+} \frac{1}{\Delta} \mathrm{pr}\{v \leq V \leq v$$

$$+ \Delta \mid V \geq v, U = u, K(x): x \geq u\} = \sum_{j=1}^{K(v)} \lambda(v)\delta(v - x_j)$$

where $x_1, x_2, \ldots$ are observed values of the contact times in the sample path of $\{K(x)\}_{x \geq u}$, and $\delta(x) = 1$ when $x = 0$ and $\delta(x) = 0$ for all other values of x. Because of the dependence on $K(v)$ and U, this hazard function is stochastic. Stochastic hazards are common in reliability theory (see, e. g., Gaver, 1963 and Rockower, 1986). Standard results from survival analysis (Cox and Oakes, 1984) show that the survival function for V can then be written, for $v \geq u$,

$$S(v \mid u, K(x): x \geq u) = \mathrm{pr}\{V > v \mid U = u, K(x): x \geq u\} = \prod_{j=1}^{K(v)} (1 - \lambda(x_j)) \quad (5)$$

Note that for $v \leq u$, $h(v \mid u, K(x): x \geq u) \equiv 0$ and $S(v \mid u, K(x): x \geq u) \equiv 1$.

Typically, as in the case of retrospective partner study data, full information on the sample paths of $\{K(x)\}_{x \geq u}$ is unavailable, and only the observed total number of contacts k and/or the rate function $\mu(\cdot)$ in the interval $[u, v]$ is known. By conditioning on this observed exposure information, deterministic survival and hazard functions for V can be obtained from (5) for both of these situations.

First, taking the expectation of (5) with respect to the sample path of $\{K(x)\}_{x \geq u}$, conditional on the total number of contacts $K(v) = k$ and the rate function $M(\cdot) = \mu(\cdot)$ gives, for $v \geq u$,

$$S(v \mid u, k, \mu(\cdot)) = \text{pr}\{V > v \mid U = u, K(v) = k, M(x) = \mu(x); u \le x \le v\}$$

$$= \int_u^v \cdots \int_u^v \prod_{j=1}^k [(1 - \lambda(x_j))\mu(x_j)/\mu^*]dx_1 \cdots dx_k$$

$$= \prod_{j=1}^k \left[\int_u^v (1 - \lambda(x_j))\mu(x_j)/\mu^* dx_j \right]$$

$$= \left[\int_u^v (1 - \lambda(x))(\mu(x)/\mu^*)dx \right]^k, \quad \text{where } \mu^* = \int_u^v \mu(x)dx \quad (6)$$

This derivation uses a standard result for Poisson processes, that given the total number of events in an interval $[u, v]$, the (unordered) times of jumps in the interval are independent and identically distributed with density $\mu(\cdot)/\mu^*$ (Cox and Isham, 1980). This survival function depends on $\mu(\cdot)$ unless the latter is constant. In addition, (6) depends on the number of contacts k, indicating that the probability of the event "infection" depends on both k and v. In fact, (6) affords two interpretations: the first, as the conditional survival function for V. In this interpretation the number of contacts can be regarded as a time-dependent covariate. Alternatively, (6) has the form of a discrete time survival function, with the number of exposed contacts $K(x)$ serving as the (random) time scale.

Now consider the survival function for V when the associated number of contacts in $[u, v]$ is not observed directly; only information on $\mu(\cdot)$ is available. From (6), for $v \ge u$,

$$S(v \mid u, \mu(\cdot)) = \text{pr}\{V > v \mid U = u, M(x) = \mu(x); u \le x \le v\}$$

$$= \sum_{k=0}^{\infty} A^k (\mu^*)^k e^{-\mu^*}/k! \quad \text{where } A = \int_u^v [1 - \lambda(x)](\mu(x)/\mu^*)dx$$

$$= e^{\mu^*(A-1)} = \exp\left\{ -\int_u^v \lambda(x)\mu(x)dx \right\} \quad (7)$$

This implies that, marginally, V, the time from infection of the index case until infection of the partner, follows a survival distribution with associated deterministic hazard function that is zero until time u (by definition, the beginning of exposure) and is given by $\lambda(\cdot)\mu(\cdot)$ thereafter. Note that, for long-term partnerships ($U = 0$), (7) becomes

$$S(v \mid \mu(\cdot)) = \exp\left\{ -\int_0^v \lambda(x)\mu(x)dx \right\} \quad (8)$$

If $\mu(x) \equiv \mu$, (7) and (8) specify Cox proportional hazards models (Cox and Oakes, 1984) with baseline hazard function given by $\lambda(\cdot)$ (defined to be zero prior to u) and a fixed offset $\log \mu$ (i. e., a covariate given by $\log \mu$ with slope identically one). For example, the proportional hazards form of (7) can be written

$$S(v \mid u, \mu) = \exp\left\{-\int_u^v \lambda(x)dx\right\}^{e^{\log\mu}}$$

Both (7) and (8) thus provide a means of linking the infection time distribution with the rate function and additional covariates, and will be used as a basis for estimation of $\lambda(\cdot)$ in the next section. Becker (1989) provides a derivation of (7) for the case of constant contact rates, referring to $\lambda(\cdot)$ as the infectiousness function.

We note that a similar expression to (7) can be obtained for the probability that the partner remains infection-free following k contacts, by margining out the random variables U and V. However, unless $\lambda(\cdot) \equiv \lambda$, the form of the resulting survival function is quite complex, with further development requiring restrictive assumptions.

4.1.2. The Constant Infectivity Case

When the infectivity function $\lambda(\cdot) \equiv \lambda$, the expressions above simplify considerably, in most cases yielding familiar failure time models from survival analysis. For example, in the general model (6), this assumption leads to the constant infectivity model (3):

$$S(v \mid u, k, \mu(\cdot)) = (1 - \lambda)^k \qquad (9)$$

Thus, assuming a constant infectivity function has the result that only the number of contacts is relevant, and information on variation of the contact rate function is unnecessary. This makes sense intuitively, but is, of course, critically dependent on the constancy of the infectivity.

On the other hand, if the contact rate function $\mu(\cdot) \equiv \mu$ and $\lambda(\cdot) \equiv \lambda$, then (7) leads to a special case of the proportional hazards regression model:

$$S(v \mid u, \mu) = \exp\{-\lambda(v - u)\}^{e^{\log\mu}} \qquad (10)$$

Here, the time between first exposure u and partner infection v is exponentially distributed with parameter $\lambda\mu$.

4.1.3. Applications to Retrospective Partner Study Data

For retrospective partner studies, the observed data ($Y = y$, $T = t$, $U = u$, $K = k$, $M(\cdot) = \mu(\cdot)$) provide only partial information about the time of partner infection. In fact, this random variable is never observed directly for any partnership. First, observation of partnerships ceases at time $U + T$ following K contacts. Second, even if the partner is infected prior to this time (i. e., $V \leq U + T$), the only information observed is the indicator Y that this event has occurred. Thus, observing ($Y = 1$, $T = t$, $U = u$, $K(t + u) = k$) implies that $u \leq V \leq u + t$. Similarly, observing ($Y = 0$, $T = t$, $U = u$, $K(t + u) = k$) implies that $V > u + t$. In survival analysis language, every observation of V is *interval censored.*

The data on $M(\cdot) = \mu(\cdot)$ provide additional information that, as is clear from examining (6) and (7), is critical in linking the survival distributions to the underlying infectivity function. Since retrospective data rarely contain detailed information about the contact rate function, constant rates are usually assumed.

4.2. Representations of the Infectivity Function

By now it has become evident that the calculation of probabilities associated with transmission (and hence estimation and inference) depend critically on the form of $\lambda(\cdot)$. This section reviews some possible models for $\lambda(\cdot)$, several of which also appeared in Kim and Lagakos (1990).

The simplest representations of infectivity assume that $\lambda(\cdot)$ changes deterministically in time following infection of the index case. In fact, the development of survival functions in Section 4.1 essentially assumed a deterministic $\lambda(\cdot)$. Special cases of deterministic $\lambda(\cdot)$ include the constant model

$$\lambda(\cdot) \equiv \lambda$$

and the model obtained by restricting $\lambda(\cdot)$ to be a step function taking values in [0, 1], with jumps at fixed time points:

$$\lambda(t) = \lambda_j \qquad \text{for } t \in [t_{j-1}, t_j); j = 1, 2, \ldots, p$$

Biologically more plausible models are obtained by allowing $\lambda(\cdot)$ to depend on factors associated with the disease process in the index case. For example, there is limited epidemiologic evidence indicating that index cases in later symptomatic stages of infection (e. g., diagnosed with AIDS) transmit the virus more efficiently (Longini *et al.,* 1989; Kim and Lagakos, 1990). This leads to the consideration of stochastic models for $\lambda(\cdot)$. Assume the disease progression in the index case can be represented as a stochastic process $\{X(t)\}_{t\geq 0}$, where $X(t)$ gives the stage of disease at time t and there are p stages. Let λ_j be the infectivity associated with the jth stage. Then $\lambda(\cdot)$ can be written

$$\lambda(t, X(t)) = \lambda_j, \qquad \text{when } X(t) = j; j = 1, 2, \ldots, p$$

Longini *et al.* (1989) considered a similar model assuming $X(t)$ was a homogeneous Markov process. The following more general expression for a stochastic infectivity function is related to models for stochastic hazard functions considered by Rockower (1986) and Jewell and Kalbfleisch (1992):

$$\lambda(t, X(t)) = \lambda_0(t) + \beta X(t), \qquad \beta > 0$$

Here, $\lambda_0(t)$ represents a "background" infectivity function that is modified by the disease status process $X(t)$ in an additive fashion. The previous equation for $\lambda(t, X(t))$ can be considered a special case of this model.

Validation of stochastic infectivity models will require a better knowledge of the biology of HIV transmission and disease progression. Because of the retrospective nature of most available partner study data, information on disease stage of the index case, especially during the period of contact with the partner, is very sparse. For this reason, the remainder of this chapter emphasizes deterministic infectivity functions $\lambda(\cdot)$. If the infectivity is assumed to be stochastic, then estimates of $\lambda(x)$ can perhaps be interpreted as approximations to the average of the underlying infectivity at time x.

4.3. Regression Models for Additional Explanatory Covariates

In applications of the models developed above, it is desirable to incorporate partnership variation in infectivity that can be attributed to observed covariates. Covariates may include information on the index case or the partner (e. g., age, presence of concomitant sexually transmitted diseases or other infections) or information on the type and nature of the partnership (e. g., use of condoms in sexual intercourse, mode of sexual intercourse). As demonstrated in the previous section, the proportional hazards model is naturally linked to several transmission models. For example, if $(y, u, t, \mu, \mathbf{z})$ are observed, and $\mathbf{z}$ denotes the observed value of an m-dimensional covariate vector, the assumption of proportional hazards (Kalbfleisch and Prentice, 1980) leads to the model

$$S(v \mid u, \mu, \mathbf{z}) = [S_0(v \mid u, \mu)]^{\exp(\beta \cdot \mathbf{z})} \tag{11}$$

where β is a $1 \times m$ vector of regression covariates, and $S_0(v \mid u, \mu)$ represents the baseline survival function defined in (7) when $\mathbf{z} = 0$. An analogous regression model can be defined for $S(v \mid u, k, \mathbf{z})$ in (6). The constant infectivity versions of (6) and (7) in equations (9) and (10) are special cases. The above assumes that the covariate $\mathbf{z}$ does not change over time; handling time-dependent covariates is more complex.

5. ANALYSIS OF PARTNER STUDY DATA

This section provides a brief overview of methods for analysis of partner study data, including a review of available statistical models, estimation methods and inference techniques. The emphasis is on data from retrospective partner studies; modifications for data from other study designs are straightforward. Most of what is discussed is treated in greater detail in Jewell and Shiboski (1990) and Shiboski and Jewell (1992).

5.1. Data Analysis Strategies

As outlined in Section 3.2, the basic data provided by partner studies consist of exposure variables (e. g., number and/or rate of contacts and duration of exposure), the serostatus of the partner at a certain point in time (denoted by Y), and covariates relating to demographic characteristics, behavior, and clinical status of both members of the partnership. The fact that the "outcome" variable Y of interest is dichotomous suggests that statistical methods for analysis of binary data can be used to examine the relationship between covariates and transmission probabilities. In particular, logistic regression and contingency table methods based on measures of association such as the odds ratio may provide useful tools for a preliminary assessment of this relationship (see, e. g., De Gruttola et al., 1989). However, for a more complete understanding of how transmission risk depends on exposure and on the underlying infectivity, statistical methods linking the transmission models presented in Section 4 to the observed data are desirable. The regression framework introduced in Section 4 provides this link.

As discussed in Sections 4.1 and 4.3, the basic transmission model (7) is a form of the ubiquitous proportional hazards model (11). One well-known property of this model is that a complementary log–log transformation applied to (11) yields a linear relationship between the survival probability, the baseline survival function, and the covariates. Applying this transformation to (7) leads to the equation

$$\log[-\log S(u + t\,|\,u, \mu)] = \log \int_{u}^{u+t} \lambda(x)\mu(x)dx$$

which, in the special case where contact rates are constant (as must be assumed for most data collected from retrospective study designs), becomes

$$\log[-\log S(u + t\,|\,u, \mu)] = \log \int_{u}^{u+t} \lambda(x)dx + \log\mu \qquad (12)$$

The complementary log–log transformation of the transmission probability yields a regression model that is a special case of (11) in linearized form, the intercept term being a function of the infectivity function $\lambda(\cdot)$, and the "independent variable" the logarithm of the contact rate with slope fixed at unity. Under the further assumption of constant infectivity, the previous expression simplifies [via (10)] to

$$\log[-\log S(u + t\,|\,u, \mu)] = \log\lambda + \log\mu t \qquad (13)$$

Similarly, under the assumption of constant infectivity, the transmission model (6) simplifies to the linear model

$$\log[-\log S(u + t\,|\,u, k)] = \log[-\log(1 - \lambda)] + \log k \qquad (14)$$

which is a transformed version of the classical constant infectivity model (9). This model applies to situations in which the contact count k is observed rather than the rate μ.

Both (13) and (14) are generalized linear regression models (McCullagh and Nelder, 1989) for the binary response Y with complementary log–log link functions. The difference between these models is quite subtle, involving the dependence of the transmission probabilities derived in Section 4.1 on the underlying exposure variables. However, for most available partner study data they yield almost identical results. In the sequel, we will focus on model (14) in investigating the constant infectivity assumption rather than the closely related model (13), mainly because of the greater familiarity of the former as a form of the classical constant infectivity model [(9) and (3)].

A vector z of additional covariates can be incorporated into all of the above models, giving [in the case of (12)] the more general model

$$\log[-\log S(u + t\,|\,u, \mu, z)] = \log \int_{u}^{u+t} \lambda(x)dx + \log\mu + \beta \cdot z$$

where β represents the associated vector of regression coefficients as in (11).

5.2. Estimation Methods

Recall the "partnership" version of the chain binomial transmission model (2) presented in Section 2. Given a form for the transmission probability P (or equivalently for $S = 1 - P$), (2) specifies the likelihood function for a single partnership. Using this basic result, the likelihood functions for a variety of data structures are easy to write down. Consider a sample of n partnerships from a retrospective design, each providing an observation on the random variables (Y, U, T, M) of the form (y_i, u_i, t_i, μ_i). As shown in Shiboski and Jewell (1992), the conditional likelihood (conditioning on U, T, and M) for the sample is given by

$$L = \prod_{i=1}^{n} (1 - S(u_i + t_i | u_i, \mu_i))^{y_i} S(u_i + t_i | u_i, \mu_i)^{1-y_i} \tag{15}$$

where S is the survival function (7), or a simplified version thereof. The likelihood functions for other data structures considered in Section 3 can be derived in an analogous fashion to (15).

Parameter estimates for the models presented above can be obtained by substituting the chosen form for $S(u_i + t_i | u_i, \mu_i)$ into (15) and applying iterative maximum likelihood methods. For the constant infectivity models (13) and (14), this yields a standard parametric likelihood, and software for generalized linear models such as GLIM (Baker and Nelder, 1978) and S (Pregibon and Hastie, 1991) will provide parameter estimates and associated standard errors. Estimation for the more general time-dependent model (12) is complicated by the intercept term, which, unless the infectivity $\lambda(\cdot)$ is given a parametric form, is a nonparametric function of the observed values of the random variables U and T that define the interval of exposure. Shiboski and Jewell (1992) adopt a semiparametric approach to estimation of this model, allowing the intercept term to remain unspecified, and applying maximum likelihood techniques based on the EM algorithm to estimate $\lambda(\cdot)$. By assuming a certain degree of smoothness in the underlying infectivity, estimates with better numerical properties are obtained. The smoothness is incorporated directly into the estimation procedure using a penalized likelihood modification of the EM algorithm proposed by Bacchetti (1990). In this procedure, a smoothing parameter (referred to as θ in the examples in Section 6) and a roughness penalty are incorporated into the maximization step of the EM algorithm. By varying the value of this parameter, a range of smoothness in resulting infectivity estimates can be explored.

In the case where all partnerships are long-term [see (8)], estimation for the time-dependent models is somewhat simplified by noting that the integral in the intercept term must satisfy monotonicity constraints. In fact, for long-term partnerships, (12) (with $u = 0$) is an example of a binary generalized additive model (Hastie and Tibshirani, 1986) and is also a special case of the additive isotonic models studied by Bacchetti (1989). Estimates of $\log \int_0^t \lambda(x)dx$ and the additional parameters β are obtained using a modification of the "backfitting" procedure for generalized additive models using isotonic regression and weighted least-squares estimation in an alternating projection algorithm proposed by Dykstra (1983). This procedure has the advantage that the EM algorithm and smoothness assumptions are unnecessary, and leads to faster convergence than in the general case.

5.3. Inference Techniques

5.3.1. Evaluating the Constant Infectivity Assumption

As discussed in Section 2, most descriptions of infectious disease transmission are based on the premise that the infectivity is a constant common to all infective–susceptible interactions. Although the constant model never provides a completely accurate description of transmission for any disease, it has the advantages that it is easily interpretable, can be readily fit to data using existing techniques, and provides a simple means of linking transmission risk to exposure information and other covariates. Beginning an analysis with examination of the constant model provides a null model against which more complex models can be compared. Detailed examination of observed deviations in fit from the constant model may lead to evidence for partnership heterogeneity in infectivity and/or variation in infectiousness and susceptibility with time following index case infection. For these reasons, most analyses of partner study data begin with an evaluation of the plausibility of constant infectivity.

By suppressing the dependence of the transmission probability $P_i = 1 - S_i$ on the underlying exposure variables, setting $\alpha = \log[-\log(1 - \lambda)]$, and letting k refer to the observed number of contacts in (9), the constant infectivity model (14) can be written:

$$\log[-\log S_i] = \alpha + \log k_i \tag{16}$$

assuming that the number of contacts k_i is measured for each individual. Note that a similar equation follows from (10) and (13), corresponding to a version of the constant infectivity model appropriate for data in which only the (constant) contact rate function μ, rather than the number of contacts, is observed [see (13)]. The goodness of fit of model (16) can be checked graphically by grouping the data over $\log k$, and plotting observed grouped values of

$\log[-\log S]$ against $\log k$. A natural alternative to (16) allowing for a more flexible relationship between the transmission probability and the exposure is given by

$$\log[-\log S_i] = \alpha + \gamma \log k_i \tag{17}$$

Tests of the null hypothesis $\gamma = 1$ (i. e., the adequacy of the constant model) can then be based on estimates of γ, the score vector, or the likelihood ratio method. For values of γ that differ from one, (17) gives transmission probabilities that increase faster or slower in k than predicted by the constant model (16).

Although model (17) generalizes (16) to allow for the possibility of a nonconstant infectivity function $\lambda(\cdot)$, many other deviations from constant infectivity are clearly possible and may be biologically more relevant. Still, model (17) has several advantages as a preliminary alternative to the constant model: first, it provides a simple means of detection of infectivities that increase with the number of contacts in a faster or slower fashion than predicted by a constant infectivity function; second, it is easily fit with available software for generalized linear models. Finally, membership in the same family of generalized linear models as (16) allows assessment of the impact of heterogeneity in infectivity, selection bias, and measurement error in independent variables on interpretations of infectivity estimates using existing methods, as discussed below and in Section 6. In addition, the effects of other fixed covariates can be easily incorporated. For model (17), addition of a vector $\mathbf{z}$ of covariates yields the regression model

$$\log[-\log S_i] = \alpha + \gamma \log k_i + \beta \cdot \mathbf{z} \tag{18}$$

5.3.2. Heterogeneity of Infectivity

As discussed in Section 2.1, one explanation for lack of fit of the constant model is variation in the infectivity λ across partnerships. This allows for the assumption of a constant infectivity function within a specific partnership, but is more flexible than (16) in that the infectivity constant may be different for different partnerships. Random heterogeneity in infectiousness as an alternative to the assumption of constant infectivity across partnerships has been explored extensively in the context of the chain binomial model (Becker, 1989) and for HIV transmission between sex partners by Wiley et al. (1989) and De Gruttola et al. (1989).

Heterogeneity can be naturally introduced into the constant model (16) by allowing λ to be an (unobserved) random effect with some distribution $G(\lambda)$ across partnerships; i. e.,

$$\log[-\log S_i] = \log[-\log(1 - \lambda_i)] + \log k_i = \alpha_i + \log k_i \qquad (19)$$

with α_i ($i = 1, \ldots, n$) representing an (unobserved) i.i.d. sample from a probability distribution induced by G. The impact of heterogeneity can be evaluated by assuming a form for this distribution, and considering the consequence of fitting model (17) to data that are actually generated from a population following model (19). This is considered in detail by Jewell and Shiboski (1990), who show that the unit slope associated with the variable $\log k_i$ in (19) is underestimated in fitting model (17), which ignores the heterogeneity. That is, the estimate of γ based on (17) will typically be less than 1 as in (19). They also show that the size of this attenuation depends primarily on the variance of the distribution G, which is directly related to the degree of heterogeneity present. If substantial attenuation is observed in the estimated coefficient $\hat{\gamma}$ from model (17), it seems reasonable to expect that the estimate of the intercept α would be affected as well. This is indeed the case. As shown in Jewell and Shiboski (1990), heterogeneity in infectivity as defined above will result in an estimate $\hat{\alpha}$ that systematically overestimates the location of the distribution of α (and hence the distribution of λ), if model (17) is fit when (19) in fact holds.

5.3.3. Measurement Error in Exposure Data

The development so far has assumed that the exposure variables U, T, M, and K are measured without error. Errors may arise because these variables are retrospectively ascertained, or in situations where the infection date of the index case is not known exactly. Clearly from Fig. 2, errors in this date have the effect that estimates of the duration of exposure T and number K or rate M of exposed contacts will be subject to considerable error. Even in cases where the index infection dates are known precisely (e. g., transfusion-associated infections), it can be expected that the rate (M) or count (K) of contacts is inaccurately measured.

When fitting model (16) or (17), there is no effect of fixed systematic overestimation (underestimation) of $\log k$ in estimating the regression coefficient of $\log k$ although the intercept, and thus infectivity, will be underestimated (overestimated). Jewell and Shiboski (1990) consider the effects of random measurement error in the contact counts in the context of model (16) adapting methods developed for generalized linear models by Stefanski (1985). The results show that ignoring random measurement error can lead to attenuation in estimated regression coefficients, analogous to the effect of ignoring heterogeneity of infectivity discussed above. In the context of model (16), measurement error in the observed number of contacts will cause the regression coefficient for log$k$ to be attenuated from 1, the true regression coefficient. The approximate attenuation in $\hat{\gamma}$ from fitting (17) can be calculated using Stefanski's approach. By calculating attenuations from a range of possible measurement error variances and comparing with attenuations observed in $\hat{\gamma}$ from fitting (17), it is possible to assess the extent to which measurement error explains the observed deviation from the constant infectivity model (16). In a similar fashion to the effect of heterogeneity discussed in the previous section, measurement error may also lead to substantial overestimation of the intercept α (and hence the infectivity).

5.3.4. Selection Bias in Retrospective Studies

Another condition that may lead to biased estimates of regression coefficients is differential selection of partnerships with infected partners ($Y = 1$) and those with uninfected partners ($Y = 0$). As discussed in Section 3.4, retrospective partner studies often consist of volunteers, and selection probabilities may be influenced by factors such as recruiting practices, length of the incubation period of the index case and/or partner, and partners' knowledge of their HIV status. Dependence of selection probabilities on the partner's serostatus can lead to biased estimates of regression coefficients in binary regression models. This phenomenon has been studied extensively in the context of case–control studies in epidemiology: it is well known that regression coefficients from the logistic regression model applied to case–control data are not subject to bias from unequal recruitment probabilities for cases and controls (Breslow and Day, 1980). However, binary regression models based on link functions other than the logistic, such as the complementary log–log in models (12)–(18), will yield biased estimates of regression coefficients when sampling probabilities for the two types of partnerships differ (McCullagh and Nelder, 1989). This bias can be approximated and expressed as a function of the (true) regression coefficients, and the ratio of the sampling probabilities for infected ($Y = 1$) and uninfected ($Y = 0$) partners, respectively. Figure 3 displays approximate values of the bias in an estimated slope coefficient for a range of values of the ratio of sampling probabilities (on the horizontal axis) and intercept coefficients, assuming the regression model (17). The vertical axis can be interpreted as giving the expected value of the estimated regression coefficient $\hat{\gamma}$ from model (17) under different assumptions about the sampling probabilities and underlying infectivity. Figure 3 illustrates that, unlike bias resulting from measurement error and heterogeneity, selection bias can either attenuate or inflate estimates of regression coefficients from their true values. Attenuation results when the selection probability for infected partners is greater than that for uninfected partners, the effect becoming more extreme for larger values of the intercept [corresponding to larger infectivity in (17)]

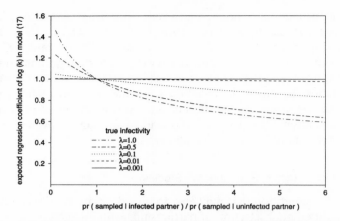

Figure 3. Approximate bias resulting from differential selection probabilities for partnerships with infected versus uninfected partners. The vertical scale gives the expected value of the estimate of the coefficient γ in model (17) as a function of the ratio of selection probabilities and the magnitude of the underlying infectivity λ, assuming that the true model is given by (16), with $\alpha = \log\left[-\log\left(1 - \lambda\right)\right]$.

and larger ratio of selection probabilities. A considerably more problematic version of selection bias will arise if selection depends on both the serostatus of the partner Y, *and* the independent variable $\log k$, or if selection operates through an unobserved variable that is correlated with both the outcome variable Y and the number of contacts K (such as, potentially, a variable that measures the health status of the index case). That is, for example, if partners who are already infected are over or underselected.

5.3.5. Inference for Time-Varying Infectivity Models

Another possible source of lack of fit of the constant infectivity model is variation of infectiousness and susceptibility with time following infection of the index case. There is biological evidence (discussed in Section 2) that HIV infectivity does vary in this manner. It is of course also possible that HIV infectivity varies between partnerships *and* with time. Model (12) allows these issues to be investigated in a regression framework paralleling that developed above for the constant infectivity case. However, formal inferential comparison of various models is difficult because of the nonparametric nature of the estimates of $\lambda(\cdot)$. For example, the deviance (-2 maximized log-likelihood) can be computed and compared across models, but changes in deviance cannot be compared directly to a χ^2 distribution as is the standard practice for parametric generalized linear models (McCullagh and Nelder,

1989). Ad hoc tests for deviance reductions can be based on simulations, or on permutation or randomization distributions. Some examples of this will be illustrated in Section 6. Alternatively, pointwise confidence intervals for $\lambda(\cdot)$ or other parameters can be calculated using the bias-corrected percentile method of Efron (1985), based on replicate bootstrap samples with replacement from the original data.

Similar to the constant infectivity case discussed above, sources of lack of fit of model (12) include (i) heterogeneity in the infectivity function $\lambda(\cdot)$ across partnerships that is not accounted for by covariates and (ii) random measurement error in the self-reported μ_i's. Random variations in $\lambda(\cdot)$ may arise from biological heterogeneity in the infectiousness of the index case, susceptibility of the partner, or the nature of the contacts. Recall that in the constant infectivity case, the consequence of both (i) and (ii) is a dilution of the slope of the fixed offset (in this case, $\log\mu$) from one toward zero and a bias in estimation of the infectivity, λ. For the time-dependent model (12) the effects of heterogeneity and measurement error have no simple interpretation. Shiboski and Jewell (1992) argue that ignoring such heterogeneity should result in a dilution of the slope of the covariate $\log\mu_i$ down from one, and bias in estimation of the value of $\int_u^{u+t} \lambda(x)dx$. As a result, the estimated shape and scale of $\lambda(\cdot)$ will be distorted by heterogeneity. A possible check for the existence of heterogeneity is to fit model (12) with an arbitrary slope γ attached to the covariate $\log\mu$. Then, analogous to (17), (12) becomes

$$\log[-\log S(u + t \,|\, u, \mu)] = \log \int_u^{u+t} \lambda(x)dx + \gamma \log\mu \qquad (20)$$

A positive estimate $\hat{\gamma}$ from this model that is significantly less than one may therefore indicate evidence of heterogeneity or the presence of measurement error.

In a similar fashion, if $\log\mu$ is measured with error, the slope of $\log\mu$ is diluted from one toward zero, and estimates of the general level of $\lambda(\cdot)$ will be biased. Furthermore, the estimated shape of $\lambda(\cdot)$ (and estimates of other covariate effects) may be altered, possibly even involving changes in direction. In addition, for many partner studies, the variables U and T defining the exposure interval may be observed with substantial error, caused by uncertainty regarding the date of infection of the index case. As $\log\mu$, this error may lead to distorted estimation of the regression coefficients of $\log\mu$ and other covariates, as well as the level and shape of $\lambda(\cdot)$. Thus the presence of a significant amount of either heterogeneity in infectivity properties or measurement error in contact rates severely limits interpretability of either the scale or shape of an estimated infectivity function $\lambda(\cdot)$.

In cases where the infectivity function $\lambda(\cdot)$ is not assumed to be constant, a further complication arises if the contact rate function $\mu(\cdot)$ is assumed constant as in (12). In general, as illustrated in Section 5.1, the transmission probability S, and hence the likelihood function, depends on $\lambda(\cdot)$ and $\mu(\cdot)$ solely through their product $\lambda(\cdot)\mu(\cdot)$. Hence, if $\mu(\cdot)$ is incorrectly assumed to be constant, systematic deviations from this assumption will be "picked up" in estimates of $\lambda(\cdot)$. Thus, declines of $\hat{\lambda}(\cdot)$ over a certain period of time may simply reflect a systematic decline of $\mu_i(\cdot)$ from a constant value over that same period. Time-varying observation of $\mu_i(\cdot)$ over the exposure period would overcome this difficulty, but this may be impossible for data collected retrospectively. In the absence of such data, systematic time variations in $\lambda(\cdot)$ are essentially confounded with systematic variations in $\mu(\cdot)$.

Finally, we note that the effect of additional covariates can be examined by generalizing (18) as follows:

$$\log[-\log S(u + t \mid u, \mu)] = \log \int_u^{u+t} \lambda(x)dx + \gamma \log\mu + \beta \cdot \mathbf{z} \qquad (21)$$

Of course, as in all observational studies, unobserved confounding variables can influence estimates of $\lambda(\cdot)$, γ, and β in (21).

5.3.6. Summary

To summarize the results regarding bias in regression coefficients for models presented above, deviation from constant infectivity as indicated by either the constant model (17) or the more general time-dependent model (20) in the form of observation of an estimated γ less than one can be explained in (at least) three ways: there may exist partnership heterogeneity in the underlying infectivity, random errors in measurement of the exposure data, or differing selection probabilities for partnerships with infected and uninfected partners (or all three may be present to varying degrees). To the extent that measurement error and selection bias can be ruled out or accounted for, then heterogeneity can be postulated and investigated further as a potential explanation of the lack of fit. On the other hand, if any of these factors remain as possibilities, then it is essentially impossible to use the data to partition the deviation from the assumed model into these three components without further information regarding the variability of the infectivity distribution, the distribution of random errors in contact counts, or the sampling probabilities. It is also important to note that ignoring any of these factors, even when fitting more general models [such as (17) or (20)], leads to biased estimates of the infectivity, and biased estimates of the effect of other independent variables [z in (18) and (21)].

6. EXAMPLES

6.1. Description of Studies Used

6.1.1. The California Partners' Study

This study is an ongoing investigation of heterosexual HIV transmission in partners of previously infected index cases (Padian *et al.*, 1987). A sample of 212 female partners of male index cases will be considered here. In this study, dates of infection of index cases can only be determined inaccurately. Thus, counts of contacts must be considered as estimates of the true number of contacts since infection of the index case. The eligibility criteria for a woman include (1) prior sexual contact with a man known to be seropositive for HIV, and (2) no other known means of infection. Thus, for example, a woman with a history of intravenous drug abuse is automatically excluded from consideration. In addition, the partnership must be monogamous on the woman's part, i. e., the index case must be the only sexual partner in the relevant period. This aspect of the study was aimed at ensuring that the infected partners of index cases could not have been infected prior to the infection of the index case or from any other mode of transmission during contact with the index case. Aside from self-referral, participants were recruited through referrals from physicians, research studies, and local departments of public health. Upon entry, serum samples were drawn from study subjects to determine status with regard to HIV infection. Furthermore, detailed medical, contraceptive, and behavioral histories were obtained in order to confirm eligibility. As a confirmation of the serostatus of the partners at recruitment, subsequent serum samples were drawn from all subjects who could be followed-up. There were no cases of subsequent seroconversion after the original determination of infection status. The date of infection of the index case was estimated based on interview data and detailed knowledge of the epidemic curve of HIV infections in California. Finally, rates of contact and contact counts were calculated according to interview information relative to the period of the partnership after the infection of the index case.

The California Partners' Study shares limitations common to many retrospective partner studies that must be considered in interpreting results of analyses. First, since the infection date of the index case could only be inaccurately determined, the number of exposed contacts is subject to mismeasurement. Second, most information (including the number of relevant contacts) was collected through interviews, making the data subject to the usual errors associated with interview techniques used to obtain behavioral and sexual activity histories. Finally, the sample of women obtained is clearly not representative of the general population of women at risk for infection through heterosexual contact.

6.1.2. The Peterman Study

This study considers HIV transmission from men to women with repeated vaginal sexual acts where the index case (the male) was originally infected by blood transfusion (Peterman *et al.,* 1988). This data set consists of 55 partnerships, all of which are long-term since each partnership was in existence at the time of the index case's transfusion. Here, the date of infection of the index case is known (or assumed) to be the date of transfusion. Thus, the relevant intervals in which to count contacts are clear. In this study, exposure periods and associated contact rates were ascertained both before and after AIDS diagnosis for index cases who developed AIDS. Here we consider the data from the exposure period prior to an AIDS diagnosis.

6.1.3. Description of Data

The first data set to be considered in the examples is from the California Partners' Study. As discussed above, the dates of infection for the index cases in this study are not known precisely. Therefore, interview information on rates of contacts and length of relationship does not necessarily accurately reflect exposure. This is particularly a problem for long-term partnerships that were formed prior to the time of the index case's infection. To help correct for the problem in the examples, a common infection date for all index cases is assumed. Several dates were chosen in the period 1980–1983, when the rate of new infections in California was known to be at a peak. The analyses reported here assume an infection date of January 1, 1982. Other choices did not change the results substantially. Even in cases where the exposure period is known to have occurred after the index case's infection, inaccuracies in the sexual history data are to be expected because of the retrospective nature of the interview data. Thus, there is a clear need to control for the possible impact of measurement error in the analyses.

Observations on the random variables (Y_i, U_i, T_i, M_i) are available for 212 partnerships, 88 of which are long-term (i. e., $U = 0$). Table 1 provides a breakdown of partnerships by serostatus of the partner at the time of observation (Y_i) and by a grouped measure of duration of exposure (T_i). Table 2 presents a breakdown of the data by serostatus Y and the observed number

Table 1. Seroprevalence Data from the California Partners' Study Grouped by Duration of Exposure

Serostatus of partner	Duration of exposure (months)										Totals
	0–10	11–20	21–30	31–40	41–50	51–60	61–70	71–80	81–90	91–100	
Seropositive	4	8	4	9	7	6	1	2	0	1	42
Seronegative	29	33	23	13	22	27	4	8	10	1	170
Totals	33	41	27	22	29	33	5	10	10	2	212

Table 2. Seroprevalence Data from the California Partners' Study Grouped by Numbers of Contacts

Serostatus of partner	Number of contacts										Totals
	1–10	11–50	51–100	101–200	201–300	301–400	401–600	601–800	801–1500	1501–3500	
Seropositive	1	5	2	3	8	4	8	6	2	3	42
Seronegative	20	24	24	27	18	13	11	15	15	3	170
Totals	21	29	26	30	26	17	19	21	17	6	212

of contacts K, grouped into ten intervals. Figure 4 graphically displays the duration of observed exposure periods of the 212 partnerships relative to the date of infection of the index case. For both the full data set and the long-term partnerships the range of t_i's observed is (1, 92) in months. Note that the majority of small values of t arise from partnerships that began some time after infection of the index case.

The second data set considered in the examples is from the Peterman partner study. For the 55 partnerships in this study, the range of observed exposure periods is (4, 67) in months; all partnerships were long-term. Unlike the California Partners' Study, the date of infection of the index case is known

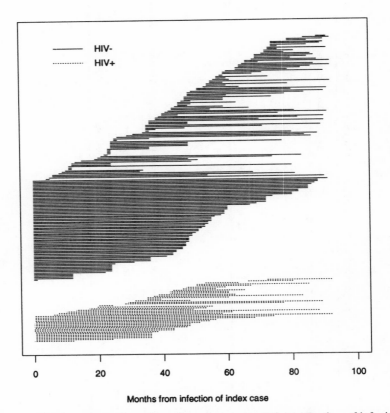

Months from infection of index case

Figure 4. Graphical presentation of durations of exposure relative to the time of infection of the index case for the California Partners' Study. The top group (solid lines) shows uninfected partners ($Y_i = 0$); the lower group (dotted lines) is infected partners ($Y_i = 1$). Here, the infection status of partners (Y_i) refers to their status at recruitment (the right-hand endpoint of the lines shown).

(or assumed) to be the date of transfusion. Thus, measurement error in exposure data for the Peterman Study is less likely to arise from uncertainty about the duration of exposure. Four partnerships were excluded because it could not be determined whether infection of the partner occurred before or after AIDS diagnosis in the index case.

6.2. Results from Fitting the Constant Infectivity Model

Figure 5 displays the fit of the constant infectivity model (16) to the California Partners' Study data. The more general model (17) is also shown. The empirical complementary log–log transformed values of the grouped proportions of seropositive partners in Table 1 are shown for reference. From Fig. 5, it is immediately apparent that the constant model fits the data poorly, whereas model (17) provides a somewhat better fit. In particular, the constant model underestimates the risk of infection after a small number of contacts. Comparison of the general model (17) to the constant model (16) shows a reduction in deviance of 21.58 yielding a p value of less than 0.0001 when compared with a $\chi^2_{(1)}$ distribution. The estimated slope coefficient for the variable $\log k$ is $\hat{\gamma} = 0.32$, indicating substantial attenuation from unity, the value consistent with the constant model (16).

Models (16) and (17) were also fit to the Peterman Study data. The reduction in deviance achieved for model (17) over model (16) was 16.98, in-

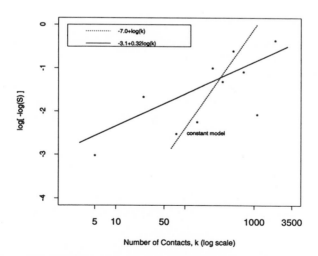

Figure 5. Plots of the fitted lines corresponding to the constant infectivity model (16) (solid line) and its generalization (17) (dotted line).

dicating a poor fit of the constant model. The slope coefficient γ from the fit of (17) was negative (-0.33), indicating decreasing prevalence of infection in partners with increasing numbers of contacts. A value of γ close to zero indicates little or no dependence of partner infection on duration of exposure (or on number of contacts). This observation has led a number of investigators to conclude that transmission probability for sexual transmission in monogamous partnerships may be unrelated to degree of exposure as measured by the number of contacts (Anderson and May, 1988; Kaplan, 1990; Wiley *et al.*, 1989). However, the coefficient here is negative; this apparent anomaly will be discussed further below in the context of time-varying infectivity.

6.2.1. Heterogeneity of Infectivity in the Constant Model

Since the observed slope in model (17) for the California Partners' Study is 0.32 (see Fig. 5), it appears that an infectivity distribution with a large variance relative to the mean must be hypothesized to explain the observed deviation of γ from 1 (Jewell and Shiboski, 1990). In particular, for heterogeneity to explain the lack of fit of the basic model, it is necessary to propose relatively extreme dispersion in infectivities associated with different partnerships, with a substantial number possessing very low or high values of λ. Finally, as shown in Jewell and Shiboski (1990), ignoring the heterogeneity of infectivity, even when fitting the more general model (17), has the consequence of overestimating infectivity properties.

6.2.2. Error in Measurement of k

To evaluate the impact of random measurement error in $\log K$ on estimates from model (17) for the California Partners' Study data, the methods discussed in Section 5 and in Jewell and Shiboski (1990) were used to estimate attenuations in $\hat{\alpha}$ and $\hat{\gamma}$ that would be expected for a range of measurement error variances in $\log K$ (i. e., multiplicative error in K). For example, for a true $\alpha = -7.00$, and $\gamma = 1$ and constant variance of the measurement error in $\log K = \sigma^2 = 0.01$, the predicted slope (intercept) when fitting model (17), ignoring the measurement error, is 0.99 (-6.85) if (16) is true.

As reported in Jewell and Shiboski (1990), the attenuations in γ remain stable over a range of α's that covers most published infectivity estimates. Thus, in order to explain entirely the lack of fit of model (16), it is necessary to invoke an enormous variance in (multiplicative) random error (i. e., an error variance in $\log k$ much larger than 0.35). For the California Partners' Study, therefore, it is likely that measurement error accounts only for a small part of the attenuation of the observed slope in model (17) from the slope 1 implicit in the constant model (16). The impact of the attenuation that occurs because of measurement error also only mitigates somewhat our statements above regarding the level of heterogeneity necessary to account for the remaining difference in the observed slope from 1. However, as shown in Jewell and Shiboski (1990), random measurement error in $\log K$ can lead to a substantial overestimation of α and thus the infectivity for relatively smaller measurement error variances.

6.2.3. Inclusion of Potential Confounding Covariates

In order to illustrate the effects of additional covariates in the California Partners' Study, a number of partnership variables were considered. Twenty partnerships were not used in this analysis since they had incomplete information on at least one covariate of interest. The first three variables analyzed were binary covariates that, respectively, assume the value 1 if (i) the partners report participation in anal intercourse, (ii) the partner reports (nonmenstrual) bleeding during intercourse, and (iii) race is nonwhite, and assume the value 0, respectively, otherwise. An additional covariate considered was the logarithm of the age of the partner. The decline in deviance when these are included in model (18) versus using model (17) was 9.54, which yields a p value of 0.05 when compared with a $\chi^2_{(4)}$ distribution. Estimated coefficients (and their standard errors) from model (18) using these three variables are reported in Table 3.

Next, a binary covariate Z that took the value 0 if the partners reported use of condoms during intercourse and 1, otherwise, was considered. A main

Table 3. Coefficient Estimates (and Standard Errors) from Fitting Two Versions of Model (18)[a]

Covariate	Coefficient (S.E.)	
	Model A	Model B
$\log k$	0.309 (0.15)	0.706 (0.41)
$\log(\text{age})$	0.864 (0.79)	0.319 (0.83)
Bleeding	1.097 (0.45)	1.063 (0.46)
Anal intercourse	0.466 (0.41)	0.435 (0.42)
Nonwhite race	0.363 (0.43)	0.280 (0.44)
No condom use		3.575 (2.54)
No condom use $\times \log k$		−0.467 (0.44)

[a] Model A includes main effect terms for $\log(\text{age})$ and covariates measuring participation in anal intercourse, experience of bleeding during intercourse, and race, in addition to $\log k$. Model B includes further terms to incorporate the main effect of use of condoms together with the interaction of this variable with $\log k$.

effect term for Z in (18) was included, together with an interaction term for Z with log$K$, together with the other four covariates discussed above. Figure 6 describes the fitted relationship between the transmission probability (P) and log$K$ for $Z = 0$ and $Z = 1$ separately, while controlling for the other covariates. The addition of these extra two terms produced a reduction in deviance of 5.84 yielding a p value 0.05 when compared with a $\chi^2_{(2)}$ distribution. Estimated coefficients from this version of model (18) are also given in Table 3. The estimated slope of log$K$ when $Z = 0$ is 0.71, which is much closer to 1 than that observed for the full set of data. That is, the constant infectivity model fits the data for condom users considerably better. Necessarily, the basic model for the noncondom users has slope of log$K = 0.24$, which is fairly similar to the results obtained above for the full set of data before adjustment for Z. It may be plausible to suggest different measurement error distributions in the two groups as an explanation for this difference in slopes. A more appealing interpretation suggests that the use of condoms removes much of the heterogeneity in infectivity that may affect noncondom users. The observed attenuation in slope for condom users is compatible with the impact of measurement error as discussed in Section 5.3. Note that, as expected, estimates of infectivity for condom users based on the models of Fig. 6 and Table 3 are much lower than those for nonusers. Finally, we reiterate the remarks of Section 5.3, which indicate that the estimated regression coefficients given in

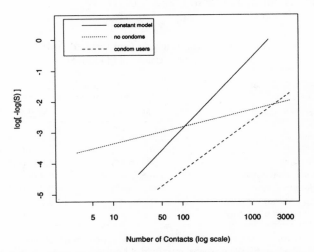

Figure 6. Plots of the fitted lines corresponding to the generalized constant infectivity model (17) applied to condom users and nonusers separately. The basic constant infectivity model (16) applied to the complete set of data has slope 1 by definition and is also shown for comparison.

Table 3 are distorted estimates of the true effects of the associated cofactors if either heterogeneity or measurement error is operating.

6.2.4. Selection Bias

The fit of model (16) to the California Partners' Study data yields an estimated intercept of -7.0 (or an estimated λ of 0.001). Figure 3 then suggests that the ratio of sampling fractions for partnerships with an infected partner to those with an uninfected partner would need to be very large to induce any noticeable influence on the observed slope of $\log k$ in (17). Thus, this kind of retrospective sampling phenomenon, even if present in the collection of data for the California Partners' Study, is unlikely to explain the observed deviation of $\hat{\gamma}$ from unity when model (17) is fit.

6.3. Results from Fitting Time-Dependent Infectivity Models

For the California Partners' Study, Fig. 7 gives estimates of $\lambda(\cdot)$ based on data from all partnerships on (Y_i, U_i, T_i, M_i) using the penalized likelihood method of Section 5. Estimates corresponding to differing smoothing parameters (θ) are shown. Note that these estimates of $\lambda(\cdot)$ correspond to fitting model (12). The corresponding estimates of the cumulative infectivity function, $\int_0^t \lambda(x)dx$, are also shown. Note that estimates of the cumulative function are quite robust to varying the amount of smoothness desired in estimates of $\lambda(\cdot)$.

Figure 8 illustrates pointwise 95% confidence intervals for $\lambda(\cdot)$, arising from (12) with smoothing parameter $\theta = 5000$, and using the bias-corrected percentile method based on 1000 bootstrap samples as discussed in Section 3.5. A summary of the information on $\lambda(\cdot)$ that can be inferred from Figs. 7 and 8 is that the infectivity function remains relatively flat until around 40 months when it begins to decline. Of course, the decline can be attributed to a general decline in the contact rate function $\mu(\cdot)$, in the partnerships at the same time rather than any change in the infectivity function as discussed in Section 5.3.5. Note the uncertainty surrounding estimation of $\lambda(x)$ for $x < 20$ months, which arises from the paucity of partnerships with both data values $(u, u + t)$ in this range. It is therefore not possible to rule out a rapid decline in the infectivity function over this period (consistent with the laboratory observations discussed in Section 2), although the "point estimate" itself does not reflect this characteristic.

We now turn to consider the effects of partnership heterogeneity and measurement error in the contact rates. As discussed in Section 5, one simple approach to investigating the presence of these effects is to fit model (20) and examine the estimate $\hat{\gamma}$ for attenuation. Figure 9 shows estimates of $\lambda(\cdot)$ and $\int_0^t \lambda(x)dx$ for both models (12) and (20) using smoothing parameter $\theta = 5000$

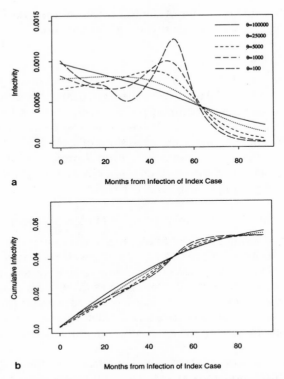

Figure 7. Estimates of the (a) infectivity, $\lambda(\cdot)$ (the monthly per-contact infection hazard for uninfected partners of infected index cases), and the (b) cumulative infectivity, $\int_0^t \lambda(x)dx$, based on fitting model (12) to the California Partners' Study data (displayed in Fig. 4), using penalized maximum likelihood methods, and various values of the smoothing parameter θ.

in both cases. Figure 10 gives the pointwise 95% confidence interval for $\lambda(\cdot)$, based on (20), using 1000 bootstrap samples as before. As noted, the point estimate of γ from (20) is given by $\hat{\gamma} = 0.40$ for the California Partners' Study. From the bootstrap samples, the 95% bias-corrected confidence interval for γ is (0.04, 0.86).

   The fact that $\hat{\gamma}$ differs significantly from 1 suggests the existence of heterogeneity and measurement error (and, possibly, the effects of other confounding partnership covariates). Although it is extremely difficult to distinguish the relative impact of these sources on goodness-of-fit, the results presented above for the constant model indicate that partnership heterogeneity is likely to be the most plausible explanation of the difference between $\hat{\gamma}$ and

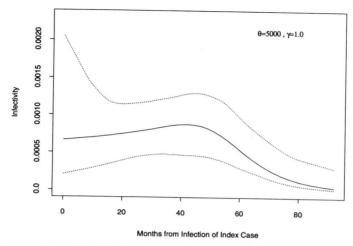

Figure 8. An estimate of $\lambda(\cdot)$ based on (12) with smoothing parameter $\theta = 5000$. The solid line is the estimate and the dotted lines are pointwise 95% confidence intervals estimated by the bias-corrected percentile method using 1000 with replacement samples from the data set.

unity. However, as discussed in Section 5, a substantial amount of heterogeneity is required to produce values of $\hat\gamma$ that are as low as 0.40.

Since $\hat\gamma$ is much less than 1, inclusion of $\log\mu$ with an arbitrary slope makes a substantial difference in estimation of the scale of $\lambda(\cdot)$ and $\int_0^t \lambda(x)dx$. We caution, however, that the presence of heterogeneity and measurement error induces bias in estimation of $\lambda(\cdot)$ and $\int_0^t$ even when based on model (20). In either case, the scale of the estimated curves for $\lambda(\cdot)$ and $\int_0^t \lambda(x)dx$ from (20), given in Figs. 9 and 10, tends to overestimate the values of the infectivity and cumulative infectivity function. Thus, it is inappropriate to interpret the vertical scales of Figs. 9 and 10 without additional adjustment. Note, however, that the shape of the estimate of $\lambda(\cdot)$ based on (20) is similar to that based on (12). Since heterogeneity has been postulated as an explanation of the value of $\hat\gamma$, the decline of $\hat\lambda(\cdot)$ after 40 months can also be attributed to the effects of heterogeneity of a true constant infectivity function $\lambda(\cdot)$ (that varies across partnerships), as discussed in Section 5.3.5.

Analyses of data from long-term partnerships will be considered next. Since all partnerships in Peterman's data are long-term, this data set will be analyzed here. Figure 11 shows estimates of $\int_0^t \lambda(x)dx$ based on (12) for both the California Partners' Study and the Peterman data. As discussed in Section 5.2, estimation of the infectivity function is somewhat simplified for long-term partnerships. Because no smoothing is necessary in this case, the estimates take the form of "step functions" as displayed in the figure. In addition,

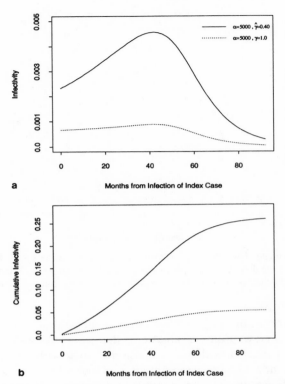

Figure 9. Estimates of the (a) infectivity, $\lambda(\cdot)$, and the (b) cumulative infectivity, $\int_0^t \lambda(x)dx$, based on (12) (dotted line) and (20) (solid line) with smoothing parameter $\theta = 5000$ in each case.

estimates are also given for model (20) for the long-term partnerships. For the California Partners' Study $\hat{\gamma} = 0.26$, whereas for the Peterman data $\hat{\gamma} = -0.37$.

For the California Partners' Study, the curves in Fig. 11 are very similar to those shown in Figs. 5 and 6, although they are plotted as unsmoothed step functions. This suggests that there is no inherent difference in infectivity properties and/or data behavior between long-term and other partnerships; this is most appropriately examined by comparing Fig. 11 with the analogues of Figs. 7 and 9 with the long-term partnerships removed. The curves for the Peterman data are similar to those for the California Partners' Study. Again, there is significant evidence of heterogeneity and/or measurement error. Furthermore, the negative sign of $\hat{\gamma}$ for the Peterman data cannot be explained by heterogeneity or measurement error. It may be the result of the effect of unaccounted confounding partnership covariates as discussed in Jewell and

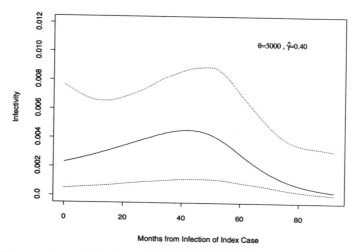

Figure 10. An estimate of $\lambda(\cdot)$ based on (20) with smoothing parameter $\theta = 5000$. The solid line is the estimate and the dotted lines are pointwise 95% confidence intervals estimated by the bias-corrected percentile method using 1000 with replacement samples from the data set.

Shiboski (1990). Unfortunately, no covariate information was available for the Peterman data. For these reasons, extreme caution must therefore be used when interpreting the vertical scale of Fig. 11 for either study.

Tables 4 and 5 give the values of the deviance for a variety of models based on the full data set and the long-term partnerships, respectively. For models 2 and 3 in Table 4, the smoothing parameter θ was set at 5000. Where given, the changes in "dof" refer to changes in degrees of freedom from the previous model as computed by approximating degrees of freedom of a smoother, according to procedures outlined in Buja et al. (1989). The p values associated with changes in deviance are calculated either by referring to a χ^2 distribution with the noted degrees of freedom, or by use of a simulation test. The latter is illustrated by the comparison of models 1 and 2 in Table 4. Here, model 1 refers to (12) with the infectivity function $\lambda(\cdot)$ assumed constant [i.e., model (13)].

From the estimated constant value of λ ($\hat{\lambda} = 0.0007$) from model (1), 100 independent data sets were generated (holding fixed the observed values of u_i, t_i, and μ_i). For each of these data sets, models 1 and 2 were fit and a change in deviance computed. This procedure thus provides an approximate sampling distribution with which the observed change in deviance can be compared. In this case, the change in deviance, 7.62, was larger than that observed for 96 of the 100 simulated data sets [where, of course, the constant $\lambda(\cdot)$ model is correct].

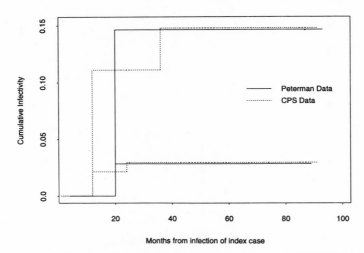

Figure 11. Estimates of the cumulative infectivity, $\int_0^t \lambda(x)dx$, for the California Partners' Study (dotted lines) and the Peterman data (solid lines) based on models (12) (lower curves) and (20) (upper curves).

The results of Tables 4 and 5 indicate evidence of a nonconstant $\lambda(\cdot)$. However, as indicated, this may be explained by either systematic variation in the contact rate function $\mu(\cdot)$ from a constant, or heterogeneity of the infectivity function. In fact, comparisons of models 2 and 3 in either Table 4 or 5 indicate the possibility of significant heterogeneity as discussed above. From Table 5, it appears that a linear function of $\log\mu$ provides an adequate assessment of the role of μ in (20) versus a more general smooth function of μ. Finally, the comparison of models 4 and 5 in Table 5 suggests that the assumption of a monotone function of t on the right-hand side of (20) appears reasonable for both studies.

The same five covariates considered in the constant infectivity case were analyzed using the time-dependent model. Complete information on all five

Table 4. Results of Fitting Models Based on (Y_i, U_i, T_i, M_i), California Partners' Study Data

Model no.	Model	Deviance	Change in deviance	Change in "dof," p value
1	(12), constant $\lambda(\cdot)$	232.36		
2	(12), arbitrary $\lambda(\cdot)$	224.74	7.62	—, $p < 0.05$
3	(20), arbitrary $\lambda(\cdot)$, $\hat{\gamma} = 0.40$	212.26	12.48	1, $p < 0.001$

Table 5. Results of Fitting Models Based on (Y_i, T_i, M_i), California Partners' Study and Peterman Data

Study	Model no.	Model	Deviance	Change in deviance	Change in "dof," p value
CPS	1	(12), constant $\lambda(\cdot)$	102.71		
	2	(12), arbitrary $\lambda(\cdot)$	92.04	10.67	—, $p \approx 0.03$
	3	(20), arbitrary $\lambda(\cdot)$, $\hat{\gamma} = 0.26$	83.69	8.35	1, $p < 0.01$
	4	(20), arbitrary $\lambda(\cdot)$, smooth function of μ	74.77	8.94	4, $p \approx 0.06$
	5	(20), arbitrary smooth functions of t and μ on RHS	71.54	3.21	
Peterman	1	(12), constant $\lambda(\cdot)$	53.36		
	2	(20), arbitrary $\lambda(\cdot)$	50.17	3.19	—, $p \approx 0.3$
	3	(20), arbitrary $\lambda(\cdot)$, $\hat{\gamma} = -0.37$	32.67	17.50	1, $p < 0.001$
	4	(20), arbitrary $\lambda(\cdot)$, smooth function of μ	29.63	3.04	2, $p \approx 0.2$
	5	(20), arbitrary smooth functions of t and μ on RHS	29.57	0.06	

variables was available for 192 of the 212 partnerships of the California Partners' Study. Data from these 192 were fit using two versions of model (21), including the additive term $\beta \cdot \mathbf{z}$ on the right-hand side as described in Section 5.3, where $\mathbf{z}$ is the vector of covariates. The first model includes the binary covariates for participation in anal intercourse, bleeding during intercourse, and nonwhite race, as well as log(age). The decline in deviance when these four covariates are included in (21) (with smoothing parameter $\theta = 5000$) versus the corresponding model excluding the covariates is 8.16 yielding a p value of 0.09 when compared with a $\chi^2_{(4)}$ distribution. Note that the value of $\hat{\gamma}$ from this model is close to that observed when the covariates are excluded, which indicates that the covariates considered do not explain the deviation of γ from 1 that has been noted previously. The next model included a main effect term for the binary indicator of no condom use together with an interaction term for this covariate with $\log\mu$. The addition of these two terms (with smoothing parameter $\theta = 5000$) produced a further reduction in deviance of 10.26 yielding a p value of 0.006 when compared with a $\chi^2_{(2)}$ distribution. Estimated coefficients for both models (designated A and B, respectively) with associated bootstrap estimates of standard errors (based on 100 bootstrap samples) are presented in Table 6.

Inspection of the estimated infectivity functions from both models revealed shapes that were similar to the estimate obtained from fitting (20) excluding covariates. As indicated in Section 5.3, it must be stressed that estimated covariate coefficients are subject to bias in this example because of the possibility of error in measuring U and T (and μ), and potential partnership heterogeneity of infectivity properties.

The slope of $\log\mu$ for condom users is 0.67, which is closer to 1 than that observed for the full set of data, indicating that (20) may provide an adequate

Table 6. Coefficient Estimates and Corresponding (Approximate) Standard Errors from Fitting Two Versions of Model (21), Including Additional Covariates, to the California Partners' Study Data

Covariate	Coefficient (S.E.)	
	Model A	Model B
$\text{Log}\mu$	0.443 (0.22)	0.673 (0.43)
log(age)	0.559 (0.87)	0.145 (1.06)
Bleeding	0.954 (0.50)	0.947 (0.97)
Anal intercourse	0.246 (0.40)	0.256 (0.47)
Nonwhite race	0.262 (0.44)	0.447 (0.51)
No condom use		1.563 (1.14)
No condom use $\times \log\mu$		−0.306 (0.53)

fit to the data for this group of partnerships. The slope of $\log\mu$ for noncondom users is 0.37, which is similar to the value obtained for the full data set. As before, a possible interpretation of the interaction is that condom use removes some of the heterogeneity in infectivity that may affect nonusers. To examine differences in shape and scale of $\hat{\lambda}(\cdot)$ between groups, (20) was fit separately to the data from condom users and nonusers. As expected, the estimate of $\lambda(\cdot)$ for condom users is uniformly smaller than the estimate for nonusers. The shape of the two estimates is very similar to the curves presented in Fig. 9 for the full data set.

7. DISCUSSION

This chapter reviews study design and data analysis issues for studies of sexual HIV transmission in monogamous partnerships. By restricting attention to simple exposures involving a single partner and index case, the methods presented allow estimation of the infectivity, or per-contact probability of virus transmission, and provide a framework for investigating how transmission probabilities depend on duration of exposure and factors associated with infectiousness and susceptibility. In addition, techniques are provided for assessing the impact of heterogeneity of infectivity, measurement error in exposure data, and selection bias on estimates and inferences.

Despite the potential relevance of these methods, the discussion of the methodology and its application to examples indicates the extraordinary difficulty of extracting even the simplest infectivity information, even from partner study data of high quality. Lack of information on the variation of the rate of contacts, the disease status of the index case, and other confounding variables, the possibility of partnership variation in infectiousness or susceptibility, and the presence of measurement error in key variables all restrict the usefulness of partner study data in providing definitive answers to many key questions regarding HIV transmission. These issues are particularly germane to retrospective data but also persist to some extent with prospective data. Further statistical difficulties with prospective designs are related to the probable absence of observed transmissions in partnerships followed prospectively, and the fact that these designs are unlikely to provide data for the period of time immediately following index case infection.

Nevertheless, the examples illustrate that some information on transmission is available from partner study data, even though quantification of the infectivity presents many challenging technical problems. In particular, by comparing results of analyses across partner studies that differ in recruitment strategies, risk characteristics of the index case, and modes of contact, useful information on how HIV transmission varies among subgroups of the population can be obtained. For example, it is possible to compare male-to-female with female-to-male heterosexual transmission using partner study data (Padian *et al.*, 1991).

Several important topics are not addressed, including applications to investigations of transmission in situations where multiple partners and several modes of infectious contact are possible, and incorporation of information on disease stage of the index case into transmission models and infectivity estimates. Although the first of these topics is critically important in describing the dynamics of the AIDS epidemic, the inherent complexity of exposure data in situations where several index cases are possible sources of infection for a given susceptible makes formulation of transmission models and estimation of infectivity a formidable task. Indeed, the difficulties encountered in obtaining reliable infectivity information in the monogamous partnership setting summarized above indicate that extensions of the methods presented here to more complicated exposures would require data of a much higher quality than any that are presently available.

Another type of transmission data that has not been considered is partner information where only the HIV status of both partners is available, but no index case can be identified. Although such data carry information about transmission probabilities, they are of limited utility in investigating risk factors for transmission and cannot be used to provide estimates of the infectivity. Magder and Brookmeyer (1991) investigate statistical methods for data of this kind.

Finally, the analysis of partner study data for purposes other than studying transmission has not been considered. For example, examination of longitudinal data on behavioral characteristics of each partner may provide valuable information on how individuals respond in the presence of HIV infection in either or both partners. This type of knowledge may be of significance in the design of effective intervention and counseling strategies. Statistical methods for the design and analysis of longitudinal studies may be useful in drawing conclusions from such data.

REFERENCES

Anderson, R. M. (1988). The epidemiology of HIV infection: Variable incubation plus infectious periods and heterogeneity in sexual activity. *J. R. Stat. Soc. A* **151**:66–93.

Anderson, R. M. (1989). Mathematical and statistical studies of the epidemiology of HIV [Editorial review]. *AIDS* **3**:333–346.

Anderson, R. M., and May, R. M. (1988). Epidemiological parameters of HIV transmission. *Nature* **333**:514–519.

Anderson, R. M., Gupta, S., and May, R. M. (1991). Potential of community-wide chemotherapy or immunotherapy to control the spread of HIV-1. *Nature* **350**:356–359.

Bacchetti, P. (1989). Additive isotonic models. *J. Am. Stat. Assoc.* **84**:289–294.

Bacchetti, P. (1990). Estimating the incubation period of AIDS by comparing population infection and diagnosis patterns. *J. Am. Stat. Assoc.* **86**:1002–1008.

Bacchetti, P., and Moss, A. R. (1989). Incubation period of AIDS in San Francisco. *Nature* **338**: 251–253.

Bailey, N. T. J. (1975). *The mathematical theory of infectious diseases and its applications.* London: Griffin.

Baker, R. J., and Nelder, J. A. (1978). *The GLIM system,* Release 3. Oxford: Numerical Algorithms Group.

Becker, N. (1989). *Analysis of infectious disease data.* London: Chapman & Hall.

Blythe, S. P., and Anderson, R. M. (1988). Variable infectiousness in HIV transmission models. *IMA J. Math. Appl. Med. Biol.* **5**:181–200.

Breslow, N. E., and Day, N. E. (1980). *Statistical methods in cancer research,* Vol. 1. Lyon: IARC.

Buja, A., Hastie, T., and Tibshirani, R. (1989). Linear smoothers and additive models (with discussion). *Ann. Stat.* **17**:453–555.

Cox, D. R., and Isham, V. (1980). *Point processes.* London: Chapman & Hall.

Cox, D. R., and Oakes, D. (1984). *Analysis of survival data.* London: Chapman & Hall.

De Gruttola, V., Seage, G. R., Mayer, K. H., and Horsburgh, C. R., Jr. (1989). Infectiousness of HIV between male homosexual partners. *J. Clin. Epidemiol.* **42**:849–856.

Dietz, K., and Schenzle, D. (1985). Mathematical models for infectious disease statistics. In S. Feinberg (ed.): *A celebration of statistics: The ISI centenary volume.* Berlin: Springer-Verlag, pp. 167–204.

Dykstra, R. L. (1983). An algorithm for restricted least squares regression. *J. Am. Stat. Assoc.* **78**: 837–842.

Efron, B. (1985). Bootstrap confidence intervals for a class of parametric problems. *Biometrika* **72**:45–58.

European Study Group. (1989). Risk factors for male to female transmission of HIV. *Br. Med. J.* **298**:411–415.

Frost, W. H. (1976). Some conceptions of epidemics in general. *Am. J. Epidemiol.* **104**:141–151.

Fusaro, R., Jewell, N. P., Hauck, W. W., Heilbron, D. C., Kalbfleisch, J. D., Neuhaus, J. M., and Ashby, M. A. (1989). An annotated bibliography of quantitative methodology relating to the AIDS epidemic. *Stat. Sci.* **4**:264–281.

Gaver, D. P. (1963). Random hazard in reliability problems. *Technometrics* **5**:211–226.

Goedert, J. J., Eyster, E., Biggar, R. J., and Blattner, W. A. (1987). Heterosexual transmission of human immunodeficiency virus: Association with severe depletion of T-helper lymphocytes in men with hemophilia. *AIDS Res. Hum. Retrovir.* **3**:355–361.

Grant, R. M., Wiley, J. A., and Winkelstein, W. (1987). Infectivity of the human immunodeficiency virus: Estimates from a prospective study of homosexual men. *J. Infect. Dis.* **156**:189–193.

Greenwood, M. (1931). On the statistical measure of infectiousness. *J. Hyg. Cambridge* **31**:336–351.

Hastie, T. J., and Tibshirani, R. J. (1986). Generalized additive models (with discussion). *Stat. Sci.* **1**:297–318.

Ho, D. D., Moudgil, T., and Alam, M. (1989). Quantitative of human immunodeficiency virus type I in the blood of infected persons. *N. Engl. J. Med.* **321**:1621–1625.

Holmberg, S. D., Horsburgh, C. R., Ward, J. W., *et al.* (1989). Biologic factors in the sexual transmission of human immunodeficiency virus. *J. Infect. Dis.* **160**:116–125.

Holmes, K., and Kreiss, J. (1989). Heterosexual transmission of human immunodeficiency virus: Overview of a neglected aspect of the AIDS epidemic. *AIDS* **1**:602–610.

Isham, V. (1988). Mathematical modeling of the transmission dynamics of HIV infection and AIDS: A review (with discussion). *J. R. Stat. Soc. A* **151**:5–30.

Jewell, N. P. (1990). Some statistical issues in studies of the epidemiology of AIDS. *Stat. Med.* **9:**1387–1416.

Jewell, N. P., and Kalbfleisch, J. D. (1992). Marker processes in survival analysis and applications to issues associated with AIDS. In N. Jewell, K. Dietz, and V. Farewell (eds.): *AIDS epidemiology: Methodological issues.* Boston: Birkhäuser-Boston, pp. 211–230.

Jewell, N. P., and Shiboski, S. C. (1990). Statistical analysis of HIV infectivity based on partner studies. *Biometrics* **46:**1133–1150.

Kalbfleisch, J. D., and Prentice, R. L. (1980). *The statistical analysis of failure time data.* Wiley, New York.

Kaplan, E. H. (1990). Modeling HIV infectivity: Must sex acts be counted? *J. AIDS* **3:**55–61.

Kim, M. Y., and Lagakos, S. W. (1990). Estimating the infectivity of HIV from partner studies. *Ann. Epidemiol.* **1:**117–128.

Longini, I. M., Clark, W. S., Haber, M., and Horsburgh, R., Jr. (1989). The stages of HIV infection: Waiting times and infection transmission probabilities. In C. Castillo-Chavez (ed.), *Mathematical and statistical approaches to AIDS epidemiology.* Berlin: Springer, pp. 111–137.

McCullagh, P., and Nelder, J. A. (1989). *Generalized linear models* (2nd ed.). London: Chapman & Hall.

Magder, L., and Brookmeyer, R. (1993). The analysis of infectious disease data from partner studies with unknown source of infection. *Biometrics* (to be published).

Padian, N., Marquis, L., Francis, D. P., Anderson, R. E., Rutherford, G. W., O'Malley, P. M., and Winkelstein, W. (1987). Male-to-female transmission of human immunodeficiency virus. *J. Am. Med. Assoc.* **258:**788–790.

Padian, N., Shiboski, S., and Jewell, N. P. (1991). Female-to-male transmission of human immunodeficiency virus. *J. Am. Med. Assoc.* **266:**1664–1667.

Peterman, T. A., Stoneburner, R. L., Allen, J. R., Jaffe, H. W., and Curran, J. W. (1988). Risk of HIV transmission from heterosexual adults with transfusion-associated infections. *J. Am. Med. Assoc.* **259:**55–63.

Pregibon, D., and Hastie, T. J. (1991). Generalized linear models. In T. J. Hastie and J. M. Chambers (eds.), *Statistical Models in S.* Pacific Grove: Wadsworth & Brooks/Cole.

Rockower, E. B. (1986). Reliability in a random environment. *Naval Postgraduate School Technical Report NPS55-86-018,* Monterey, Calif.

Shiboski, S. C., and Jewell, N. P. (1992). Statistical analysis of the time dependence of HIV infectivity based on partner study data. *J. Am. Stat. Assoc.* **87:**360–372.

Stefanski, L. A. (1985). The effects of measurement error on parameter estimation. *Biometrika* **72:**583–592.

Weiss, R. A. (1991). Will therapy spread disease? *Nature* **350:**276.

Wiley, J. A., Herschkorn, S. J., and Padian, N. S. (1989). Heterogeneity in the probability of HIV transmission per sexual contact: The case of male-to-female transmission in penile–vaginal intercourse. *Stat. Med.* **8:**93–102.

Index